Dietary Influences on Cancer: Traditional and Modern

Editors

R. Schoental, Ph.D., D.Sc.
Department of Pathology
Royal Veterinary College
University of London
England

T.A. Connors, Ph.D., D.Sc.
Director
Toxicology Unit
Medical Research Council
Carshalton, Surrey
England

CRC Press, Inc.
Boca Raton, Florida

Library of Congress Cataloging in Publication Data
Main entry under title:

Dietary influences on cancer.

Bibliography: p.
Includes index.
1. Cancer—Nutritional aspects. 2. Nutritionally
induced diseases. I. Schoental, Regina. [DNLM:
1. Carcinogens. 2. Diet—Adverse effects. 3. Neoplasms—Etiology. 4. Mycotoxins. QZ 202 D565]
RC262.D52   616.99:4071   81-4948
ISBN 0-8493-5647-4   AACR2

This book represents information obtained from authentic and highly regarded sources. Reprinted material is quoted with permission, and sources are indicated. A wide variety of references are listed. Every reasonable effort has been made to give reliable data and information, but the author and the publisher cannot assume responsibility for the validity of all materials or for the consequences of their use.

Direct all inquiries to CRC Press, Inc., 2000 N.W. 24th Street, Boca Raton, Forida 33431.

International Standard Book Number 0-8493-5647-4

Library of Congress Card Number 81-4948
Printed in the United States

THE EDITORS

Regina Schoental is currently attached to the Department of Pathology of the Royal Veterinary College, University of London, England. Dr. Schoental received her Ph.D. From the University of Cracow, Poland, and her D.Sc. from the University of Glasgow, Scotland. She has done extensive research on various aspects of chemical carcinogenesis at the William Dunn School of Pathology, University of Oxford, the Department of Chemistry, University of Glasgow, and from 1954 until her retirement, she was on the Scientific Staff of the Medical Research Council, at the Toxicology Research Unit, Carshalton, Surrey, England.

Dr. Schoental has written over 200 publications dealing mainly with the biochemical and biological aspects of carcinogenesis by polycyclic aromatic hydrocarbons, alkylnitroso compounds, pyrrolizidine alkaloids, mycotoxins, and certain other "natural" products which may be involved in human and animal cancer.

Her present research interests are concerned with the mechanisms by which vitamins and coenzymes can modify the biological effects of environmental carcinogens.

Tom Connors, Ph.D., D.Sc. is Director of the Medical Research Council's Toxicology Unit. He was formerly Head of the Department of Experimental Cancer Chemotherapy of the Institute of Cancer Research and a Reader in Biochemical Pharmacology in the University of London. He is currently Visiting Professor at Brunel University and the Universities of Aston in Birmingham and Surrey.

Dr. Connors' research interests are concerned principally with studies on the mechanism of action of anticancer agents, chemical carcinogens, and other chemicals with selective toxicity.

CONTRIBUTORS

M. Gelfand, M.D., F.R.C.P.
Professor
University of Zimbabwe
Mount Pleasant, Salisbury
Zimbabwe

Iwao Hirono, M.D.
Professor
Department of Carcinogenesis
    and Cancer Susceptibility
Institute of Medical Science
University of Tokyo
Shirokenedai Minato-ku, Tokyo
Japan

L. J. Kinlen, F.R.C.P., D.Phil.
University of Oxford
Department of Regius
Radcliffe Infirmary
Oxford
England

Gert L. Laqueur, M.D.
Retired
Formerly Chief
Laboratory of Experimental Pathology
National Institutes of Health
Bethesda, Maryland

Philip M.D. Martin, Ph.D.
Reader in Plant Pathology
University of Botswana and Swaziland
Malkerns
Swaziland

Hiromu Matsumoto, Ph.D.
Professor
Agricultural Biochemistry
University of Hawaii at Manoa
Honolulu, Hawaii

Minako Nagao, Ph.D.
Section Head
Biochemistry Division
National Cancer Center
    Research Institute
Chuo-ku, Tokyo
Japan

Takashi Sugimura, M.D., Dr. Med. Sc.
Director
National Cancer Center
    Research Institute
Chuo-ku, Tokyo
Japan

Hiroyuki Toyokawa, M.D., Dr. Med. Sc.
Associate Professor
Department of Epidemiology
School of Health Sciences
Faculty of Medicine
Tokyo University
Bunkyo, Tokyo
Japan

A. Olufemi Williams, M.D., F.R.C.P.
Professor of Pathology
University of Ibadan
Ibadan
Nigeria

TABLE OF CONTENTS

INTRODUCTION

Despite the great efforts directed towards the finding of cancer cures, the achievement of this goal is not yet in sight. "Curability" has been claimed for less than 3% of the more rare of human cancers. Neoplasias of the digestive tract and of the sex organs, which together account for more than half of all the human cancers — remain the most challenging problems: without clues to their etiology, prevention cannot be attempted, and significant progress still eludes their treatment.

These human cancers were common before the industrial developments of the last 50 years, and before the introduction into the human environment of synthetics. The agents which in preindustrial times were responsible for tumors must have largely been present in the "natural" environment.

Radiation, oncogenic viruses, as well as a number of small molecular chemical compounds have been found in the last 50 years to be able to induce in experimental animals tumors similar to those which occur "spontaneously" in man. The chemical agents include estrogens, certain plant constituents (cycasin, pyrrolizidine alkaloids, derivatives of allylbenzene, of hydrazine, etc.), and some of the secondary metabolites of microorganisms (aflatoxins, sterigmatocystin, streptozotocin, elaiomycin, ochratoxin, T-2 toxin, zearalenone etc.) which induce tumors in various target organs (the liver, the digestive tract, the kidneys, the mammary glands, the pituitary, the genital organs etc.) The mechanism(s) by which the various tumors are induced are still not clear.

In addition, it has been demonstrated that tumors can develop in animals as a result of the formation of highly carcinogenic nitroso compounds in the body by nitrosation from nitrite and some precursor secondary or tertiary amines. Carcinogenic substances can also be formed in the course of the preparation of food (broiling, frying, fermentation, etc.) adding to the "embarras de richesse" of potential causes of tumors, and to the difficulties when trying to trace agents of significance for the etiology of particular cancers in man and animals.

However, extrapolation to humans of the results obtained in rodents and other experimental animals may not necessarily be justified. This is especially so when the agents represent precarcinogens, and require metabolic activation by specific, genetically determined enzyme systems. The variations in the pathways and rates of biotransformations may be responsible for species differences in response to known carcinogens; thus, e.g. aflatoxin B_1 or retrorsine which are effective hepatocarcinogens in rats, are not usually carcinogenic in adult mice, while dieldrin and phenobarbitone appear to induce liver tumors mainly in mice. Epidemiological studies of human communities have been mostly successful in providing evidence for the etiology of certain unusual or industrial cancers but have their limitations. These have been recognized following the demonstration that a single or a few exposures to carcinogenic agents when occuring at a critical stage of tissue growth may be sufficient to induce tumors.

The Relative Difficulties of Tracing Etiological Agents of Fetal Abnormalities and Those that are Responsible for Tumors

The latent period between the exposure to a carcinogen and the time of the appearance of recognizable tumors can be very long; in experimental animals under conditions of "optimal" dosage it may take more than a quarter of their respective lifespans to develop neoplasias. In man the latent period for most cancers is estimated to be 20 to 30 years.

How is it then that occasionally tumors occur in newborns? This applies not only to humans but also to livestock. However, as yet no experimental models exist for the purposeful induction by carcinogens of tumors in newborn animals. Transplacental exposure of the early embryo to carcinogenic agents leads mainly to its death, resorption, or abortion, while exposure of the fetus during midgestation, results in developmental abnormalities. Tumors have been found after transplacental treatments during the last stages of pregnancy, but these usually develop after latent periods not much shorter than when the treatment starts soon after birth.

Many of the carcinogenic agents are teratogenic and though not all teratogens are able to induce tumors, more efforts should be directed to the tracing of the teratogenic agents which are responsible for human fetal abnormalities. This would be easier to achieve than tracing etiological agents of cancers as the effects may become obvious in less than 9 months. Particular attention should therefore be focused on women during pregnancy by monitoring daily so that no significant factors should escape detection. This could be achieved if the pregnant women were encouraged to register daily themselves (possibly on electronic registration gadgets) any events out of the ordinary, or ill health which followed some of the food consumed, unseasonal weather conditions, psychological upsets etc. Such records could be computerized for evaluation with the outcome of pregnancy and would facilitate the identification of nongenetic factors involved in the etiology of neonatal abnormalities. The same records would be of great value for tracing some of the agents possibly involved in certain neoplastic, cardiovascular, and other chronic disorders, which may develop later in life, and open the ways for their prevention (see Appendix 1).

In recent years it has been assumed that transformation of normal into neoplastic cells involves changes in the nuclear chromatin akin to mutation; a number of in vitro and in vivo procedures have been developed which allow detection of whether a substance has mutagenic effects on certain microorganisms, on mammalian cells in culture etc. These procedures, which require very small amounts of the test material, and give results within a short time, have been used for the screening of materials suspected of carcinogenic potentialities; about 90% of known carcinogens show indeed mutagenic activity in some of such tests, which however, show also false positives. Even more disturbing were the findings that important carcinogenic agents and promoters gave negative results. These included estrogens (steroidal as well as diethylstilbestrol and zearalenone), cycasin, urethane, pyrrolizidine alkaloids having retronecine as the basic moiety, benzene, dioxin, griseofulvin, T-2 toxin, and certain other mycotoxins etc. The screening of unknown materials by the mutagenicity tests used to date are therefore not reliable as evidence for carcinogenic potentialities of unknown agents.

Experimental use of rodents, though expensive and time-consuming, remains at present irreplaceable for the testing of new materials for pathological potentialities (teratogenic, carcinogenic, and others).

Congenital abnormalities, like tumors, have been known from prehistoric times to occur in animals and man. Dietary factors are often involved, such as starvation, vitamin deficiencies and excesses, (especially of vitamin A) etc. Supplementation with B vitamins of the diet of pregnant women at high risk of giving birth to abnormal offspring has been reported to be effective in the prevention of spina bifida and anencephaly.

Not all body deficiencies of vitamins need be nutritional; they could be secondary, and result from the action of various toxic substances. Aflatoxin B_1 is known to deplete the liver of vitamin A; azaserine, heliotrine, streptozotocin, and a number of nitroso and other compounds deplete nicotinamide, and the NAD coenzymes; retrorsine, estrogens, and certain other carcinogens deplete cytochrome P.450 etc. The mechanisms of depletion of vitamins and cofactors, and their relation to the initiation of the carcinogenic processes are fascinating problems, which require elucidation.

The present book deals with geographic epidemiology and with certain dietary factors, which may be involved in the incidence of idiopathic tumors, but which till now have not received adequate attention. Problems related to conventional nutrients, their imbalance and the way they can modify the action of carcinogens have been extensively discussed elsewhere by other authors.

The epidemiological data, which indicate that certain foods may contribute to higher incidence of specific cancers in certain geographical areas than in others, is discussed by Kinlen (Chapter 6). The epidemiology of cancers among communities which retained the traditional ways of life is discussed by Williams (Chapter 1) in relation to Nigeria, by Gelfand (Chapter 2) in relation to the Mashona in Zimbabwe and by Toyokawa (Chapter 3) in relation to Japan where the introduction of Western foods is changing the traditional patters. However, foodstuffs, in the course of their preparation (cooking, frying, etc.) undergo modifications; the formation of mutagenic substances, some of which may be carcinogenic, is discussed by Nagao and Sugimura (Chapter 10).

In many countries, plants used as food or herbal remedies may contain toxic and carcinogenic agents (Schoental, Appendix 2). These include plants containing the hepatocarcinogenic pyrrolizidine alkaloids; other, as yet unknown carcinogens are present in bracken used as food in Japan, as discussed by Hirono (Chapter 4). The pathological lesions and tumors induced by the plant carcinogen, cycasin, are described in detail by Laqueur and the biochemical changes by Matsumoto (Chapter 5).

Mycotoxins which can present health hazards to livestock and man are only recently receiving increased attention, though moldy foodstuffs have been traditionally considered unwholesome. Of the existing 100,000 species of molds, relatively small numbers have as yet been adequately examined. Not all are toxigenic, and some have been used for the production of valuable industrial products, foods, and medicines. However, a number of microfungi produce secondary metabolites which have toxic, teratogenic, carcinogenic, estrogenic, and/or other pathological effects (Schoental, Chapter 7). Till recently the sporadic presence of mycotoxins in food or otherwise in the environment remained mainly unrecognized, though these could contribute to ill health, and to various reproductive and neoplastic disorders in animals and man, when the climatic conditions are conducive to their production (Martin, Chapter 9; Schoental, Chapter 8).

Recently, a sensitive, accurate, and reproducible radioimmunoassay of T-2 toxin in biological materials has been developed. This permits the detection and the estimation of this mycotoxin when it is present in cereals at levels of a few ppb,* in blood serum at levels of 0.5 ppb, and in milk, or urine at levels of 2.5 ppb.** This relatively simple procedure should facilitate the detection of this carcinogenic mycotoxin in foodstuffs, and make it possible to evaluate its role in various human and animal disorders.

Certain of the secondary metabolites of microorganisms which have been used for medicinal purposes proved of value as antitumor agents, and for the treatment of childhood leukemias. However, among the patients who survived 10 to 20 years after the treatment, some developed tumors unrelated to the neoplasias originally treated. This may indicate that the "natural" tumor growth inhibitory substances, as well as the synthetic ones, could have carcinogenic potentialities (Connors, Chapter 11).

From the accumulating evidence it is clear that though in the present century great changes occurred in medications, the traditional herbal remedies having been mostly replaced by pure substances, which lend themselves to exact dosimetry, yet, iatrogenic chronic diseases, including cancer have not been eliminated.

For various reasons some of the originally planned additional chapters have not been received. We apologize to our contributors and publishers and are grateful for their consideration and patience in face of the unfortunate delays that ensued. I also thank Mrs. N. Brewster for her valuable help.

R. Schoental
T.A. Connors

---

* Lee, S. and Chu, F. S., Radioimmunoassay of T-2 toxin in corn and wheat, *J. Assoc. Off. Anal. Chem.*, 64, 156, 1981.
** Lee, S. and Chu, F. S., Radioimmunoassay of T-2 toxin in biological fluids, *J. Assoc. Off. Anal. Chem.*, 64, 684, 1981.

APPENDIX 1

Pregnant women, in selected areas of high and of low incidence of perinatal mortality and fetal abnormalities, should be asked (in addition to the questions included in the usual questionnaires) about the geographical position of their homes in relation to a possible source of dampness:

1. How close they live to a river or other water reservoirs
2. Whether their living room or kitchen faces North or is in the basement
3. Is the food kept in a scullery, kitchen, refrigerator, etc?

The pregnant women should be asked to tick off (or otherwise to record) every day during pregnancy the absence, or the occurrence of unusual events, such as:

1. nothing unusual
2. severe cold weather
3. rain
4. sore throat
5. influenza
6. indigestion
7. severe vomiting
8. miscarriage
9. accident
10. other illness

Did any of the ill effects follow consumption of specific food, e.g.

11. herbal remedies
12. sausages or other meats, which appeared moldy
13. bread or cereals, which might have become moldy
14. fruit or vegetables, which might have become moldy
15. cheese
16. beer
17. cider
18. spirits
19. other food or drink
20. psychological upset

The data could then be computerized and statistically evaluated at the end of pregnancy in relation to the observed perinatal mortality and neonatal anomalies. The data may also be used in relation to the development of chronic disorders of the mothers and offspring in later life.

Chapter 1

DIET AND CANCER IN TROPICAL AFRICA

A. Olufemi Williams

TABLE OF CONTENTS

I. INTRODUCTION

The potential role of diet in the causation of diseases is well recognized. There is considerable evidence that dietary indiscretion either through ignorance, poverty, or sociocultural practices may be of etiological importance in the epidemiology of diseases including certain types of cancer. The qualitative and quantitative aspects of dietary intakes are important in the etiology of certain diseases. These aspects of dietary intake may influence or dictate whether diet acts in a uni- or multifactorial setting in the pathogenesis of a lesion. In the case of malignant tumors, there is no evidence to suggest that diet alone can cause cancer except in the case of betel nut and tobacco chewers in India, who develop submucous oral fibrosis[1] with subsequent development of cancer of the buccal mucosa.[2] Although diet is an accepted environmental etiological factor in carcinogenesis, the objective evaluation of its role as a sole operating factor in any part of the world, including Nigeria, must be considered difficult for at least two reasons. The first is that the diet may be deficient in the well-recognized nutrients before its consumption or the diet may be malabsorbed as a result of intestinal parasitosis. This is further complicated by the addition of "indigenous potions" to diet for medicinal or cultural purposes. The inherent variation in metabolism of dietary foodstuffs with different kinds of indigenous potions is a significant factor that makes evaluation difficult. However, when potions are prepared and presented for consumption, they could be in a pure form, which for this paper will be referred to as "simple potions", or in a mixture which will be referred to as "mixed potions". The pure potion may be animal or vegetable derived, while the mixed potion may be a mixture of animal, mineral, and vegetable products or a mixture of several vegetable products. These potions can be added to food either in the dry pulverized form or in the wet or suspension state. These potions could be taken with or without food, either before or after a meal, or at times related to the severity of symptoms. The frequency of administration, therefore, varies and quantities ingested also vary. In discussing the role of diet and cancer in tropical Africa, including Nigeria, three separate systems of the body are preeminent. These are the gastrointestinal, the hepatobiliary, and the reticuloendothelial systems.

II. GASTROINTESTINAL SYSTEM

The two organs which are highly susceptible in this system are the stomach and colon, including rectum. Cancer of the stomach is not uncommon in certain parts of Nigeria which have been studied using conventional methods. Mulligan, working in Ilesha, a town in the western region of Nigeria, showed that this was the most common form of cancer encountered in a collection of surgical cases in a hospital over several years.[3] This is in contrast to what was observed in Ibadan, a town which is only 60 mi away.

The Ibadan Cancer Registry, which has amassed data over several years, reported that cancer of the stomach was the fifth most common form of cancer encountered in Nigerian Africans living in Ibadan and its environs.[4,5] In these areas, the most frequently consumed items of diet of the indigenous population are yams, cassava, and maize. These food items are consumed two or three times a day and more important, they are consumed from very early life. Meat and fish are consumed in moderate to large quantities. Palm oil, which consists mainly of unsaturated fats, is used more often for preparation of most meals, while animal fats are rarely used for cooking. Fish and meat when taken are usually in the roasted, dried, or barbecued state, because this is the only way of preservation in the absence of refrigeration in rural areas. Vitamin B_{12} deficiency is distinctly rare in these population groups, and the classical pernicious anemia with atrophic gastritis is relatively uncommon. Folate deficiency, however, with megaloblastic erythropoiesis, is not uncommon. The role of folate deficiency in patients with gastric cancer is poorly understood in these population groups but requires further studies. The role of potential cocarcinogens or carcinogens in the staple foods consumed, particularly those containing cyanides, as has been shown in the case of cassava, also requires further study.[6] Autoimmune phenomenon which may either result or be associated with atrophic gastritis is relatively rare in Nigeria.[7] HLA-B$_8$, which is associated with certain autoimmune dieseases, also appears to be relatively infrequent in the population.

It would therefore appear that certain nondietary but specific antecedent or associated lesions of gastric carcinoma are relatively uncommon in the African. Further, there are no known parasites which inhabit the stomach which may be carcinogenic or cocarcinogenic and for which food may be its vehicle. There is, however, a fish tapeworm called *Eustoma rotundatum* which inhabits the duodenum and produces an eosinophilic duodenitis, but not malignancy. An analysis of data from Ibadan Cancer Registry has failed to reveal any specific etiological pointer for gastric cancer among those who were known to take certain medicinal potions. The question which requires clarification, however, is whether these medicinal potions have any etiological importance, or whether they were in fact taken as therapeutic measures for the complaints.

A. Colon and Rectum

The relationship between diet and bowel habit has been well recognized since the days of Hippocrates, but the possible relationship between diet and bowel on one hand and colorectal diseases on the other hand has been highlighted relatively recently.[8] The astute observations of Burkitt revealed that certain diseases of the bowel, including benign and malignant tumors, were related to the bulk, content, and transit times of stools in different population groups. Although there are minor areas of disagreement with the Burkitt hypothesis, there appears to be epidemiological support in certain parts of Africa including Nigeria, where benign or malignant colorectal tumors are relatively uncommon,[4,5,9,10] when compared with frequency or incidence data in other population groups living in the developed and industrialized countries. This relatively low incidence may be due to the composition of the diet which is rich in fibers, to the bulk of the stools which produces a faster transit time, and to the frequency of stools passed per diem, which is higher in the African than in the Caucasian. In a comparative study of colorectal polyps and cancer between Nigerian Africans and American blacks living in Washington, D.C., who have adopted a Western type of diet, it was evident that the frequency of neoplastic benign polyps and cancer of colon and rectum in the American blacks was significantly different from what occurred in their ethnologically related Nigerians living in Africa.[9,10]

Recent studies have incriminated the role of high intake of animal fat in the etiology of colon cancer. Furthermore, the alterations in the fecal bacterial flora and production of carcinogenic substances by bacteria from bile steroids have also been implicated in colorectal carcinogenesis. The fast transit time in subjects on high fiber diet will minimize or reduce the duration of contact between carcinogens produced and colonic mucosa, while the corollary of these features has been shown to be true.[11-14] Dietary consumption of animal protein such as meat, beef, eggs, fish, and milk is relatively low in Nigerians, but there is a noticeable increase in consumption of these animal proteins in economically affluent Nigerians inhabiting the urban areas. If these dietary factors are of any etiological significance, a significant increase in colorectal neoplasms can be predicted for the higher socioeconomic groups in urbanized Africans in the very near future. It would appear that a temporal factor is also very important in the pathogenesis of colorectal cancer.[9] If the period of exposure to the carcinogen is relatively short or shortened by reduced life expectancy, the incidence of colorectal cancer will be low as the peak average

age incidence for the tumor may be higher than the life expectancy of the population group. For example, the frequencies of colorectal tumors in the American blacks and Nigerian Africans are similar under the age of 40 years, but over the age of 40 years, the frequency is much higher in the American blacks with a longer expectation of life. Age specific curves, therefore, revealed low rates for the Nigerian throughout life while there is a significant increase after the age of 40 years for the American blacks. This observation will suggest that a genetic factor is perhaps not important, but that environmental factors and the duration of exposure to significant etiological factors are important.

Experimental evidence indicates that certain reduced bile salts may have carcinogenic properties.[15,16] Furthermore it has been shown by Hill et al. that there is a close correlation between the geographical incidence of colonic cancer and fecal deoxycholate concentration.[17] Recent studies of bile salt metabolism in the Nigerian revealed a reduced level of deoxycholate conjugates in bile but increased cholates and a larger total pool of bile salts.[18] Deoxycholate, which is a dihydroxy bile salt, is produced in the intestinal lumen when circulating bile comes in contact with the bacterial flora of the intestinal lumen. The reduced level of deoxycholate in the Nigerian would either suggest reduced bacterial dehydroxylation of bile salts or interference with dehydroxylation by high cellulose fiber in their diets, which is not present in the refined, fiber-depleted diets of Caucasians in the developed countries. It has been suggested that in countries where a high fiber diet is consumed, there is alteration in bile salt metabolism by dietary fiber. The mechanism whereby colonic mucosa undergoes malignant change may be as a result of long exposure to high concentrations of dehydroxylated bile salt metabolites in the presence of low residue fiber-depleted diet as occurs in Western countries. The role of bile salts in the etiology and pathogenesis of cholelithiasis will be dealt with in the following section.

III. HEPATOBILIARY SYSTEM

The role of diet in the etiology and pathogenesis of hepatobiliary neoplasms is well recognized in experimental animals, but its significance in humans remains poorly substantiated and understood. The role of dietary deficiencies in the etiology of liver cell carcinoma is still to be clarified. In humans, consumed diet may be contaminated by mycotoxins in which case, the toxin, such as aflatoxin, may be the hepatocarcinogen. In other instances, diet may be contaminated by parasites such as *Chlornorchis sinesis* which may result in hepatic chlornorchiasis with attendant biliary (bileduct) cholelithiasis and carcinoma. It has been suggested that the fluke produces a toxin which is cholangiocarcinogenic. There is experimental and indirect evidence that diets deficient in certain essential amino acids may predispose to fatty change of the liver. This makes the liver more susceptible to subsequent insults which may act as promoters in carcinogenesis, while malnutrition may be an initiator. Such secondary injuries which may promote carcinogenesis include aflatoxin, senecio alkaloids, sterigmatocystin, or infection by hepatitis B antigen. By the time the neoplasm develops, the footprints of malnutrition or other causative factors are usually not evident or not easy to identify.

The field studies on dietary aflatoxins and primary liver cell carcinoma suggest an association between the mycotoxins and liver cancer,[19] but the role of malnutrition either as an initiator or a cocarcinogen has not been critically evaluated in that setting. Liver disease in the alcoholics may be due to dietary inadequacies or be a result of the alcohol, or its metabolites, or incidental contaminants. There is no evidence that the effects of malnutrition on the liver alone predispose to liver cancer or to cirrhosis, which is very often an antecedent lesion. However, liver cancer is not uncommon in population groups which are known to have a high incidence of malnutrition in early life, but in addition have high frequencies of hepatitis B antigenemia,[20-22] are exposed to increased levels of dietary aflatoxins,[19] and are also exposed to pyrrolizidine alkaloids.[23] Malnutrition, therefore, may exert its pathogenic role either by its effects on hepatic metabolism and morphology or by its effect on the immune system.

IV. RETICULOENDOTHELIAL SYSTEM

Tumors of the reticuloendothelial tissues are not uncommon in children living in tropical Africa including Nigeria.[24] The frequency of certain types of tumors, particularly solid lymphomas, is greater in African children living in Africa than in Caucasian or American black children.[25] The reason for the relatively high observed frequency of lymphomas in African children may be related to a number of factors including malnutrition, which predisposes them to altered immunological status. Numerous studies have shown that malnutrition and stress in early life interfere with cell mediated immunity (T-cell). There is also an established relationship between T-cell levels and the onset of neoplasia. Persistent infections, particularly in early life, appear to lead to atrophy of the thymus with secondary T-cell deficiency. This is usually followed by B-cell stimulation with subsequent development of B-cell hyperplasia and lymphoma. The incidence of neoplasia alone, with atrophy of the cell mediated immune system, increases with age. This altered immunological profile appears to be of great importance in the development of lymphoma of the upper gastrointestinal tract[26] and lymph nodes. In tropical Africa and in several developing countries, malnutrition and multiple parasitism and other bacterial infections are relatively common in early life. Infantile gastroenteritis, which is one of the very common infections, may lead to thymic atrophy and persistent cell mediated immune deficiency state.[26] It is therefore not surprising that the incidence of intestinal atrophy and intestinal lymphoma is relatively high in those countries where infant feeding is frequently complicated by enteritis when compared with countries where infantile enteritis is relatively uncommon.[27] The combination of malnutrition and enteritis, which is not uncommon in several developing countries, usually leads to severe marasmus. Repeated bouts of enteritis in children with malnutrition predispose these children to secondary immune deficiency states with highly probable development of malignant disease of tissues of the reticuloendothelial system. With the reduction of infantile enteritis in a country like Iran, due to improved hygiene and introduction of modern infant care methods, the relatively high frequency of duodenojejunal lymphomas reported from that country has shown a downward trend.[26,28] It would therefore appear that cancer may result from inadequate intake of a balanced diet potentiated by persistent depletion of the cell mediated immune system.

The exposure of the unborn child to "natural" toxic substances, including carcinogens, is considered to be a real problem, but there is a lack of studies on this aspect of vertical carcinogenesis in the tropics. It is well-known that certain chemicals of plant origin are mutagenic and/or teratogenic, and it is also known that certain plant products are carcinogenic in experimental animals. The more common types of cancer encountered in the African child, which include lymphomas and retinoblastoma, have not been reported or shown to be used by or associated with ingestion of substances of plant origin or other toxic chemicals. Liver tumors are relatively uncommon in early life in the African child, but the fact that there is a significant increase in the number of liver tumors in adolescence may suggest early exposure to hepatocarcinogens.[29] A prospective study of pregnant women in several parts of Africa, where ingestion of "native medicine" occurs, should be carried out to find out the nature of the constituents of such medicines and the subsequent fate of the offspring, especially in relation to the development of cancer early in life.

REFERENCES

1. **Rosenfeld, L. and Callaway, J.,** Snuff dippers cancer, *Am. J. Surg.,* 106, 840, 1963.
2. **Pindborg, J. J. and Sirsat, S. M.,** Oral submucous fibrosis, *Oral Surg.,* 22, 764, 1966.
3. **Mulligan, T. O.,** Burkitt's lymphoma in Ilesha Western Nigeria, *Br. J. Cancer,* 25, 52, 1971.
4. **Edington, G. M. and Maclean, C. N. U.,** A cancer rate survey in Ibadan, Western Nigeria, *Br. J. Cancer,* 19, 471, 1965.
5. **Williams, A. O. and Edington, G. M.,** Malignant disease of the colon, rectum and anal canal in Ibadan, Western Nigeria, *Dis. Col. Rectum,* 10, 301, 1967.
6. **Osuntokun, B. O.,** *Plant Foods for Human Nutrition,* 2, 215, 1972.
7. **Williams, A. O. and Nwabuebo, I. O. E.,** unpublished data.
8. **Burkitt, D. P.,** An epidemiological approach to gastrointestinal cancer, *Cancer,* 20, 146, 1970.
9. **Williams, A. O., Chung, E. B., Agbata, A., and Jackson, M. A.,** Intestinal polyps in American negroes and Nigerian negroes, *Br. J. Cancer,* 31, 485, 1975.
10. **Williams, A. O. and Prince, D. L.,** Intestinal polyps in the Nigerian African, *J. Clin. Pathol.,* 28, 367, 1975.
11. **Goldstein, F. J.,** Diet and colonic disease, *J. Am. Diet. Assoc.,* 60, 499, 1972.
12. **McGregor, J. L.,** Carcinoma of the colon and stomach. A review with comment on epidemiologic associations, J.A.M.A., 227, 911, 1974.
13. **Modan, B., Barell, V., Lubin, F., Modan, M., Greenberg, R. A., and Graham, S.,** Low fibre intake as an etiologic factor in cancer of the colon, *J. Natl. Cancer Inst.,* 55, 15, 1975.
14. **Wynder, E. G. and Shigenatsu, T.,** Environmental factors of cancers of the colon and rectum, *Cancer,* 20, 1520, 1967.
15. **Cook, J. W., Kennaway, E. L., and Kennaway, N. M.,** Production of tumours in mice by deoxycholic acid, *Nature (London),* 145, 627, 1940.
16. **Badger, G. M., Cook, J. W., Hewett, C. L., Kennaway, E. L., Kennaway, N. M., Martin, R. H., and Robinson, A. M.,** The production of cancer by pure hydrocarbons. V, *Proc. R. Soc. Br.,* 129, 439, 1940.
17. **Hill, M. J., Drasar, B. S., Hawkesworth, G., Williams, R., and Growther, J. S.,** Bacteria and aetiology of cancer of large bowel, *Lancet,* i, 95, 1971.
18. **Falaiye, J. M.,** The dietary fibre theory and bile salt pattern in Nigerians, *Afr. J. Med. Sci.,* 7, 151, 1978.
19. **Linsell, C. A. and Peers, T. G.,** Field studies on liver cell cancer, in *Origins of Human Cancer, A,* Vol. 4, Hiatt, H. H., Watson, J. D., and Winsten, J. A., Eds., Cold Spring Harbor Laboratory, Cold Spring Harbor, N.Y., 1977, 549.
20. **Williams, A. O. and Almeida, J.,** Ultrastructure of hepatitis associated antigen in Nigerians, *Am. J. Trop. Med.,* 21, 273, 1972.
21. **Williams, A. O., Gupta, G., and Fabiyi, A.,** Hepatitis B antigen in Nigerian children, *East Afr. Med. J.,* 50, 521, 1973.
22. **Williams, A. O.,** Hepatitis B antigen and liver cancer, *Am. J. Med. Sci.,* 270, 53, 1975.
23. **Williams, A. O. and Schoental, R.,** Hepatotoxicity of *Senecio abyssinicus*—experimental and ultrastructural studies, *Trop. Geogr. Med.,* 22, 201, 1970.
24. **Williams, A. O.,** Tumors of childhood in Ibadan, Nigeria, *Cancer,* 36, 370, 1975.
25. **Olisa, G., Chandra, R., Jackson, M. A., Kennedy, J., and Williams, A. O.,** Malignant tumors in American black and Nigerian children. A comparative study, *J. Natl. Cancer Inst.,* 55, 281, 1975.
26. **Dutz, W. and Kohout, E.,** 3rd Int. Symp. Oncol., Cancer Institute in Teheran, 1978, 115.
27. **Barelat, A. A., Saidi, F., and Dutz, W.,** Cancer survey in south Iran with special reference to gastrointestinal neoplasms, *Int. J. Cancer,* 7, 353, 1971.
28. **Kohout, E. and Dutz, W.,** Analysis of lymphocyte receptors (B and T cells), *Prog. Clin. Pathol.,* 7, 117, 1978.
29. **Cameron, H. M. and Warwick, G. P.,** Primary cancer of the liver in Kenyan children, *Br. J. Cancer,* 36, 793, 1977.

Chapter 2

CANCER AMONG THE SHONA IN RELATION TO THEIR TRADITIONAL DIET AND MEDICINES*

M. Gelfand

TABLE OF CONTENTS

* Since this manuscript was submitted for publication the nation of Rhodesia has become known as Zimbabwe.

I. THE SHONA NATION AND ITS DIET

The Shona nation, about 6 million in strength, occupies about three quarters of the country of Rhodesia, which lies between the Zambesi in the north, the Limpopo to the south, with Mozambique on its eastern border and Botswana on its western border. In size it is about 150,000 square miles. To the southwest of the Shona are the Zimbabwe people, a much smaller ethnic group of Zulu origin, living in an area centered around Bulawayo. The Shona all speak a common language and their customs, religion, and culture are similar in essentials in all parts of their territory. This nation is comprised of four major tribal groups: the central Zezuru, the northeastern Korekore, the eastern Manica, and the southern Karanga. Each of these is divided into a fairly large number of smaller groups or clans, each occupying an almost independent province under its own chief. The totem of the dominant group in each clan is shared by all the members of that clan.

The staple cereal is mostly determined by the rainfall of that area. For instance, in central Mashonaland the main grain is maize, whereas in the drier north and eastern regions it is mapfunde *(Sorghum caffrorum),* but the method of planting and tending crops and of preparing the food is essentially similar. There have been some change of habits, of course, due to western influence, especially in urban areas and other centers such as mission stations, boarding schools, and administrative centers. For instance, breakfast is coming into vogue more and more — consisting of a cup of tea with milk and sugar and bread and jam. Traditionally the Shona eat two main meals a day, one at midday and the other at nightfall. These two meals are much the same as they always were in both rural and urban areas. For at least 10 years I have been studying the dietary habits of the Shona and their methods of preparing their food.[1]

The Shona system of agriculture was a shifting one, which was possible because land was plentiful and the population small. Men could move to fresh spots when the land they were cultivating was no longer productive. Nowadays the position is different on account of the very large population increase. Land has become scarce and, in order to make the most of the soil on which they must remain, farmers rotate their crops — a method that is frequently new to them.

II. FEEDING THE CHILD

The baby is generally suckled from the second day of his birth or from as soon as the mother's milk appears. Thereafter, he is fed on demand during the day with no fixed feeding times so commonly in force among European mothers. As long as he is quiet the baby is not disturbed, but whenever he cries he is put to the breast. Both breasts are given; usually there is no supplementary feeding with cow's milk.

It is incorrectly held by many people that the Shona mother simply stuffs her baby with porridge (sadza) shortly after it is born. This is not true. Within a few days after birth, its mother gives the child a liquid gruel called bota. It is prepared from specially ground millet and carefully sieved. She often mixes the powdered roots of certain herbs in it for several days to prevent abdominal pains or gastroenteritis. The liquid gruel is fed to the child once or twice a day for a few months as a supplement to the breast milk. After that it is given in increased amounts, but the main supply of food is breast milk. In order to feed her child this liquid porridge, cow's milk, or perhaps a little diluted sweet beer, the mother fills the palm of her left hand with it. She then places the side of this hand along the baby's lower lip and, with a little gentle pressure, opens his mouth and directs the flow of the fluid into the mouth with the little finger of her right hand. The gruel is given as long as the child is breast fed until the crawling stage is reached. It is gradually thickened until the baby is able to eat thick porridge. Feeding bottles have come into use with increasing frequency. Traditionally the mother feeds her baby from her hand until he is just under 1 year old, after which she pours bota into a wooden spoon, and the child learns from watching her how to bring it to his own lips. Soon he finds he can take the porridge from the spoon by himself. Later when the child is ready to eat stiff porridge, she puts it into his hands and he soon discovers how to put it into his mouth. By the time the baby's teeth appear it receives not only thick porridge but relish as well, usually in the form of ground peanuts. This peanut butter is boiled in a little water, and the child is shown how to dip a piece of stiff porridge into this mixture.

Meat is not given to a child until he is 3 or 4 years old, as it is considered a special delicacy and, therefore, it is felt that the child's character and behavior will be better if he is taught from an early age that he cannot have everything he wants in life.

From about the age of 6 months the child is offered a little sweet beer (bhume). The mother fills a small calabash and holds it to the baby's mouth, allowing him to drink a little. A strong belief exists among Africans that if a baby develops diarrhea while he is on the breast, this milk supply must be withdrawn immediately, as it is held that he has been poisoned by the mother's milk. Also, after an infant has had a severe attack of diarrhea, he is not put back on the breast. An important sanction is that which forbids the husband and wife to have sexual intercourse while the baby is on the breast and before the midwife has received her final payment for delivering the baby. It is feared that if intercourse takes place before she is given her fee, the couple will develop severe backaches and the baby may be poisoned by the mother's milk.

By the time a child has reached the age of 5 to 7 years, he is ready to be handed over to his grandparents. He has learned how to behave conventionally and show regard for others; correct manners and social behavior in accordance with customary practices are fairly well inculcated in him.

Cooking is one of the daily tasks of a woman. No man cooks except when on a long journey on which he is unable to have his meals brought to him and he cannot carry sufficient supplies with him. Every Shona husband expects his wife to cook for him, but he has no right to interfere or even make suggestions on these matters. He knows that at least twice a day he will receive food.

Every boy and girl must learn how to plant the various seeds grown in the lands. When a girl is about 9 years old she is taught how to use a small hoe. First she is shown how to weed and then how to scatter millet seed. At 15 she is initiated into the art of brewing beer. Usually when a mother prepares the evening meal she puts aside a small portion of the stiff porridge she has just cooked, on a plate or in a small basket, with a little relish for the younger children to eat in the morning.

When the meal has been cooked the men are served at the dare (the meeting place in the village reserved for men). The young children sit around their mother in the house waiting for their food. The women do not sit in separate groups like the men, but if grown-up women and young girls are with her the mother may give the former a plate of stiff porridge to share and the young girls another. A daughter is allowed to help herself from the same plate as her mother until she has reached the age of 14 or 15 years when she is given her own. She may then help her mother by giving the smaller children pieces of food from it. She may not leave either, until the children are finished. After the mother has taken a piece of porridge from her plate, she is followed by her eldest daughter and then each of the rest according to his age. Infants and toddlers are not permitted to help themselves to any food from their mother's plate. It is her duty to take a suitably sized portion of stiff porridge from it, dip it into the relish, and hand it to the child to eat, while she is eating herself until they are both satisfied. When she has more than one child to feed, she is careful to give the first morsel to the youngest child to prevent him from crying or becoming restless. No preference is shown either to sex or age among the other young children she feeds. When one of them has finished his portion and is ready for more, if the mother has not noticed this, the child should say "pepapi", which denotes that he is ready for more. When he is satisfied he remains silent, indicating that he has had enough. Hands are washed after the meal.[2]

At about 8 o'clock in the morning the mother washes the younger children's faces, warms on the fire the stiff porridge left over from the previous night, and divides it among them. It is accepted that a child cannot wait as long for food as an adult, therefore the mother usually leaves a little of the porridge prepared for the midday meal to give the younger children if they are hungry at about three in the afternoon. Those between the ages of 6 and 10 years old, herding cattle in the fields, must be remembered as they require more than merely the edible fruits and plants they find in the bush. Before setting off with the cattle, each of these children is given some stiff porridge to eat outside the house. When the midday meal is ready the mother sends one of her daughters to the fields to take her brothers their porridge and relish. If she is planning to be working elsewhere at that time and thus unable to prepare the children's midday meal, she makes them a special dish the evening before, known as mutakura. She boils maize seeds and leaves them to cool. In the summer, when the maize is still young, the children are given green cobs to roast in the fields. Boiled pumpkin is also popular with the little cattle herders.

No girl is allowed to go to the mens' meeting place unless she is taking food there or has to report to her father some mishap, such as loss of cattle. Usually a boy is permitted to eat there when he begins to herd cattle. He sits near his father who leaves some stiff porridge on his plate for the child to eat when he has finished. When a boy is about 15 years, his mother sends or brings his own plate of food. A girl eats from the same plate as her mother untils she reaches puberty (mandara). When her breasts have developed she shares one with other young girls. She is not allowed her own until she marries and leaves the village.

Youths from the age of 15 years are treated as responsible men but eat in a separate group from their fathers. Nowadays this has changed a good deal. Parents may have their meals together in the house with their children, but do not eat from the same dish. The father has his own and the children theirs. The mother eats with her daughters and father with his sister's son or his grandchild. A mother treats her grown-up son as a senior man according him the same degree of respect. She kneels when she hands him his food in the same way as she does before her husband. Married men and youths are not permitted to talk or make a noise until the meal is over, when they resume their conversation. There are a few avoidance rules (or taboos) with regard to food that must be observed by unmarried girls and boys. For example, they may not eat the mouse called shana *(Steatomys praternisis)* as it lives in a hole by itself. The fish called ramba is also forbidden to unmarried people.

III. CULTIVATION OF CROPS

The minda (lands) are usually chosen close to the homestead, but their distance from it varies. The amount of land cultivated depends on the man's needs. In addition, several families graze their cattle on communal pasture land. When a field had been used for 3 or 4 years consecutively, it was changed for a new one on the same allotment (shifting agriculture), as rotation of crops was not a feature of traditional agriculture. Each field is between half an acre and an acre, and the soil is traditionally turned with hoes. The best time to plant is in November, by which time the grass and leaves on the ground from previous crops have had a chance to decay and fertilize it. The members of the family scatter the seed over the surface of the soil, generally during the 15 days after the new moon has appeared.[3]

The most important crops are finger millet (zvivo or rukweza), the primary grain grown on the high veld and used extensively for making beer. Sorghum (mapfunde), may be the principal crop in the low veld. Bulrush millet (mhunga) grows mostly in the low veld. It is used widely for making beer as well as for food. Maize (chibabwe) is grown wherever possible and rice (mupunga) is a common crop, especially in wetter regions.

Finger millet seed is scattered, but those of maize are planted by hand—three seeds in a small hole, dug with a mattock the morning after a fall of rain and then covered with soil. Pumpkins are planted in the same field as the two main crops (maize and millet). The wife's field or those of the co-owners are generally near or next to that of the husband. The next planting season, peanuts are sewn in the fields formerly occupied by millet and maize. Rice (mupunga) is planted in wet soil. The most popular legumes are vembi *(Vigna unguiculata),* several varieties of which are grown. Groundnuts or peanuts are also very well liked and used as a relish. The bambara groundnut is also very popular. Sweet potatoes are grown extensively in more humid areas and several kinds of pumpkins and squash all over the country. Another popular crop is watermelon. Cassava is planted mostly in the lowveld, but is not eaten much unless there is a famine. Bananas are grown extensively throughtout the warm and humid areas. Red peppers are also cultivated and used as a condiment.

The traditional way of planting has just been described, but since the advent of the white man, new ways have been adopted. Each field often contains only one crop and the plow has been introduced. The wife's field is prepared in the same way as her husband's, but is usually smaller and contains many different crops such as groundnuts, rice, bambara groundnuts, cowpeas, and sorghum.

Weeding is essential in order to have good crops. This is done by hand or with a hoe as soon as the seed has germinated. Husband, wife, and children all help and friends and neighbors are invited to join in as well. They work all day until the weeding is completed and they are provided with food and beer. Thus the working party becomes a social gathering known as hoka.[4]

The millet is picked in May and placed in a heap on a flat rock, where it is dried ready for threshing. Again friends are asked to share the work. Groundnuts are also spread out to dry in a winnowing basket on the ground.

Many people in rural areas employ medicines, possessing a magical connotation, to ensure good, bountiful crops. These are mixed with the seed and such preparations are known as divisi.

As a close association exists between the Shona religion and the various agricultural pursuits and produce of the land, it is worth referring briefly to some of the more common religious practices connected with them. No work is permitted on the lands on certain days of the lunar cycle. Such a ritual day is knows as chisi. The tribal spirit, the founder spirit of the family lineages, is believed to play a vital part in ensuring good crops. This spirit is responsible, too, for the rain in its area. Therefore it is customary for the clansmen of a ward (dunhu) to gather together at specified times of the year when the spirit enters its medium and addresses the people.

IV. THE PREPARATION OF FOOD

A. Methods of Making Meal From Grain

The preparation of food is in the hands of the woman, who is also responsible for stamping and grinding the grain. Finger millet, bulrush millet, and rice can be stored in a granary for years, but maize can only be kept for several months, as it is liable to be invaded and destroyed by insects. Sorghum keeps for about a year. These grains are ground to flour by a variety of utensils, such as the mortar and pestle, the small and the large grinding stone, and the winnowing basket.

1. The Preparation of Stiff Porridge

Stiff porridge, eaten by all Shona people with every meal, is its bulky item and consists largely of starch. It is consumed with the relish or meat. To cook it a woman places a clay pot of water on a fire, and when the water is warm she adds a little meal to it, stirring until there are no lumps in the pot. She puts in more from time to time until the mixture is thick, smoothing out lumps by rotating a wooden spoon. She still adds more meal until the porridge is of the desired consistency. She then dishes it out into wooden or clay pots. No salt whatever is added.

Sorghum and bulrush millet porridge are eaten in the cold season after these grains are harvested, before the main cereals are used. Maize is next exployed and millet eaten last, usually in the spring, because it stores well and also because it can be cooked relatively quickly, as it needs less preparation than the others. Rice porridge is cooked mainly in the rainy season, as it is harvested early, and if kept is liable to be destroyed by borers.

2. The Preparation of Mealie Meal

After harvesting, the maize is taken to a flat rock with a depression and spread out to dry for 2 or 3 weeks or even longer. A more popular method of drying the cobs is to place them on a drying platform where they are left for 2 or 3 months. When they are dried they are left in a corner of the house for a couple of weeks, after which they are threshed with the handle (mupinvi) of a hoe or with a stamping pole to separate the grain from the cob. The former is collected and stored in the granary. Meal can be prepared from maize in several ways. The woman may take what she requires to the stamping block. First she pours a little water into the maize seeds until it is a quarter full. Then she stamps them and pours the stamped grain into a winnowing basket, winnowing it to remove the chaff. The crushed maize is then put into a little clay pot, water added, and these seeds soaked overnight. The next morning the water is removed and the wet maize spread on a flat rock. When it is almost dry it is placed in the stamping block again, winnowed once more and left to dry in the sun for about half an hour. After that it is finally ground into fine meal on the grinding stone.[5]

3. The Preparation of Liquid Gruel

Thin or liquid gruel is cooked in the same way as stiff porridge, except that more water is added in order to make it into a very thin mixture. It is poured into a wooden plate and eaten with a wooden spoon. A popular method of administering a liquid medicine is to add it to the gruel as it is being cooked.

B. Some Food Sources

Groundnuts — The plants are pulled up by their roots and the seeds removed. In order to prepare relish from the nuts they are dried, shelled, and roasted for 3 to 5 min. Then they are spread out in a winnowing basket to cool and the red skins removed by hand. The nuts are now ground into peanut butter in a stamping block. This is stored in a calabash, and, when relish has been cooked in a little clay pot, some of the peanut butter is poured on it and the mixture stirred with a stirring stick until it is ready to eat. The relish is put into a small clay pot and is consumed with stiff porridge.

Bambara groundnuts — When the nuts are ripe the plants are up-rooted and washed with the nuts still attached to them. The bulk of the crop is stored on the drying platform, but some may be taken out, stamped gently with a stamping pole, winnowed, and then cooked with a little salt.

Beans — Beans are planted in the same field, at the same time as maize and millet. They may be cooked in their shells with green maize, pumpkin, round nuts, or ground-nuts, but may be cooked alone when they are boiled in a clay pot and served on plates. Each person shells his own by hand. However, there are several ways of preparing beans.[6]

Pumpkin — Pumpkin seeds are planted in November in the same field as other crops and are tended only by women. The green leaves of pumpkin are very popular for use as relish and also can be cooked, dried, and stored for winter when fresh vegetables are not available.

Mushrooms — Mushrooms are gathered in the rainy season, especially after the first rains. Great care is taken culling them as some varieties are edible and others highly poisonous.

Relish — Relish, provided at each meal, is an essential part of the diet. Pumpkin leaves have already been mentioned in this connection. Those of wild vegetables are also gathered and used for relish. The most popular vegetables in Mashonaland are cowpeas and pumpkin leaves. Pumpkin leaves are cut into small pieces and eaten cold. When mixed with groundnuts this relish is called nhope. Spinach leaves and bean leaves are prepared similarly. There are several recipes for making savory relish. First comes peanut butter made by shelling roasted peanuts and grinding them into a fine powder in a bowl. This is then moistened with water and cooked until it forms a paste (dovi). Another savory relish consists of boiled locusts dried and eaten with stiff porridge. Flying ants and caterpillars are prepared the same way. These relishes and side dishes are excellent complementary foods to the staple cereal, and the addition of peanut butter results in an appreciable increase in the calorific value of the diet.[7]

Fruit — Different kinds of fruit are eaten whenever they are available. Some are found throughout the year, as in every season certain types are ripe. Their variety and quantity depend on the situation of the village and its proximity to woods, hills, rocky places, and streams. Each kind of fruit grows best in its particular location, but hardly any villages are without one or two indigenous fruits close at hand. The hacha *(Parinari caratellifolia)* is a very common fruit that can be eaten immediately as it is picked. Generally it is stamped and when the hard skins have been removed, it is served in plates. An alcoholic beverage is made from it. Another popular fruit is the mazhanje *(Uapaca kirkiana)*. Its outer shell is broken, the seeds discarded, and its sweet contents eaten. In the lower-lying country the fruit of the boabab tree *(Adensonia digitata)* is well liked. The large oval shaped fruit is broken, open, the seeds discarded, and the powdery substance remaining is mixed with water and cooked with the thin porridge of one of the cereals. It may also be mixed with honey and eaten in this form. Only a few of the fruits growing in Mashonaland have been mentioned, as it would be difficult to incorporate in this chapter the very long list of fruits growing there. Wine is also made from the fruit of certain trees; for instance mukunyi is one prepared from that of the mapfura *(Sclerocarva caffra)*. A pot is half filled with the fruit and cold water is added. This is allowed to stand for 3 days, after which the scum is skimmed off the top and the beverage is ready to drink. By the fourth day it is very intoxicating.[8]

Tobacco and snuff — Tobacco was grown in Mashonaland before the arrival of the European, and smoking and snuff taking are common practices. A pipe made from the wood of the tree, called mutara *(Gardenia resiniflua)* was used only by men. Many people smoked through reeds. A third type of pipe consisted of a reed fitted into a hole in the lower end of a maize cob filled with tobacco. Traditionally women did not smoke but frequently took snuff.

Salt — In the last 25 years all salt eaten by the Shona has been imported, but traditionally a potassium salt is used by burning to ashes the grass, called mangora, in a broken clay pot and sieving the ashes until white salt is formed.[9]

C. Sources of Protein

The Shona people are great lovers of meat in most of its forms; their only problem is that it is often difficult to obtain an adequate quantity in their daily lives. Avoidance of the flesh of a particular animal because it is a symbol of a particular totem is of little moment. Each clan is subject to the avoidance of the meat or fat of its symbolic or eponymous animal, but such restrictions do not really affect the protein intake of its members to any significant degree. In any event the majority of animals, representing the various totems, are eaten very rarely or not at all, and those who may not eat certain foods find these restrictions of no particular importance. All Shona groups still firmly accept the totem cult, no matter what level of education their individuals may have reached.

The avoidance of eggs by traditional Africans should be mentioned although they are being eaten in urban areas and by those who have adopted a more western way of life. They were and still are not eaten by the most traditional practicing Shona, especially by children and by women with babies, as it is feared that if a woman (not so much a man) eats an egg she might become sterile through an antagonistic action of the egg on her own ova.

Except for these two avoidances the Shona are most sensible consumers of a wide range of protein foods, indeed probably wider than those of Europeans, since they eat mice, caterpillars, and big game such as elephant. Further they readily eat the heart, lungs, intestines, and other parts of an animal's body at which many Europeans look askance. An important drawback, however, is that many of these sources of protein are seasonal. This applies particularly to fish, game, caterpillars, and even to a certain extent to milk.[10] Practically no village in Mashonaland lacks its own cattle pen.

1. The Slaughtering of Cattle

A rope is looped over the animals's horns and its head is tied close to the trunk of a tree. A man lifts an axe and cracks the base of the head, just behind the horns, with heavy blows. The animal sinks to the ground senseless from the blow. Quickly its neck is cut across the front with sweeps of a knife. The blood that flows is caught in a receptacle and cooked with omentum fat. Next the meat of the front of the abdomen is removed, then inner organs including the liver, intestines, heart, and lungs are taken out to be boiled or roasted, but not dried. Next the stomach is given to the boys who herd the cattle and they boil or roast it at the mens' meeting place and eat it then and there. The meat from the front of the abdomen is roasted with a little of the animal's liver at the spot where it was killed. It is eaten there by the men. The rest of the liver is given to boys to roast for themselves. The lungs are discarded. Some of the meat is taken to the main hut where it is cooked and eaten and the rest is dried for future use. The blood that was collected when the animal was killed is put in a clay pot and covered with fat from the abdominal cavity and a little salt. It is dished out on plates and known as musiya.

2. Preparing Dried Meat

Most of the meat is dried. It is cut into strips which are placed on a drying platform. In the center, underneath this platform, a fire is made. The meat is left there until only embers remain below. The process is slow and the meat may take 2 or 3 days to dry thoroughly. When it is removed from the platform, it is placed in the sun for another day to ensure that it is completely dry. It is then cut up and stored in pots in the main hut to be used for relish in the winter months when food is scarce. It is usually cooked in a pot with water, a little salt, and often with peanut butter.[11]

3. Milk

The Shona are fond of milk, but its supply is so variable that many people in rural areas seldom drink it. Traditionally it is consumed "soured". Sour milk is prepared by pouring the fresh milk into a clay pot and leaving it to stand overnight. The cream is not skimmed off the milk. The next day it is poured from the clay pot into a calabash, where it remains, and more is added each day until the calabash is full. After 2 or 3 days the milk becomes thick with lumps suspended in a watery liquid (whey). This is poured into a small pot and given to the children to drink. The curds are mixed with the fat and served as a relish with thick porridge, which is dipped into it as it is eaten. This is consumed mostly in the summer.[12]

4. Goats

Although they are not as highly prized as cattle, goats have a real place in the village. Their meat provides a useful form of protein and is less expensive than beef. A goat is often killed as an offering to the ancestral spirit. An average family may kill three or four goats a year, whereas an ox is slaughtered much less often, probably not more than one a year if any at all. The choicest part of the goat is the meat of the foreleg. When a goat is killed its blood is collected in a plate and covered with some of the omental fat in order to make musiya. Formerly the skin of the animal was eaten. The large intestine is washed and cooked for the family, the shoulder often cut into pieces and eaten raw by the children. Some of the lungs is given to the small boys who roast and eat it. The rest is reserved for the adults who roast it. The men also receive a small piece of liver which they cut into pieces and roast on the fire. The wife cooks the rest of the liver in the main hut.

The meat itself is cut into portions. Some is cooked and eaten, but the greater part dried and kept for when it is needed. When required the wife cuts the strips of dried meat into small pieces and cooks them in water. When ready they are removed with a large spoon, leaving a little of the watery soup in which they were boiled in the pot. This is poured into a smaller pot, some peanut butter added to it, cooked until it is well mixed, and poured back into the big pot. The meat is stewed in it and a little salt added.[13]

Fresh meat is usually available in the spring. Formerly a fair amount was obtained in this season by hunting and trapping, and the dried meat was kept in reserve for winter when green vegetables would not be procurable. It was eaten during the planting season and until late in the rainy season.

5. Sheep

In many areas of Rhodesia there are no sheep, but in others, such as the Mount Darwin district, they are plentiful. A sheep is killed the same way as a goat, and its fresh blood is collected when it is slaughtered and used to make musiya, which is given to children, as adults are not permitted to eat it. The stomach also goes to boys and girls and the rest of the meat is divided and prepared in the same way as goat's meat.

Pork is usually eaten fresh, as its fat content is so high, and when dried, it keeps only a month. The intestines of the pig are not eaten.

6. Hunting and Snaring Game

Formerly hunting was an everyday affair in the life of the Shona, and game was an important source of protein. The flesh of buck (deer), dassies (wild rabbits), guinea fowls, and doves is popular.

7. Mice

In rural areas the women and their daughters catch mice at the beginning of the cold season by digging in the woods. The one most sought after is the Shana *(Steatomys praternisis),* which is eaten by adults but not by children. The woman takes home the dead mice, cleans them in cold water, and throws away the internal organs. They are then placed in a clay pot and boiled with water and a little salt. Then they are dried at the fire and are ready to eat. They may also be grilled. Another type, the gerbil, lives underground and is caught in large numbers. However, the supply of mice tends to be seasonal. In a good season a woman may catch as many as 200, but although they are a useful source of protein, they are not specially favored as a dish. When they are available, a woman may eat on the average one mouse every few weeks.[14]

8. Fowl

It is difficult to assess the exact importance of the fowl as a source of protein in the Shona diet. Although flesh is eaten regularly, it seems that fowls are not killed as often as we might expect from visits to a village, largely because there is a limit to the number of birds a small village can maintain. On enquiry, it appears that a family may eat one or two fowls a month if they are plentiful.

9. Fish

Although Shona are fond of fish, it does not comprise an important source of protein for them. On European farms and mines the laborers are often given a ration of dried fish, but the supply of fresh fish tends to be seasonable. Also smaller rivers tend to dry up in the dry season.

A fish is prepared by scraping off the scales, opening it, and throwing away the intestines. It is then cooked. Fish, particularly the smaller varieties, are often dried. After being cleaned and their intestines removed, they are placed on rocks to dry in the sun for an hour a day for two successive days. Dried fish is kept in a pot and boiled when required. It is eaten as a relish with stiff porridge.[15]

10. Insects

Bees — The Shona use honey made by several different types of bees. Its supply is not greatly important in the diet as it is seasonal, sporadic, and only obtained locally. Further it is not easy to collect.

Locusts — Locusts are looked upon as a delicacy rather than a food on account of their sporadic seasonal appearance.

Flying ants — Flying ants, inhabiting the ant hills, are available in the summer at the beginning of the rains.

Caterpillars — Various kinds of caterpillars are eaten as a delicacy when they are fully grown. Again they are seasonal, also mostly appearing at the beginning of the rains. They are gathered from the branches of trees, their intestines squeezed out and discarded, and the remainder roasted in a little water. They can be dried and kept for relish to be eaten throughout the year.[16]

D. Beer

Beer, prepared from one of the cereals such as finger millet, bulrush millet, and maize, is usually consumed by adult men and to a much lesser extent by women. The traditional Shona woman does not drink strong beer, at least until she has passed the climacteric, when she may drink a stronger variety.[17] An unmarried man is not permitted to drink the stronger form of beer with an alcoholic base of about 3%. But all Shona — men, women, and children are allowed to have the sweet preparation of beer. This is perfectly safe as it contains only 0.5% of alcohol. Millet is the cereal of choice for the preparation of beer, but maize or bulrush millet can be used instead and the brewing procedure is the same, no matter what grain is used. Normally beer is prepared only for special occasions. There are a number of these occasions but only three main ones. The first is for hoka, the occasion on which friends and relations come to help a man weed or reap his crops, and the second for a party or gathering of people who dance and play musical instruments. The third is the ritual occasion when it is made specially for a ceremony at which the spirit elders and alien spirits are remembered and praised.

To make beer, some grain is soaked overnight on a flat rock. It ferments after 2 or 3 days and is then called chimera. This is spread out in the sun for a day to dry and then ground into meal, and later boiled on a fire to make into thin porridge called bota. It stands until the next day when it has acquired a sweet taste. It is then boiled again and is now called manga. This is poured into pots and, when it is cold the next day, plates are put on top of the pots. These stand for 5 days and on the sixth the lids are removed and a handful of grain added to each pot. This causes the beer to ferment. By the following day it has become strong. Finally it is strained with a beer strainer and is now ready to drink.

E. Special Features of Shona Eating

When considering the diet of the African one should remember the manner in which the food is prepared, served, and eaten. There are several factors which may have a bearing on the development or unlikelihood of developing a pathological state. It is difficult to assess their exact influence, but it may be helpful to take cognizance of them. The Shona have two main meals a day, and in traditional society breakfast was not eaten. Today, however, a small breakfast is becoming common in both towns and rural areas.[18] Normally water, other drinks, or soups are not taken with meals. Water is drunk between them.

A meal consists of one course — a cereal mixture and a relish or meat. They are eaten at the same time, that is, the porridge is dipped into the gravy and put into the mouth and this is followed by a portion of the meat. Meals are served lukewarm — neither hot nor cold.

Another interesting feature of Shona meals is that they are never eaten standing. Traditionally it is correct to sit on the ground. This gives one a relaxed feeling and also one of safety as no one can attack another if all are seated. It is striking, too, that in traditional society and often even in urban homes today, all those gathered for a meal eat from a common plate. Each person waits for his turn to take his portion. This gives him a feeling of sharing the food, as no one receives a bigger portion than another. It is not done to talk during a meal; thus there is no so-called polite conversation and everyone eats with his mind on his food.

Men and women eat apart, the men at a special place outside the house set apart for them, and the women and their young children in a room inside it. Thus an argument between husband and wife is unlikely to occur during a meal.

V. PATTERN OF DISEASE IN RELATION TO DIET

Field studies on Shona food in rural (traditonal) and urban areas revealed that peptic ulcer was more commonly encountered in the urban African.[19] it was difficult to attribute the increase to the diet, as the pattern of diet in the towns was still based on the traditonal one. There may have been other reasons for the change. Perhaps the tension might be greater in town life. The incidence of acute appendicitis was also higher in town where some clinicians held that those who were employed as cooks were affected by acute appendicitis more often than farm laborers who ate in a traditional way. This condition was certainly less often encountered in the rural areas studied.

It is difficult to know the exact position with regard to the appearance of carcinoma of the stomach. There was a period recently when there seemed to be an increase in the frequency of this disease, as compared with 30 or 40 years ago, but again it is not as common as might be expected. I cannot link this disorder with a preexisting gastritis or gastric ulcer. Many African men tend to drink heavily, but cancer of the stomach seems not to be related to this habit. On the other hand, leiomyosarcoma of this organ is an interesting tumor met now and then in the African, but there seems not to be any evidence of any connection between it and the diet.

Cancer of the stomach — Cancer of the stomach is common in Japan and this has been atrributed to the high intake of fat of the Japanese. But in contrast, on the whole the diet of the African tends to be low in animal fats. Carcinoma of the esophagus is very common in Shona men and appears to be becoming more frequent. Women are seldom affected by it, but unfortunately we have not been able to establish a definite relationship to any one factor, although alcohol is suspected. There are areas in Africa in which the disease is uncommon, and yet alcohol is consumed with apparently the same frequency and regularity as in Mashonaland. A study conducted in Salisbury by Wapnick et al.[20] seemed to indicate a combination of alcohol consumption and cigarette smoking as responsible, the individual swallowing his saliva, which contains large amounts of irritant such as nicotine.

Hypochromic anemia — Hypochromic anemia is common in Rhodesia, but there does not appear to be any increased liability of these patients to develop cancer of the stomach. When salt is added to food, this is done only in the cooking, and, as far as I know, condiments and spices are not used. Food is eaten with the fingers; portions of stiff porridge are rolled with them to the right size in the palm of the hands. This may be an important point as it is not always easy to judge the correct size to suit the individual when eating European food with a knife and fork.

On the whole, their lips and mouth appear to be freer of cancer than those of people of other races with whom I have been in contact, but then smoking is perhaps rarer. However, deficiency disorders such as cheilosis and angular stomatitis are very common, due to ariboflavinosis. Glossitis, too, as a result of pellagra, is encountered fairly often. In the eastern part of Cape Province carcinoma of the floor of the mouth was not uncommonly seen among Africans, and this was attributed to tobacco irritation through chewing it or possibly through the use of long wooden pipes by men and women.[21]

The small bowel — It would seem that vegetable bezoar is formed in some way in the stomach and revolves around the high fiber content of the African's diet. Thus two diseases, very uncommon in the Shona, are ulcerative colitis and diverticulitis. The rarity of the latter in Africans has been attributed to the high fiber content of their diet, which encourages more daily motions than the western one which tends to be of low bulk and more liable to produce constipation. Why ulcerative colitis is rare is not clear. It may be due to the high fiber content of the diet. Similarly Crohn's disease is seldom met with in Africans in Rhodesia, but it is very doubtful whether the diet is a factor leading to this condition which is now being linked in a common etiology with ulcerative colitis.

Carcinoma of the colon — Carcinoma of the colon, too, is rarely seen in African society in contrast to European communities. This is held to be due to dietetic differences in the two races. It is suggested that because of the more refined diet of the white man, carcinogens remain longer than normal in the intestine, where they come into contact with the mucosa, thus, after some years, rendering it more susceptible to malignant changes. On the other hand, because of the diet of the African, in whom two or three motions a day are normal, the carcinogens are moved along more swiftly and so do not come into such intimate contact with the mucosal cells. Another suggestion is that the white man's diet, which is richer in saturated fatty acids, may be a precipitating factor in leading to malignant degeneration in the cells of the mucosa. However, carcinoma of the rectum in Africans is more common than in the colon itself.

Primary carcinoma of the liver — Primary carcinoma of the liver is an interesting disease seen very commonly in Rhodesia, mostly in men and generally in those over the age of 45 years, but comparatively rarely in the younger age groups. It is not clear, however, whether a toxic agent, such as aflatoxins, plays a role in its production. The Shona eat groundnuts in the form of bota or peanut butter. We have little evidence to show whether one of the folk doctor's remedies with a hepatoxic action is responsible. We know that many Shona people take herbal medicines frequently and regularly, but it is extremely difficult to find any particular agent that could be held responsible.

Malnutrition and gastroenteritis — There seems to be general agreement that an individual, especially a child, who is in a state of malnutrition, is liable to develop gastroenteritis.

VI. TRADITIONAL TREATMENT OF DISEASE

The traditional medical practitioner in Rhodesia is known as the n'anga. Generally an illness is attributed to the upset of an ancestral spirit or to the evil of a witch. In order to prevent the affected person from suffering continually or perhaps dying, a twofold treatment is instituted. First, the particular spirit or evil force causing the illness must be discovered and placated so that no further damage is inflicted on the patient or his family. Secondly, a medicinal preparation, usually prepared from a plant, is given to neutralize the "poison" already introduced into the body. Thus the n'anga has knowledge of many plants that he believes will cure or relieve the symptoms of which the patient complains, such as headache, vomiting, diarrhea, constipation, mental confusion, abodminal pains, menstrual disturbances, infertility, impotence, etc.

Each herbalist tends to guard his roots and other medicines closely, and there is no attempt to correlate the results with those of others. A serious drawback to the success of the herbalist is that he treats symptoms and not disease, thus failing to recognize the many different causes of headache, cough, diarrhea, and other symptoms. All types of headache are treated in the same way. An offended ancestral spirit or an evil one can cause headache, backache, cough, diarrhea or any other symptom it pleases. On the other hand, the African herbalist probably, over many years, has come to recognize the medicinal properties of certain roots, which when taken internally, are followed by certain beneficial or disastrous results. He will have learned whether certain herbs have a cathartic, emetic, or aphrodisiac effect and which ones relieve cough, indigestion, or pain in various parts of the body. The value of counter irritation in the relief of pain is appreciated. Cupping and making incisions in the skin into which an ointment is rubbed are almost universal. The same effect is produced by practitoners who suck the affected part with their mouths, and by so doing they gain a reputation equal to that of any specialist in western society, especially when they produce a piece of animal bone, a stone, or thorn from their mouths as proof that the evil has been safely removed.

Incisions are made with a razor blade or any other sharp instrument possessed by the n'anga. He may employ a sharp metal instrument known as chitso. Irritant powder is rubbed into the cut producing an increased blood supply to the diseased part. When he has done this the doctor may also apply suction with his mouth or more probably with his murimiko, a small horn from which the tip has been removed and the gap covered with beeswax. He pierces the wax with a pin and then applies the opposite end of his murimiko to the skin at the swelling, sucking hard through the pinhole to create a vacuum. When this is over he squeezes closed his wax and relaxes his lips so that the murimiko remains attached to the patient. This is left for about 20 min. It is said to suck out impure blood from a swelling or bruise due to an injury.

The powder rubbed into an incision is prepared by burning roots to charcoal in a broken clay pot over a fire, or else by placing a burning ember into the pot with the roots and a little water and castor oil or fat. It is stored in a horn until required.

A very popular treatment is drinking an infusion in which the root, or occasionally a leaf or bark, is soaked in water for several hours or sometimes boiled in it. The extract is then mixed in a thin liquid finger millet *(Elusine indica gaertn)* or maize porridge and given to the patient once, twice, or three times a day according to instruction. Only occasionally is it mixed in stiff porridge. Usually the root is preferred to the bark or leaf for this purpose. It is stamped in a stamping block and then ground to fine powder, which is usually diluted with water and then added to a thin porridge. Not uncommonly, two or more portions of different insects or animals are mixed together to produce a medicine. There is no end to the possible combination that may be used.[22]

A great number of different plants are used as herbal medicines by traditional folk practitioners. It is impossible to mention all, but the popular ones found by us (Mavi, Drummond, and Gelfand) have been selected.

VII. HERBAL PLANTS USED BY N'ANGA FOR MEDICINAL PURPOSES

Acalypha senensis — This is widely used for a variety of children's ailments such as depressed fontanelle, dysentery and abdominal pains, and as a tonic.[23] In adults it is employed for pulmonary and dermatological complaints as well as for an aphrodisiac. A cold infusion of its crushed roots is administered by one of the large Shona tribes, the Karanga, for rheumatic and neuralgic pain.

Albizzia antunesiana — This is frequently prescribed for different ailments, the more common of which are abdominal, gynecological, pulmonary, and venereal, and it is also used for depressed fontanelle. It is also employed as an aphrodisiac, its root being sold to patrons in beer halls. The bark contains tannin and saponin. In Zambia an infusion of this herb is favored as a lotion for cuts and is applied to wounds. Its sap is used as eyedrops for ophthalmic inflammation. A cold infusion of the roots serves as a remedy for gonorrhea and as an aphrodisiac. The roots are chewed to cure coughs and colds.[24]

Alepidea amatymbica — This is used for various complaints and is known as a charm to drive away evil spirits as well as one for bringing good luck.[25] The root is employed for divination. Before a n'anga begins to divine with his wooden bones, he chews the root of *Alepidea* and spits it on his bones. Newly purchased bones are boiled with the root. It is believed that only n'anga can obtain this root from the bush. It is said that if any other person tries he will become mad. The n'anga must be naked when he digs out this plant. Besides its magical uses, it is considered of value for abdominal complaints and as a bee repellant. Watt and Breyer Brandwijk mention that the Zulu employ it as an enema for children with coryza and cough and also as a snuff for colds and influenza. The Sotho chew the roots for chest disease and the Xhosa employ the plant for abdominal complaints.

Aloe sp. — These are often prescribed by African folk practitioners for a variety of ailments. They are popular remedies for abdominal, gynecological, and venereal disorders. It has been noted that some n'anga favor it for diarrhea, while others prefer it as a purgative for constipation.[26] In many records of the medicinal use of the aloe in Rhodesia, it is not known which species is concerned. It is likely that several are used indiscriminately, as there is little or no distinction between species in their vernacular names. Apparently the most commonly used species are *A. chabaudii, A. greatheadii* and *A. excelsha.*

A. greatheadii — Aloes may also be employed for nonhuman disorders. N'anga give *A. greatheadii* to chickens to cure them of disease. The roots are crushed and soaked in water which is then given to them to drink.

A. chabaudii and *A. globuligemma* — There are records of death following the taking of aloe leaf as medicine, although in most cases the evidence is only circumstantial. In one, three cups of an extract of *A. chabaudii* were given to a patient living in Inyanga, about 120 mi northeast of Salisbury. After taking it, he was unable to move his limbs, developed convulsions, and died. Over the past few years a number of cases of alleged poisoning by *A. globuligemma* have been reported in the Nyamandhova and Bulalima-Mangwe districts of Matabeleland. The histories of the latest two cases are worth recording in detail. On June 1, 1974, a storekeeper on the Botswana border south of Plumtree complained to his wife of stomach pains, for which he took "liver salts", but as the symptoms continued, he left his home in his car at 4 p.m. 2 days after their onset, saying he was going out on business. He returned at about 5:30 that afternoon with a quantity of aloe leaves, which he had picked himself. They were cut up and placed in a 2-pt saucepan of water and boiled at the same time as the family supper was being cooked. The mixture was removed from the fire after supper and allowed to cool. When he had had his bath the man poured some of this liquid into a cup and drank it. About 8:40 p.m. that night he complained to his wife that he was "powerless" and that the medicine he had drunk was no good. He died shortly afterwards. The only abnormal signs noticed had been slight salivation and twitching of his right leg. He had neither vomited nor purged. No other member of the family was ill. An autopsy was performed, but nothing of note was found in the viscera. The remains of the liquid in the saucepan in which the leaves had been cooked were taken to a government analyst, who fed some of it to a guinea pig. The animal died 10 min later. Yet the leaf of *A. globuligemma* growing in the Botanic Garden was fed to another guinea pig without any ill effect. This medicine, called icena by Africans, is used by them for disorders of the stomach, including constipation, and is normally harmless. Efforts to find a toxic aloe in this neighborhood proved unsuccessful.

In the Plumtree area on January 30, 1975, two African women requiring a purgative scooped out the inside of one leaf of *A. globuligemma,* boiled it in a tin of water, and drank the liquid at 10 a.m. By 2 p.m. one of the women had died and the other was taken to hospital in a serious condition, from which she fortunately recovered. A large plant from which the leaf was taken was submitted to the Herbarium for examination. Several young plants from its immediate vicinity were also sent there. The large ones smelled strongly of rats and proved toxic to guinea pigs; the small plants did not have the rat-like smell and were not toxic. The plant is in cultivation in Salisbury, where it has almost lost its unpleasant smell but not its toxicity.

A. orthlopha — Another example of aloe poisoning occurred when two women, employed as weeders in the Botanic Gardens in Salisbury, took an infusion of the leaves of *A. orthlopha* (an endemic plant of the serpentine of the Great Dyke in Rhodesia). They drank this at 8:30 a.m. and by 9:30, one of them was in a state of collapse, appearing drunk. She could not stand on her own. They were rushed to the hospital, where the second woman became ill. Both had recovered completely by 4 p.m. A guinea pig, dosed with the leaf, survived.[27]

Annona sp. — *Annona* sp. are used for a variety of complaints, including gynecological, venereal, pulmonary, and dermatological ones, as well as for generalized body pains. Its use as a repellent is well known. It is also employed as a good-luck charm and to purify the blood. This plant contains a glycoside which is not deleteriously affected by boiling.

Aristolochia heppii — The root is a remedy for a variety of complaints, including abdominal ailments, swollen legs, and depressed fontanelle. Most n'anga mentioned that if it is taken by a pregnant woman, it could cause abortion. A related species *A. petersiana,* is suspected of causing abortion in Rhodesia when used with *Indigofera arrecta.* In East Africa, this plant is a well-known poison, and Hardcourt and Trump consider it poisonous to man and animals. They mention that it has been used by some tribes as an ingredient in arrow poison.

Asparagus spp. — *Asparagus* spp. are popular with African practitioners for several disorders. The most common ones treated with this herb are pulmonary, abdominal, liver, gynecological, venereal, bilharzial, and ophththalmic, as well as those of the nervous system and depressed fontanelle. It is also used for magical purposes. Most species seem to be harmless. The cultivated *A. officinalis* is apparently excreted in the urine and has a diuretic effect. Poisoning by this species may consist of minor temporary irritation of the skin or painful irritation and inflammation with vesicles or blisters. A dermatitis of this nature may persist for weeks if the infection is severe and the patient susceptible.

Aspilia pluriseta — *A. pluriseta* is used for many different disorders, including those of an abdominal, gynecological, hepatic nature as well as those of the nervous system and for swollen legs. The plant has also been recommended as a panacea and is said to stop rain when it is pointed towards rain clouds.

Blumea aurita — *B. aurita* is employed for pulmonary, heart, nervous, and abdominal complaints, and for fever and painful legs. The plant is well known for its aromatic smell which, it is believed, drives away bad spirits and removes bad luck. It is also used as a remedy for bed wetting and as a tonic for infants.

Boophane disticha — A variety of ailments, especially edema and dizziness, are treated with *B. disticha.* It is also employed for magical purposes, such as helping a football team to play well. It is well known to n'anga for its power to induce possession. In most cases no drug is required for this, except for a bewtiched patient, when this will help the n'anga's spirit to possess him. In order to obtain this effect the bulb is crushed in water, boiled, and then mixed with the powdered roots of *Zanha africana* and those of mukundagona (the identity of which is not yet known). The patient is given only a teaspoon of this decoction.

Boophane is a well known human and stock poison, producing a hallucinatory state.[28] A patient 24 years of age was advised by a n'anga to drink the juice of a boophone bulb if he developed abdominal pains and felt weak. On January 18, 1952, after suffering great discomfort, he cut off the root of one of these bulbs, allowing a few drops of its juice to collect on a plate. This he mixed with cooked porridge of which he ate only 2 spoonfuls. Within minutes his mouth became very painful and he felt a burning pain running down to his epigastrium. He became dizzy and fell to the ground unconscious. He regained consciousness 20 hr later in the hospital, talkative and restless. He displayed an intense photophobia, his skin was dry, and his temperature 99.6°F, pulse 77, and respirations 18/min. His pupils were widely dilated but reacted to light. The next morning he was still irrational, talkative, and inclined to resist examination. His pupils were still dilated, but equal, and reacted to light. Tests proved no parasites were present in the peripheral blood and no protein or sugar in the urine. He soon improved and made an uninterrupted recovery.

In the Chiota district on February 21, 1974, a boy 17 years of age, who, with other boys, had drunk an infusion prepared from a bulb of boophane, was found drowned in a river near his home, after having wandered by himself in an apparently hallucinatory state. His companions had also been intoxicated. The pulp of the tuber had been soaked in water for 30 min. The first and second infusions were thrown away and the third consumed.

The characteristic signs of boophane poisoning in nonfatal cases are

1. Rapid development of staxia and giddiness
2. Impaired vision
3. Talkativeness or quietness and depression
4. Stupor
5. Coma

Four alkaloids are isolated from the bulb:

1. Buphanine (resembling hyosine in pharmacological action)
2. A weak basic alkaloid (with convulsive action)
3. A water soluble alkaloid (similar in action to colchicine)
4. Narcissine

It is claimed that a fifth alkaloid, hemanthine (resembling atropine in action), has also been isolated from it. When this was applied in a 2% solution to the conjunctivae, a burning sensation with lachrymation and mydriasis was produced.

Carissa edulis — Several complaints are treated with this herb, including pulmonary, abdominal, ophthalmic, and nervous system ailments. It is also given for venereal disease, general body pains, and for magical complaints. The root powder is mixed with that of blister beetle *(Mylabris pustulata)* as a remedy for gonorrhea. The mixture works as a diuretic. The root is said to contain a cardiac glucoside carissin.[29]

Cassia abbreviata — *C. abbreviata* is well known as a remedy for abdominal, venereal, and gynecological disorders and for backache. It is also used as an aphrodisiac. Many n'anga mention that the infusion can cause abortion when taken by mouth. It has also been used in the management of blackwater fever, both by African and European practitioners.

C. singueana — *C. singueana* is popular for gynecological, abdominal, venereal, ophthalmic, and cardiovascular complaints. It was also recommended to induce the cord to drop off an infant's navel and as a panacea for all ills. Its bark contains tannin.

Chenopodium ambrosioides — This plant is well known for use in nervous system disorders including convulsions, madness, and delirium. It is also employed for high fever, as a tonic, and for gynecological complaints. It has an aromatic smell which is believed to drive away bad spirits and snakes and is used as a treatment for people worried by ghosts. In modern medicine this plant is used as an anthelmenthic to expel hookworms, tapeworms, and roundworms. Chenopodium poisoning seems not to have been recognized by n'anga, as they have not used it internally except for the insertion of its leaves into the vagina as a treatment for a painful uterus. According to European sources its poisonous properties are well known. Its oil may cause headache, vertigo, tinnitus, nausea, vomiting, temporary deafness, gastroenteritis, and, in severe cases of poisoning, kidney and liver damage, jaundice, and complete prostration with death. Cumulative effects may be produced by small doses given several days apart.

A case of alleged chenopodium poisoning was recorded in the Marandellas law court. On Thursday, June 6th that year an African woman, aged 22 years, was suffering from dizziness and chest pains. The next day she went into the bush and collected leaves of *C. ambrosioides* of which she drank an infusion. The following day she was feeling better but on the next afternoon she became quite ill. She vomited frequently and was dizzy; she could not keep her balance and started to shiver and shake. By eight in the evening she was worse, lost consciousness on her way to the hospital, and on arrival there was certified as dead.

Cissampelos mucronata — C. mucronata is well known as medicine for a variety of complaints including abdominal, hepatic, gynecological, and ophthalmic disorders, bilharziasis, sore throat, backache, and venereal disease. In Tanzania its root is used in pregnancy.

C. molle — *C. molle* is a popular remedy for abdominal, gynecological, and nervous system complaints as well as for depressed fontanelle, backache, and difficulties in walking caused by witchcraft. It is popular, too, as an aphrodisiac and for abdominal pains, and even laymen know of its uses.

Combretum platypetalum — This is perhaps best known as a medicine to dilate the vagina to procure an easy passage for the birth of a baby. It is used for several abdominal complaints such as pain, diarrhea, and vomiting. An infusion of roots is generally preferred but very rarely the fruits, flowers, or leaves are employed. Its seeds are known to be highly poisonous. Severe illness was recorded in two adults with stomach pains and vomiting after eating some of the seeds. School children have frequently been ill from eating them.[30]

Croton megalobotrys — This is popular for constipation and is also used as an emetic and for a variety of abdominal complaints, especially for dropsy. Its bark is well known as a human and fish poison. Two n'anga have stated that it can cause abortion. In the early 1950s this plant was used in a trial by ordeal by a visiting herbalist from Malawi, and was later nicknamed Muchape (the Malawi vernacular name of *C. megalobotrys*). In Mozambique and South Africa, it is employed as an antimalaria remedy and also as a fish poison. Its bark and seeds are known to cause an intense sensation in the throat, salivation, nausea, and purging.[31]

Cyphostemma sp. — This is a remedy for many gynecological complaints and also for backache, wasting disorders, and goiter. The plant is taken to prevent lightning from striking and to drive away bad luck. It is said to be poisonous if taken by mouth.

Datura stramonium — This is used for venereal, abdominal, and pulmonary disorders and for goiter, boils, and chitsinga (a pain believed due to a foreign body stationery or moving inside the patient). Among other uses, *Datura* is employed in divination. Before starting to divine, the n'anga sniffs tobacco snuff mixed with the powdered leaves of Datura. He then chews its roots and spits them on his hakata (bones) as he commences to throw them. When determining the cause of death the n'anga chews the leaves of *Datura* before he starts to divine. This we were told helps him to communicate more easily with his spirits. *D. stramonium* is used by n'anga to relieve bronchial spasm in asthma. The patient burns the prescribed dried leaves in a broken clay pot (chayenga) and inhales the smoke. This plant may cause posioning in man, the patient becoming confused, incoherent, ataxic, and stuporose.[32] Physical signs include flushing, widely dilated pupils, dryness of mouth, pyrexia, tachycardia, and exaggerated reflexes. A case of *Datura* poisoning was described in an African male by Thomas and Gelfand.[33] The patient, aged 20 years, was brought to the hospital in a state of mental confusion. It transpired that he had consulted an African doctor for urinary frequency for which he had been given the leaves of a *Datura* plant. On admission, he was healthy in appearance but restless and disorientated. He thought it was daytime and that the doctor examining him was at first a policeman, then a native commissioner, and lastly even his employer, but definitely not a person. He attempted to catch imaginary objects on the orderly's sleeves and searched his bed for fictitious articles. He was frequently found threading imaginary needles or industriously mending tears in the blankets. He was obviously not frightened and was constantly smiling and laughing for no apparent reason. He often undressed and tried to wander around the ward naked. On examination, there was no localized weakness, and he was able to move his limbs freely, although he staggered when he walked. His pupils were widely dilated and reacted sluggishly to light. The tendon reflexes were equal and brisk and the plantar responses flexor. Of interest was the presence of a large tumor extending from just above the symphysis pubis to just below the umbilicus. The pulse was full and regular, its rate 120/min. His blood pressure was 128/70. As the cause of his condition was not recognized at the time, he was admitted and symptomatic treatment was instituted. A gastric lavage was performed and 5 cc paraldehyde administered subcutaneously because of the restlessness. After 12 hr he had improved greatly, and he gradually recovered and several hours later became normally orientated. He could then recall what had happened. His pupils, however, remained dilated several hours longer.

Dichrostachys cinerea — This is popular with n'anga in Rhodesia. Analysis showed that neither its fruit nor bean contain hydrocyanic acid. In South Africa it is given for a great diversity of complaints, such as toothache, abdominal, chest, syphilis, and skin diseases.

Dicerocaryum zanguebarium — This is a popular remedy for measles in Rhodesia. It is also used during labor when an infusion is continually instilled in the vagina to allow an easy passage for the baby. It is also drunk as an aid to the parturition. The infusion is used by laymen as a substitute for soap. The Sotho in South Africa give an infusion of the leaf to women and animals to expel a retained placenta. In East Africa it is used in the treatment of hydrocele and gonorrhea.[34]

Dicoma anomala — This is a well known panacea to n'anga and even laymen are aware of it. It is employed for a variety of disorders, including the prevention of witchcraft, abdominal, gynecological, and pulmonary disorders, as well as for venereal diseases. It is common to see babies with the root of this plant suspended from around their necks as a charm to prevent witchcraft. The infusion is used for most of the treatments with it.

Diospyros lycioides — This is used for abdominal, pulmonary, and gynecological complaints and is an antidote for snake bites and poisoning.

Elephantorrhiza goetzei — A variety of disorders are treated with *E. goetzei*. These include abdominal, rheumatic, venereal, and heart complaints and depressed fontanelle. One n'anga mentioned that an infusion of its roots is drunk to purify the blood.

Eriospermum abyssinicum — This is a remedy for depressed fontanelle in babies, hence its vernacular name is chipande (fontanelle). Babies are often seen with a root of this plant, or that of *Dicoma anomala,* hanging from their necks to prevent depression of their fontanelles.

Flacourtia indica — Several conditions, varying from gynecological, pulmonary, and ophthalmic disorders to teething in babies, are treated with *F. indica*. To ensure a good harvest its seeds are soaked in its root infusion and planted in the field. A n'anga recommends drinking its root infusion to stop noisy bowel sounds.

Gardenia sp. — *Gardenia* sp. is widely used by n'anga to prevent witches from entering a home or a village. Twigs are pegged around it as a protection against evil. The ladle in a n'anga's special calabash (gona) is cut from this species. As with many other remedies it is also employed for pulmonary, gynecological, and nervous disorders. In tribal areas of Rhodesia, when the ground is being cleared near houses, these bushes are not cut down as they are thought to ward off lightning.

Gnidia kraussiana — N'anga often recommend *G. kraussiana* as a purgative and emetic, but an overdose is known to be highly poisonous. Its tuber root is used to prepare this medicine. The fresh root is applied to ulcers, boils, and to draw pus out of wounds. From time to time it has been responsible for the death of Africans who have used it as medicine. Several cases of stock poisoning have also been reported in Rhodesia after animals have grazed on its leaves. *Gnidia* poisoning is said to cause loss of appetite, gastrointestinal upset, and diarrhea changing later to constipation. An increased respiratory rate with intense thirst and salivation is another symptom. The root is also well-known as a fish poison.[35]

Loranthus sp. — *Loranthus* sp. is perhaps the most popular plant used by n'anga and is included among the medicines of most of them. Most of the herbs in their medicinal calabashes are different species of loranthus from different trees. When a n'anga looks for a *Loranthus* sp. to use, he looks for one growing on a particular type of tree rather than of a particular species of the plant. In Rhodesia, the one growing on *Ficus burkei* is suspected of causing death.[36] One of the *Loranthus* sp. in East Africa is alleged to be poisonous.[37]

Maytenus sengalensis — This is another extremely popular medicine prescribed by n'anga and is taken for a variety of complaints, including nervous and pulmonary disorders, bilharzia, skin and venereal diseases, abdominal, gynecological and ophthalmic ailments, as well as being an aphrodisiac. In traditional areas, branches of the tree are used to cover graves and for other purposes in burial ceremonies. For example, if a person dies in a Salisbury hospital and is buried in a Salisbury cemetery, his relations ask to see the grave. The elder brother or the father of the deceased brings with him a small branch of chizhuzhu *(M. sengalensis)*, which he shakes over the grave. He then removes a little soil and a few stones from it saying, "I have taken you to bury you at home."[38]

Myrothamnus flabellifolia — This is given for a variety of complaints, including those of the nervous, pulmonary, abdominal, gynecological, and dermatological systems. It is also used to drive away bad spirits and to prevent bad luck. It has been recorded that the Karanga chew its leaf to treat scurvy, halitosis, and for Vincent's angina. A sick person washes himself in the water in which a dry plant has been revived and became green again. Early European settlers in Rhodesia used it to alleviate pain. Amongst white people it is colloquially known as the resurrection plant.

Mondia whitei — *M. whitei* is often employed for different complaints, especially for constipation and as an aphrodisiac. Its powdered roots are often sold in markets.

Ozoroa reticulata — This is popular for several disorders, such as abdominal and gynecological, as well as for backache and the inflamed navel of an infant. It is also favored as an aphrodisiac.

Pavetta schumanniana — Various disorders of the lung, abdomen, and uterus are treated with *P. schumanniana,* which is also given to cure venereal disease.

Peltophorum africanum — This is another herb given for many very different disorders, such as those of the abdominal, ophthalmic, and nervous system. It is used as well for edema and anemia and also for sore throat. It may be employed as a diuretic and as a diaphoretic. Many n'anga regard it as a panacea for all diseases.

Piliostigma thonningii — This has wide usage, which includes most complaints. It is a well-known remedy for menorrhagia (excessive menstruation). Its bark is used for coughs, and a mixture of the roots and tobacco has a stimulating action.

Pterocarpus angolensis — This is used for a variety of dissimilar ailments, including abdominal, gynecological, venereal, pulmonary, and dermatological ones, as well as for the treatment of bilharzia and as an aphrodisiac. Watt and Breyer-Brandwijk[39] mention that in Zambia ashes of the seed of this tree are applied to inflamed areas of the skin and to bleeding gums. Red sap from its bark is employed as a remedy for sores and for the control of ringworm. An enema of the sap is used to eliminate intestinal parasites. Decoctions of the root are employed to cure gonorrhea and the pounded leaf in enema form to treat backache.

Ricinus communis — This is taken for a number of different complaints, such as abdominal, nervous, and genitourinary ones. It is a popular plant grown by nearly every n'anga for its seeds, which are used to prepare oil for their gona. Although these seeds are highly poisonous, our n'anga do not seem to be aware of this, as they are used externally and in only very small doses. That the leaves and seed are poisonous has been mentioned as having been recorded from most parts of the world.[40] Many unwanted children have been murdered by the inclusion of the seeds of this plant in their food. The symptoms of *Ricinus* poisoning are a burning sensation in the mouth, throat, and stomach, hemorrhagic enteritis, salivations, shivering, increased temperatures, and coma. Death may ensue within about 3 days.

Securidaca longipedunculata — A number of dissimilar disorders are treated with *S. longipedunculata*. Patients with nervous, ophthalmic, abdominal, venereal, and gynecological complaints may all be given this plant, which is also used as an aphrodisiac, an antidote for snake bite, a snake repellant, or as a charm to drive away bad spirits.

Trichodesma physaloides — This is employed to prevent witchcraft as well as for a variety of ailments. Its tuber is a well-known aphrodisiac and also a cure for wounds. There is no record of its being poisonous.

Triumfetta welwitschii — This is a well known remedy for depressed fontanelle and diarrhea and is also used as an aphrodisiac.

Turraea nilotica — This plant is popular for a wide range of complaints — gynecological, ophthalmic, venereal, pulmonary, abdominal, nervous system, and dermatological. It is also regarded as an aphrodisiac and an antidote for poison. It is considered of value for depressed fontanelle.

Warburgia salutaria — This is well recommended by n'anga as a panacea for many complaints. It is also popular, as it is believed to have magical powers which, among other virtues, ends discord between relatives or friends. N'anga usually spit some of its chewed bark on their divining bones (hakata) before beginning to throw them. In South Africa it is regarded as a remedy for colds, malaria, and chest complaints. This tree appears to be extinct in Rhodesia. The only specimen in the Government Herbarium is one obtained by Mr. S. Mavi from sucker shoots from the Mutema Tribal Trust Lands near Chipinga, but no living trees were found in this locality. All had been cut down and their bark removed. The bark, however, is still used by n'anga and sold at market places for a very high price. A piece the size of a palm costs about $5.00. It is imported from Mozambique. The bark is said to contain tannin and mannitol. An unidentified alkaloid has been isolated from the dry bark. The roots, leaves, and bark have a pungent ginger-like or pepper-like taste, due to the presence of an amorphous resinous substance.[41]

Zanha africana — The root powder of the *Z. africana* is considered of great importance to n'anga in foretelling the prognosis of an illness. If the patient sneezes after sniffing this powder, it is taken that he will recover. This root, however, is suspected of being poisonous. Verdcourt and Trump mention that both the roots and the fruits are believed to be poisonous and that deaths have been reported as a result of their use.

Zingiber officinale — This is used for constipation and for depressed fontanelle. Its rhizome is a source of spice ginger, which is made available to patrons of beer halls to relieve constipation. It is also sold in markets.

Ziziphus mucronata — This is said to cure abdominal pain, bilharzia and pneumonia. Watt and Breyer-Brandwijk mention that the Zulu take powdered leaf and bark in water for chest pains and the Chuanas and Tongas use the roots as a remedy for dysentery.[42]

VIII. POISONOUS PLANTS

Drummond, Mavi, and Gelfand have listed the plants in Rhodesia said to be poisonous to humans:

- *Abrus precatorius* — Poisoning with the seed of *A. precatorius* may cause inflammation of the intestinal mucosa and hemorrhagic effusions in the body cavities and organs.[43]

- *Adenia gummifera* is said to be capable of producing acute centrilobular necrosis of the liver lobule.
- *Aloe* sp. — It has been suggested that some tobacco snuffs may contain aloe and that carcinoma of the nose and accessary sinuses in black South Africans may be due to aloe snuff.[44]
- *Boophane disticha* — At autopsy, the heart and intestines may show petechiae.
- *Bowiea volubilis* fibers, used as a purgative, may cause pronounced gastrointestinal irritation.[45]
- *Capparis tomentosa* — This plant is used widely and is believed to have poisonous properties.
- *Chenopodium ambrosioides* is employed as an infusion for a large variety of complaints and poisoning with it by n'anga must be extremely rare. Oil of *Chenopodium* was used for hookworm disease in western medical circles but not by traditional herbalists.
- *Combretum platypetalum* is alleged to be toxic in large doses, but little has been recorded about this.
- Overdose of *Courbonia glauca* may lead to death. At autopsy, hemorrhages are described in the small intestine.[46]
- *Cucumis hirsutus* is said to be a severe poison. If taken in toxic doses, it probably causes a hemorrhagic gastroenteritis. It is often used as a purgative.
- *Curcumis myriocarpus* is employed as a purgative, administered in enema form. It may perhaps cause a fatal hemorrhagic gastritis and enteritis.
- An infusion of *Dalbergia nyasse* is used for abdominal complaints. It is known to be fatal, but little in the way of gross lesions seems to be recognized at autopsy.
- *Datura stramonium* is used for various disorders including dysentery. Overdoses of its root are said to be poisonous.
- *Dichapetulum cymosum* is very poisonous to domestic animals in whom autopsy reveals dilatation of the heart with intracardiac hemorrhages. The animal staggers and then becomes comatose within a few hours of eating the plant.[48]
- *Dioscorea* sp. — Its tuber may be toxic; the main effect of an overdose is on the nervous system. It is employed for diarrhea and as a diuretic.
- *Encepharlartos* sp. — Its seed is known to be toxic to rabbits, producing an effect on the liver with icterus and hemorrhages in the intestines and heart.
- *Erythrophleum africanum* — The bark of this tree may be used for trial by ordeal, hence its name, the ordeal tree. The bark is poisonous. In humans it produces a bradycardia and dyspnea and death from an acute cardiac affection is described in animals.
- *Euphorbia ingens* may cause death in humans if overdosed. It is an irritant to the skin and leads to blistering.
- *Euphorbia* sp. are said to be toxic to man, but little detail of its effects are recorded.
- *Excoecaria bussei* — Its bark or root is used as a purgative. It is said to be very poisonous and may produce vomiting and intestinal upset.
- *Gloriosa superba* — Its tuber is used for different medical reasons, but it may result in a serious gastrointestinal upset with a terminal bloody diarrhea.[49]
- *Gnidia kraussiana* — This plant is poisonous, causing a fairly rapid death, characterized by gastrointestinal upset. At autopsy, congestion of the gastrointestinal tract, lung, and kidney are found.[50]
- *Indigofera demisa* — There is some doubt as to whether this plant is toxic to man.
- *Ipomoea verbascoides* — The root of its tuber is employed as a purgative and emetic. It is not certain how toxic it is.
- *Jatropha multifida* — Poisoning with this nut may be fatal. The illness that results is severe and is characterized by acute gastrointestinal upset.

- *Loranthuson ficus burkei* is used as a poison but its effects on the body are not known.
- *Manihot esculenta* is believed to be poisonous and said to cause a violent and rapid death, its main effect being on the esophagus and stomach. The root causes hallucinations and delirium.
- *Neorautanenia mitis* — This shrub is said to be a molluscicide. Little is known of its precise adverse effects on man.
- *Nerium oleander* — The leaf and stem are dangerous, especially to children. The main effect is on the gastrointestinal tract, producing an acute bloody flux. Its action resembles that of digitalis.
- *Nicotiana glauca* — Although this plant is poisonous to cattle and has been reported as poisonous to man, little is known about its effects.[51]
- *Phytolacca dodecandra* — The root is used as a purgative and may cause rapid death in humans.[52,53]
- *Ricinus communis* — It is recognized that humans may die from poisoning with the leaves or seeds of this plant. A cereal crop may become contaminated by the seeds, leading to acute poisoning. Its main effect is a severe gastroenteritis with bleeding into the heart, pleurae, liver, and kidneys.[54]
- *Securidaca longepedunculata* — The root is used as a purgative and astringent. It may be a gastric irritant causing vomiting, diarrhea, and bleeding into the gastrointestinal tract.
- *Solanum incanum* and *panduriforme* — The fruit of these species is frequently employed in the treatment of a wide range of disorders. In humans it causes headache, vomiting, diarrhea, cyanosis, fever, perspiration, and mydriasis. It is known to cause rapid death with coma, paralysis, signs of severe gastrointestinal irritation, and bleeding.[55,56]
- *Turraea nilotica* — The root and bark are employed for various symptoms, such as indigestion and intestinal upsets. It is said to be poisonous to man.
- *Urginea* sp. — The bulb of the species is extremely poisonous to cattle and sheep, producing severe diarrhea. Its effects on a fatal human case are not known.[57,58]
- *Neorautanenia mitis* — This shrub is said to be a molluscicide. Little is known of its precise adverse effects on man.
- *Splenostylis marginata* — This is a fish poison.
- *Spirostachys africana* — The latex of this tree may be an acute irritant to the eyes.[60]
- *Swartzia madagascariensis* is also a fish poison.
- *Trichilia emetica* — The leaves and bark of this tree are employed as a laxative, but it may be fatal, occasionally causing severe acute gastrointestinal irritation with vomiting, the passage of blood, and coma.[59]

Only the common plants which we found on our surveys to be used by n'anga have been dealt with in this chapter. Many of these plants have some toxic properties. I might mention two species of Senecio plants, the small and big "nyangozi" collected in 1960. The big nyangozi is used for childhood diseases by application to the skin. The small nyangozi contains pyrrolizidine alkaloids, which are hepatotoxic, whether given by mouth or applied to the skin.[61]

REFERENCES

1. **Gelfand, M.,** *Diet and Tradition in an African Culture,* Livingstone, Edinburgh, 1971, 1.
2. **Gelfand, M.,** *Diet and Tradition in an African Culture,* Livingstone, Edinburgh, 1971, 55.
3. **Gelfand, M.,** Diet and Tradition in an African Culture, Livingstone, Edinburgh, 1971, 72.
4. **Gelfand, M.,** *Diet and Tradition in an African Culture,* Livingstone, Edinburgh, 1971, 74.
5. **Gelfand, M.,** *Diet and Tradition in an African Culture,* Livingstone, Edinburgh, 1971, 79.
6. **Gelfand, M.,** *Diet and Tradition in an African Culture,* Livingstone, Edinburgh, 1971, 96.
7. **Gelfand, M.,** *Diet and Tradition in an African Culture,* Livingstone, Edinburgh, 1971, 102.
8. **Gelfand, M.,** *Diet and Tradition in an African Culture,* Livingstone, Edinburgh, 1971, 105.
9. **Gelfand, M.,** *Diet and Tradition in an African Culture,* Livingstone, Edinburgh, 1971, 113.
10. **Gelfand, M.,** *Diet and Tradition in an African Culture,* Livingstone, Edinburgh, 1971, 195.
11. **Gelfand, M.,** *Diet and Tradition in an African Culture,* Livingstone, Edinburgh, 1971, 122.
12. **Gelfand, M.,** *Diet and Tradition in an African Culture,* Livingstone, Edinburgh, 1971, 127.
13. **Gelfand, M.,** *Diet and Tradition in an African Culture,* Livingstone, Edinburgh, 1971, 132.
14. **Gelfand, M.,** *Diet and Tradition in an African Culture,* Livingstone, Edinburgh, 1971, 147.
15. **Gelfand, M.,** *Diet and Tradition in an African Culture,* Livingstone, Edinburgh, 1971, 158.
16. **Gelfand, M.,** *Diet and Tradition in an African Culture,* Livingstone, Edinburgh, 1971, 103.
17. **Gelfand, M.,** *Diet and Tradition in an African Culture,* Livingstone, Edinburgh, 1971, 211.
18. Gelfand, M., The dietary habits of the African and European with special reference to the Shona-speaking peoples, *S. Afr. Med. J.,* 47, 1501, 1973.
19. **Gelfand, M.,** The patterns of disease in Africa, *Cent. Afr. J. Med.,* 17, 69, 1969.
20. **Wapnick, S., Castle, W. M., Nicolle, D., Zanamwe, L. K. D., and Gelfand, M.,** Cigarette smoking, alcohol and cancer of the oesophagus, *S. Afr. Med. J.,* 46, 2023, 1972.
21. **Beyers, C. F.,** Incidence of surgical diseases among the Bantu races of South Africa, *S. Afr. Med. J.,* 30, 323, 1956.
22. **Gelfand, M.,** *Medicine and Magic of the Mashona,* Juta, Cape Town, 1956, 167.
23. **Watt, J. M. and Breyer-Brandwijk, M. R.,** *The Medicinal and Poisonous Plants of Southern and Eastern Africa,* Livingstone, Edinburgh, 1962, 395.
24. **Watt, J. M. and Brandwijk, M. R.,** *The Medicinal and Poisonous Plants of Southern and Eastern Africa,* Livingstone, Edinburgh, 1962, 555.
25. **Watt, J. M. and Brandwijk, M. R.,** *The Medicinal and Poisonous Plants of Southern and Eastern Africa,* Livingstone, Edinburgh, 1962, 1032.
26. **Drummond, R. B., Gelfand, M., and Mavi, S.,** Medicinal and other uses of succulents by the Rhodesian African, *Excelsa,* 5, 51, 1975.
27. **Drummond, R. D., Gelfand, M., and Mavi, S.,** Medicinal and other uses of succulents by the Rhodesian African, *Excelsa,* 5, 51, 1975.
28. **Gelfand, M. and Mitchell, C. S.,** Buphanine poisoning in man, *S. Afr. Med. J.,* 26, 573, 1952.
29. **Watt, J. M. and Breyer-Brandwijk, M. R.,** *The Medicinal and Poisonous Plants of Southern and Eastern Africa,* Livingstone, Edinburgh, 1962, 81.
30. **Shone, D. K. and Drummond, R. B.,** *Poisonous Plants of Rhodesia,* Ministry of Agriculture, Salisbury, 1965, 6.
31. **Watt, J. M. and Breyer-Brandwijk, M. R.,** *The Medicinal and Poisonous Plants of Southern and Eastern Africa,* Livingstone, Edinburgh, 1962, 399.
32. **Shone, D. K. and Drummond, R. B.,** *Poisonous Plants of Rhodesia,* Ministry of Agriculture, Salisbury, 1965, 46.
33. **Thomas, J. and Gelfand, M.,** Datura poisoning, *Cent. Afr. J. Med.,* 1, 78, 1955.
34. **Watt, J. M. and Breyer-Brandwijk, M. R.,** *The Medicinal and Poisonous Plants of Southern and Eastern Africa,* Livingstone, Edinburgh, 1962, 830.
35. **Shone, D. K. and Drummond, R. B.,** *Poisonous Plants of Rhodesia,* Ministry of Agriculture, Salisbury, 1965, 54.
36. **Blake Thompson, J.,** Native herbal medicines, *NADA,* i, 23 1931.
37. **Verdcourt, B. and Trump, W. C.,** *Common Poisonous Plants of East Africa,* Collins, London, 1969, 208.
38. **Gelfand, M.,** *Shona Ritual,* Juta, Cape Town, 1959, 198.
39. **Watt, J. M. and Breyer-Brandwijk, M. R.,** *The Medicinal and Poisonous Plants of Southern and Eastern Africa,* Livingstone, Edinburgh, 1962, 642.
40. **Verdcourt, B. and Trump, W. C.,** *Common Poisonous Plants of East Africa,* Collins, London, 1969, 59.
41. **Watt, J. M. and Breyer-Brandwijk, M. R.,** *The Medicinal and Poisonous Plants of Southern and Eastern Africa,* Livingstone, Edinburgh, 1962, 152.
42. **Watt, J. M. and Breyer-Brandwijk, M. R.,** *The Medicinal and Poisonous Plants of Southern and Eastern Africa,* Livingstone, Edinburgh, 1962, 883.

43. **Watt, J. M. and Breyer-Brandwijk, M. R.,** *The Medicinal and Poisonous Plants of Southern and Eastern Africa,* Livingstone, Edinburgh, 1962, 67.
44. **Watt, J. M., and Breyer-Brandwijk, M. R.,** *The Medicinal and Poisonous Plants of Southern and Eastern Africa,* Livingstone, Edinburgh, 1962, 685.
45. **Watt, J. M. and Breyer-Brandwijk, M. R.,** *The Medicinal and Poisonous Plants of Southern and Eastern Africa,* Livingstone, Edinburgh, 1962, 691.
46. **Verdcourt, B. and Trump, E. C.,** *Common Poisonous Plants of East Africa,* Collins, London, 1969, 23.
47. **Shone, D. K. and Drummond, R. B.,** *Poisonous Plants of Rhodesia,* Ministry of Agriculture, Salisbury, 1965, 46.
48. **Shone, D. K. and Drummond, R. B.,** *Poisonous Plants of Rhodesia,* Ministry of Agriculture, Salisbury, 1965, 8.
49. **Verdcourt, B. and Trump, B. C.,** *Common Poisonous Plants of East Africa,* Collins, London, 1969, 178.
50. **Shone, D. K. and Drummond, R. B.,** *Poisonous Plants of Rhodesia,* Ministry of Agriculture, Salisbury, 1965, 55.
51. **Shone, D. K. and Drummond, R. B.,** *Poisonous Plants of Rhodesia,* Ministry of Agriculture, Salisbury, 1965, 50.
52. **Shone, D. K. and Drummond, R. B.,** *Poisonous Plants of Rhodesia,* Ministry of Agriculture, Salisbury, 1965, 48.
53. **Verdcourt, B. and Trump, E. C.,** *Common Poisonous Plants of East Africa,* Collins, London, 1969, 29.
54. **Verdcourt, B. and Trump, E. C.,** *Common Poisonous Plants of East Africa,* Collins, London, 1969, 59.
55. **Verdcourt, B. and Trump, E. C.,** *Common Poisonous Plants of East Africa,* Collins, London, 1969, 169.
56. **Shone, D. K. and Drummond, R. B.,** *Poisonous Plants of Rhodesia,* Ministry of Agriculture, Salisbury, 1965, 49.
57. **Watt, J. M. and Breyer-Brandwijk, M. R.,** *The Medicinal and Poisonous Plants of Southern and Eastern Africa,* Livingstone, Edinburgh, 1962, 725.
58. **Shone, D. K. and Drummond, R. B.,** *Poisonous Plants of Rhodesia,* Ministry of Agriculture, Salisbury, 1965, 34.
59. **Verdcourt, B. and Trump, E. C.,** *Common Poisonous Plants of East Africa,* Collins, London, 1969, 105.
60. **Verdcourt, B. and Trump, E. C.,** *Common Poisonous Plants of East Africa,* Collins, London, 1969, 105.
61. **Schoental, R.,** Carcinogens in plants and microorganisms, in *Chemical Carcinogens,* Searle, C. E., Ed., ACS Monograph, 173, Washington, D.C., 1976, 626.

Chapter 3

A STUDY OF THE RELATIONSHIP BETWEEN DIET AND CANCER MORTALITY IN JAPAN

Hiroyuki Toyokawa

TABLE OF CONTENTS

I. INTRODUCTION

Dietary habits are important as risk factors in the incidence of cancer as well as for the prevention of cancer, especially in the alimentary canal and auxiliary digestive organs such as the liver and pancreas. Conclusive evidence of the association of dietary habits with the incidence of cancer has been obtained in only a few cases because of the many variables involved.

In order to overcome these many variables, the effects of diet should be studied from a statistical point of view since, as Dantzig[1] has pointed out, numbers are a scientific language. In this study, therefore, the relationship between the amounts and types of food consumed and cancer mortality will be dealt with statistically, in order to examine the relationship between dietary habits and cancer.

II. SOURCES OF DATA

Two sources of data are employed in this study: Nutrition Survey in Japan[2] and Vital Statistics.[3]

Data on the amount of food consumed are obtained from the Nutrition Survey, which has been carried out annually by the Japanese Ministry of Health and Welfare and authorized by the 1952 Law of Nutrition Improvement. In the survey, random samples of households were drawn from each prefecture, with the sample size determined by the population of the prefecture. Samples were chosen at the rate of 1/10,000 households. In 1971 the number of households was 3697. While this sample size is large enough to make the nutritional status of the Japanese population clear, it may not be large enough to analyze the relationship between dietary habits and cancer mortality in great detail. Since, however, there are no more reliable data anywhere than these, these data will be used to draw certain conclusions about the relationship between food and cancer.

The Nutrition Survey[2] is usually carried out during a 3-day period and is conducted by dieticians in the field who make personal visits to the homes and check the records prepared by housewives. Japanese housewives are asked to weigh precisely and to record the amounts of each of the food items used in the preparation of meals. On their visits, the dieticians check and make any corrections necessary in the records of the amounts of food items. These amounts are recorded in grams per day per capita.[2,4]

The data on cancer mortality are obtained from Vital Statistics,[3] administered and published by the Health and Welfare Statistics and Information Department, Minister's Secretariat, Ministry of Health and Welfare.[3]

III. METHODS

To present actual figures of food consumption of the population, correlation coefficients are calculated among the major food items and are shown in the correlation matrix in Table 1.[4-9]

In addition, principal component analysis is employed on the correlation matrix to identify the major food items with respect to dietary characteristics. Next, the components are estimated statistically. The major food items are divided into two categories, modern and traditional, according to their estimated values in both the first and second components. It will be explained later how this actually is done.[4,5]

In order to make the relationship in the dietary pattern between food consumed and cancer mortality clearer, multiple correlation coefficients are calculated for the combinations of mortality in cancer site compared with both the modern and traditional food groups.

Table 1
FOOD CONSUMPTION STRUCTURE, JAPAN IN 1971
(CORRELATION MATRIX)

	Rice	Wheat	Eggs	Potatoes	Sugar	Cakes	Oil and fat	Beans	Fruits	Green vegetables	Other vegetables	Milk and products	Seaweed	Meat	Fish
Rice	1.000														
Wheat	−0.314[a]	1.000													
Eggs	−0.052[a]	0.112[a]	1.000												
Potatoes	0.055[a]	0.017	0.025	1.000											
Sugar	−0.023	0.112[a]	0.146[a]	0.038[a]	1.000										
Cakes	−0.052[a]	0.058[a]	0.105[a]	0.067[a]	0.133[a]	1.000									
Oil & Fat	−0.167[a]	0.216[a]	0.230[a]	0.083[a]	0.240[a]	0.116[a]	1.000								
Beans	0.163[a]	−0.098[a]	0.052[a]	0.086[a]	0.099[a]	0.063[a]	0.013	1.000							
Fruits	−0.137[a]	0.172[a]	0.243[a]	0.094[a]	0.232[a]	0.224[a]	0.252[a]	0.031	1.000						
Green Vegetables	0.009	0.058[a]	0.118[a]	0.145[a]	0.070[a]	0.030	0.163[a]	0.097[a]	0.189[a]	1.000					
Other Vegetables	0.068[a]	0.027	0.188[a]	0.163[a]	0.161	0.129[a]	0.223[a]	0.230[a]	0.255[a]	0.147[a]	1.000				
Milk and its Products	−0.248[a]	0.231[a]	0.197[a]	0.026	0.120[a]	0.140[a]	0.235[a]	0.013	0.295[a]	0.158[a]	0.111[a]	1.000			
Seaweed	0.074[a]	−0.038[a]	0.062[a]	0.091[a]	0.047[a]	0.068[a]	0.032[a]	0.116[a]	0.090[a]	0.061[a]	0.118[a]	0.009	1.000		
Meat	−0.156[a]	0.198[a]	0.236[a]	0.098[a]	0.118[a]	0.111[a]	0.295[a]	−0.015	0.297[a]	0.153[a]	0.222[a]	0.207[a]	0.006	1.000	
Fish	0.155	−0.083	0.064[a]	0.027	0.095[a]	0.121[a]	0.033[a]	0.169[a]	0.126[a]	0.117[a]	0.191[a]	−0.014	0.125	−0.043[a]	1.000

[a] Positive and negative coefficients which are statistically significant ($\alpha = 0.05$).

IV. FOOD CONSUMPTION PATTERN

The food consumption pattern[4-9,12] in Japan in 1971 is shown in Table 1, where we find positive and negative coefficients. Those which are statistically significant (α = 0.05) are marked with a footnote. Major pairs of food items whose correlation coefficients are significantly positive form a synergistic combination in the Japanese daily diet. On the other hand, food items which are negatively correlated means that in the Japanese diet the use of one usually excludes the use of the other. In terms of Japanese dietary habits, the food consumption pattern consists of many such synergistic and antagonistic combinations of food. Thus, if one investigates the causative associations of diet to cancer or other diseases, one must bear in mind food consumption characteristics.

These facts point out clearly that one does not eat only a single food, but enjoys a great variety in meals. It is, therefore, difficult to implicate a single food item as a cause of cancer or some other disease. Dietary patterns are culture-linked, as is illustrated in the food consumption pattern. When an attempt is made to show a clear causative association of diet with cancer, one might well start from this food consumption pattern. This approach should be called a method of dietary ecology or a method of numerical dietary ecology — a means of processing quantitatively the amount of food consumed.

Let us now examine the individual correlation coefficients found in the correlation matrix (see Table 1).[4-9] The correlation coefficient for rice and wheat is −0.314. This is the most significantly antagonistic relation of all the combinations. In terms of daily diet, someone who eats a large amount of rice will naturally eat a lesser amount of wheat in the form of bread and noodles, but not cake. Also, it should be emphasized that the correlation coefficient between rice and dairy products (including milk) is −0.248 and shows a definite antagonism, even though such an antagonistic combination might seem unusual to people of the western world. In addition, there are many other interesting examples that show Japanese dietary characteristics in the correlations between rice and meat, −0.156; rice and oil (fat), −0.167; and rice and fruit, −0.137. As for the rice-fruit correlation, the influence of seasonal variation must be considered. The Nutrition Survey in 1971 was held in May when fruit was not in season, but fruit was consumed synergistically with rice in the subsequent annual Nutrition Surveys because they were conducted in November, a time when fruit was in season.[8,9] On the other hand, correlation coefficients between rice and fish, rice and pulses, rice and seaweed, and rice and other nongreen vegetables are all significantly positive. These synergistic counterparts of rice have traditionally been eaten for a long time, so they should be categorized as traditional food items.[4-9,15]

We can also find positive correlations for wheat in the following cases: wheat and egg, wheat and sugar, wheat and meat, wheat and oil (fat), wheat and fruit, and wheat and dairy products. On the other hand, we find negative correlations in the following wheat combinations: wheat and fish, wheat and pulses, wheat and seaweed, and wheat and rice. Synergistic counterparts of wheat are likely to be considered as western or modern food items in Japan where there is no distinction between westernization and modernization. Prior to 50 years ago, with few exceptions, the Japanese people did not eat meat, and even these exceptions consumed far less meat a century ago. Neither did the Japanese have milk and other dairy products. Oil and fat were precious and not obtainable by the majority at that time. Therefore, these must be considered as modern foods in present day Japan. Although there is no distinction between bread and noodles in this data, it has been shown in another paper[6,7] that combinations of bread and fish, and bread and pulses had a much more negative correlation than the combinations of wheat and fish, and wheat and pulses. Whereas noodles ("udon") is mostly a traditional food, wheat, including such noodles, has been identified as a modern food.

There are many more positive coefficients than negative coefficients in the correlation matrix. Thus we should recognize that a synergistic relation exists basically among daily food consumptions. In other words, a person who eats a large quantity of one type of food is likely to consume large quantities of other foods. If we recognize this tendency, we must realize the importance of antagonistic combinations.

V. TRADITIONAL AND MODERN FOOD GROUPS

In order to clarify the factors comprising a dietary pattern, the author has calculated a principal component analysis from the correlation matrix above (Table 1). Food pattern and weight vectors are calculated and presented in Table 2. The first component's contribution rate is about 18%, and that of the second component is about 12%. Thus the combined contribution rate in the second is about 30%. When we examine both columns, we are able to understand the meaning of each factor. In the first factor we can read the essence of common vs. noncommon to the Japanese or cheap vs. expensive on the basis of the consumer's judgment. This follows since items such as rice, having a negative score, are very important to the Japanese, and in addition, food items getting small positive scores such as pulses, fish, and seaweed are considered to be cheap by consumers at the time, even though the cost of fish might rise afterwards. Also, fruit, meat, and dairy products are considered to be expensive, even luxurious, by consumers. These products might not be given large positive scores. Thus, it might be concluded from the above scores that quite nourishing food is expensive and expensive food is good to the taste.[4,12]

The second component is interpreted essentially as traditional vs. modern. Fiteeen major food items are pictured on a graph which is plotted with the first component on the horizontal axis and the second component on the vertical axis. The author calls this graph the "Two-Dimensional Spatial Diagram of Food Consumption" (Figure 1).[5] It shows that apparently the traditional food items cluster in the direction of rice, whereas modern food items cluster in the direction of wheat. Further, it shows that rice and wheat are quite far apart in their relative positions. Therefore, we can divide food items into traditional and modern food groups. Each of the food items in the same food group is consumed in a daily meal. Thus we can see the relationship between food groups and cancer mortality.

VI. CORRELATION BETWEEN FOOD CONSUMED AND CANCER MORTALITY

The correlation coefficient between single food items and cancer mortality is calculated in terms of an average amount of food consumed and cancer site mortality (Table 3). In this table, pairs of single food items and cancer site mortality are shown only when they have significant correlations with the calculated coefficient values.[13-15]

Rice has positive correlation coefficients in a few combinations, for example rice-pancreatic cancer in males and rice-rectum cancer in males. Nevertheless, the Japanese, who eat a large quantity of rice, had a lower mortality of both diseases than the Americans and Europeans, who eat little rice by comparison. Negative correlations in combinations of rice-leukemia mortality is higher in western countries than in Japan. In addition, leukemia mortality has begun to increase recently in Japan corresponding to the westernization of dietary habits. There have been, of course, not only dietary changes, but also many other changes in, for example, environmental factors and improved medical diagnosis. Since results that are estimated are, for that very reason, not acceptable in epidemiological concensus, such results should be identified as nonspecific relations or as having possibly only superficial causality.

Table 2
STRUCTURE VECTOR AND WEIGHTING VECTOR
(3609 HOUSEHOLDS, JAPAN, 1971)

Factor no.	1	2	3	4
Contribution rate	18.31	11.90	7.15	6.51

Structure vector				
Rice	−0.277	0.633	0.068	−0.232
Wheat	0.400	−0.485	0.010	0.134
Potato	0.226	0.254	0.604	0.380
Sugar	0.433	0.112	−0.347	−0.218
Cake	0.364	0.118	−0.436	0.446
Oil & Fat	0.607	−0.116	0.049	−0.204
Bean	0.145	0.558	−0.012	−0.116
Fruits	0.660	−0.018	−0.120	0.101
Vegetable	0.382	0.186	0.450	−0.017
Other	0.498	0.412	0.095	−0.163
Seaweed	0.150	0.373	−0.033	0.517
Fish	0.173	0.538	−0.311	0.030
Meat	0.572	−0.171	0.242	−0.183
Egg	0.500	0.025	−0.072	−0.322
Milk & dairy products	0.538	−0.263	−0.045	0.135

Weighting vector				
Rice	−0.101	0.355	0.064	−0.238
Wheat	0.146	−0.272	0.009	0.137
Potato	0.082	0.142	0.564	0.389
Sugar	0.158	0.063	−0.323	−0.223
Cake	0.133	0.066	−0.406	0.456
Oil & Fat	0.221	−0.065	0.045	−0.208
Bean	0.053	0.313	−0.011	−0.118
Fruits	0.240	0.010	−0.112	0.103
Vegetable	0.139	0.104	−0.420	−0.018
Other	0.181	0.231	0.089	−0.167
Seaweed	0.054	0.209	−0.031	0.529
Fish	0.063	0.302	−0.290	0.030
Meat	0.208	−0.096	0.226	−0.187
Egg	0.182	0.014	−0.067	−0.329
Milk & dairy products	0.196	−0.148	−0.042	0.138

In considering both the columns of the traditional food group and the modern food group, there are as many significant correlations in the former as in the latter, even though cancer sites in each column are not the same. Alimentary cancer stands out in the column of the traditional food group more than any other site either in a positive correlation or a negative one. When the modern food column is examined, an opposite relationship is noted. Therefore, we can suspect that the traditional Japanese dietary patterns might predispose to alimentary cancer. This hypothesis is being followed up by a much more detailed study which will be conducted through a carefully designed investigation, since the modern food group which is protecting the Japanese against alimentary cancer is causing cancer in European and American populations. Every food item is eaten in a set, and every dietary pattern may also have been linked with specific cancers, so that we have to make clear the relationship between cancer and dietary habits in terms of multiple correlation analysis.[4]

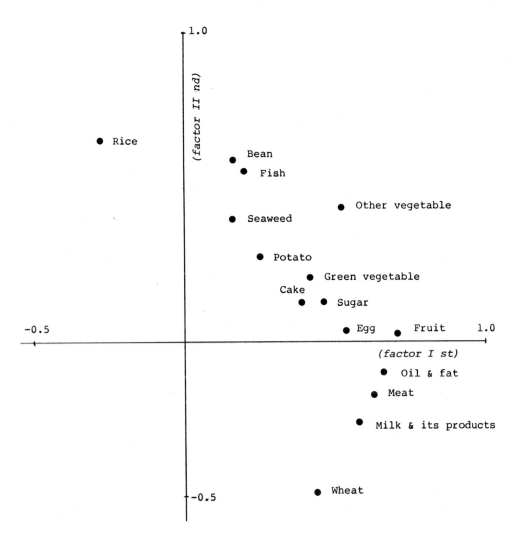

FIGURE 1. Two-dimensional spatial diagram of food consumption (3609 households examined in Japan Nutrition Survey, 1971)

VII. CORRELATION BETWEEN CANCER MORTALITY AND CLUSTERED FOOD ITEMS (TABLE 4)

Here 15 major food items are paired into two subgroups — traditional and modern. The multiple correlation coefficient is calculated for each pair of food items and cancer site mortality in both sexes (see Table 2).

Multiple correlation coefficients between cancer mortality as a whole and clustered food groups are almost the same for males, but coefficient values in combination with the traditional food group become larger than those in combination with a modern food group.

As to the mortality of mouth and pharynx cancers, it is sugguested that the wheat group (modern food group) has a more positive correlation in females than with males. Nevertheless, since neither type of cancer has a high incidence rate in Japan, we did not consider these types of cancer in this study.

Table 3
CORRELATION COEFFICIENTS BETWEEN EACH PAIR OF THE FOOD INTAKE AND SPECIFIC CANCER MORTALITY

Food	Sex	Positive correlation		Negative correlation	
Rice group (traditional food group)					
Rice	m	Pancreatic cancer	(0.305)		
		Rectal cancer	(0.289)		
	f			Breast cancer	(−0.378)
				Leukemia	(−0.348)
Potatoes	m	Cancer of gall bladder	(0.377)	Stomach cancer	(−0.306)
	f	Pancreatic cancer	(0.382)	Uterus cancer	(−0.313)
		Cancer of gall bladder	(0.288)		
Pulses	m	Cancer of gall bladder	(0.505)		
		Esophagus cancer	(0.361)		
	f	Cancer of gall bladder	(0.412)	Stomach cancer	(−0.412)
				Breast cancer	(−0.372)
				Uterus cancer	(−0.328)
Green vegetables	m	Pancreatic cancer	(0.360)		
		Colon cancer	(0.289)		
Other vegetables	m	Esophagus cancer	(0.357)		
Seaweeds	m	Stomach cancer	(0.304)		
	f	Pancreatic cancer	(0.540)		
		Colon cancer	(0.351)		
		Esophagus cancer	(0.309)		
Fish	m	Colon cancer	(0.445)	Cancer of mouth and pharynx	(−0.291)
		Pancreatic cancer	(0.398)		
	f	(Cancer of urinary organs)	(0.372)		
Wheat group (modern food group)					
Wheat	f	Breast cancer	(0.562)		
Eggs	m	Cancer of bladder	(0.355)	Cancer of gall bladder	(−0.315)
		(Cancer of urinary organs)	(0.327)		
		Cancer of trachea and lung	(0.324)		
	f	Uterus cancer	(0.336)		
		Cancer of bladder	(0.323)		
Oils and fats					
Milk and milk products	m			Lymphatic and hematopoietic cancer	(−0.314)
				Leukemia	(−0.301)
	f	Breast cancer	(0.518)	Lymphatic and hematopoietic cancer	(−0.296)
Meat	m			Cancer of gall bladder	(−0.432)
	f	Uterus cancer	(0.324)		
Sugar	m	Liver cancer	(0.329)	Cancer of gall bladder	(−0.459)
		Cancer of trachea and lung	(0.317)		

Table 3 (Continued)
CORRELATION COEFFICIENTS BETWEEN EACH PAIR OF THE FOOD INTAKE AND SPECIFIC CANCER MORTALITY

Food	Sex	Positive correlation		Negative correlation	
Oils and fats (Continued)					
Confectionery	m			Cancer of trachea and lung	(−0.378)
				Liver cancer	(−0.320)
	f	Breast cancer	(0.341)	Cancer of trachea and lung	(−0.299)
Fruit	m	Cancer of bladder	(0.379)	Cancer of gall bladder	(−0.314)
		Cancer of trachea and lung	(0.328)		
	f	Breast cancer	(0.385)	Cancer of gall bladder	(−0.450)

Note: Figures in parentheses are significant correlation coefficients ($P < 0.05$).

As to effects on the digestive organs, traditional food items have a large coefficient of multiple correlation. This implies their importance as well as a causal relation. These results are strongly supported by all epidemiological findings which have been reported, especially on stomach cancer, since it shows a large difference in the two food groups. We observe that by multiple correlation we can distinguish between the traditional food group and the Japanese dietary habits, a distinction that is not clear from using single correlations. There is not so large a difference as might be expected between traditional and modern groups where esophageal cancer is concerned. The reason for this might be that the Japanese people with a modern dietary pattern eat rice together with its synergistic food items at least once a day through habitual necessity. Although cancer of the esophagus is supposed to be connected with eating hot cooked rice, its mortality has recently decreased in Japan.

It is very interesting to note that cancer of the stomach, small intestine, rectum, and pancreas are associated with the traditional dietary pattern, while cancer of the liver and gall bladder are associated with the modern dietary food group.

As for respiratory cancer, we can find a larger synergism with the modern food group than with the traditional group. In spite of these results, the modern food group should not be blamed as the direct causes of these types of cancer because the sites are non-alimentary ones.

It is suspected that modern food items are usually consumed in a population whose environment is conducive to respiratory cancer, i.e., an environment where air pollution, heavy smoking, etc., are prevalent.[12] Therefore, the relationship calculated between respiratory cancer and the modern food group is, at best, indirect. When we study the dietary causes of cancer and other diseases, we should keep in mind both the food consumption structure and the complicated interaction of environment.

With regard to breast cancer in females, the modern food group has a much larger multiple correlation than the traditional food group whose multiple correlation, however, is also relatively large. Because of this, we do not consider that there is a direct relationship between breast cancer and the food groups, nor between respiratory cancer and food groups. Neither can we detect any specific relationship between dietary pattern and the other cancer sites.

Table 4
MULTIPLE COEFFICIENTS BETWEEN EACH PAIR OF CANCER MORTALITY AND DIETARY PATTERN

Organ or site	Dietary pattern (male)		Dietary pattern (female)	
	Rice group[a]	Wheat group[b]	Rice group[a]	Wheat group[b]
Total	0.504	0.493	0.630	0.318
Mouth, pharynx	0.424	0.505	0.293	0.580
Digestive organs	0.537	0.351	0.690	0.285
Esophagus	0.545	0.461	0.474	0.433
Stomach	0.604	0.243	0.690	0.243
Small intestines	0.610	0.200	0.478	0.539
Rectum	0.422	0.296	0.424	0.399
Liver	0.364	0.567	0.275	0.439
Gall bladder	0.561	0.678	0.568	0.673
Pancreas	0.656	0.485	0.625	0.497
Respiratory organs	0.366	0.719	0.302	0.514
Larynx	0.449	0.530	0.304	0.454
Trachea, lung	0.386	0.659	0.315	0.478
Bones	0.479	0.542	0.300	0.314
Skin	0.296	0.631	0.460	0.495
Breast	0.465	0.535	0.591	0.734
Male sexual organs or uterus	0.372	0.389	0.478	0.690
Prostate or ovarium	0.321	0.390	0.441	0.456
Urinary organs	0.525	0.432	0.594	0.513
Bladder	0.499	0.458	0.544	0.533
Kidney	0.347	0.278	0.489	0.482
Lymph, hematogenic organs	0.408	0.542	0.415	0.465
Leucocyte	0.346	0.516	0.547	0.352

Note: N = 46;
   R, 5% significance level: 0.2875;
   R, 1% significance level: 0.3721.

[a]   Rice group: rice, potatoes, green vegetables, light-colored vegetables, seaweeds, and fish.
[b]   Wheat group: wheat, eggs, sugar, confectionery, fruit, milk, milk products, and meat.

VIII. LIMITATIONS OF THE METHOD

Some dietary patterns causing cancer can be related through multiple factor analysis to the amount and type of food consumed as previously mentioned. However, there are three major weak points in the process of obtaining the factors employed in the principal factor analysis.

The first concerns the sampling process. The data utilized were obtained from the Nutrition Survey in Japan, which is planned and conducted for the purpose of obtaining information on the nutritional status of the people. For this reason, the data are not always adequate to be linked with other data such as cancer mortality from Vital Statistics. In the Nutrition Survey, sample households are randomly selected at a rate of one per each 10,000 households in the population. However, the populations of the 46 prefectures differ widely. For example, the population of the largest unit, metropolitan Tokyo, is more than 11 million, while the population of the smallest prefecture is only one million. The latter population consists of 200,000 households. This small sample size is not adequate for statistical treatment. Thus, there is a statistical weakness in this study.

The second weak point is found in the nutritional data obtained from the survey of households rather than from individuals — it is impossible to distinguish between the sexes in the amount of food consumed. Since dietary characteristics cannot be calculated by sex, it is impossible to determine correlation coefficients between dietary agents and the cancer mortality of each sex, even if cancer mortality is calculated. Since it was not possible to obtain more precise nutritional data broken down by sex, it was necessary to utilize the available data by standardizing it using a conversion factor already established in regard to energy and protein demand for males aged 19 to 39 years.

The third weak point lies in the collection of nutritional data only over a 1-year period, while the incidence of cancer is affected by food intake over a period of long duration. Even though a dietary pattern cross-sectionally examined for several days might have been maintained over a period of several years, a dietary study of 3 days is too short to pursue the association between diet and cancer. Yet, it can be argued that multiple correlation analysis between major food groups divided into traditional and modern categories and the mortality of each cancer site is better than correlations analysis between single food items and mortality of each cancer site.

Current nutritional research methods are insufficiently developed to obtain reliable and accurate data on dietary parameters. Thus, one must study not only the techniques of dietary analysis and, as a consequence, techniques of survey and statistical analysis, but one must study the concepts of dietary characteristics in order to determine the nutritional parameters in our population. Many aspects of daily living which are related to economics, behavioral sciences, and psychology must be taken into account as well as sporadic contamination of particular food items with mycotoxins and other incidental ingredients which may be carcinogenic.

IX. CONCLUSIONS

Even though there are several weak points in this investigation, the following conclusions can be drawn.

An outline of dietary influences on cancer in the Japanese was shown with regard to the traditional and modern food patterns.

Fifteen major food items were divided into traditional and modern food groups according to Japanese dietary characteristics using multiple factor analysis techniques. Multiple factor analysis was calculated from the correlation matrix, which was, in turn, calculated from the matrix of the average amounts, in grams, of these 15 major food items consumed per capita per day based on a dietary survey of 3609 households.

The relationship between the amount of food consumed and the cancer mortality at body sites was estimated in terms of multiple correlation coefficients between the traditional and modern food groups and the cancer site mortality.

It was shown that the traditional food group consisting of rice, seaweed, pulses, and certain vegetables which are all native to Japan, when considered as a group (food pattern), seemed to influence the incidence of stomach cancer, while the traditional items, considered individually, did not do so.

It was shown that, with regard to the relationship between modern food groups and the mortality from respiratory cancer, there may have been external influence, e.g., urbanization and industrialization, which played a role.

REFERENCES

1. **Dantzig, T.,** *Number: The Language of Science,* Macmillan, New York, 1933.
2. Nutrition Survey in Japan, Bureau of Public Health, Ministry of Health and Welfare, Japan, 1971.
3. Vital Statistics of Japan, Statistical Information Department, Ministry of Health and Welfare, Japan, 1971.
4. **Toyokawa, H.,** The nutritional status in Japan from the viewpoint of numerical ecology, *Soc. Sci. Med.,* 12 (6A), 517, 1978.
5. **Toyokawa, H.,** A Prospective Studying Method Based on Dietary Characteristics, Proc. Workshop U.S.-Japan Malnutrition Panel, Inoue, G. and Yoshimura, H., Eds., Osaka, Japan, December 5, 1978.
6. **Toyokawa, H.,** *Community Nutrition (Kohshuh Eiyo)* Koseikan Ltd., Tokyo, 1976.
7. **Toyokawa, H.,** *Daily Food and Health (Shokuseikatsu to Kenko)* Taishuhkan Shoten, Ltd., Tokyo, 1975.
8. **Toyokawa, H., Miyake, Y., and Itoh, M.,** Study of food consumption in Japan, *Jpn. J. Public Health,* 22, 571, 1975.
9. **Miyake, Y., Toyokawa, H., and Itoh, M.,** Study of food consumption in Japan. II, *Jpn. J. Public Health,* 23, 589, 1976.
10. **Marui, E. and Toyokawa, H.,** Methodological study of the regional structure concerning food-consumption-pattern, *Jpn. J. Public Health,* 25, 363, 1978.
11. **Marui, E. and Toyokawa, H.,** Quantitative analysis of food intake pattern similarity, *Jpn. J. Public Health,* 22, 385, 1975.
12. **Toyokawa, H. and Uezumi, T.,** A study of the analysis of regional food-structure in mean-standard deviation model. II. A trial on definition of parsmeters of food consumption, *Jpn. J. Public Health,* 19, 129, 1973.
13. **Yanai, H., Inaba, Y., Takagi, F., Toyokawa, H., and Yamamoto, S.,** An epidemiological study on mortality rates of various cancer sites during 1958 to 1971 by mean of factor analysis, *Behviormetrika,* 5, 55, 1978.
14. **Maruchi, N., Aoki, S., Tsuda, K., Tanaka, Y., and Toyokawa, H.,** A statistical examination on the relationship of food consumption to cancer mortality in Japan, *Proc. 10th Int. Congr. Nutr.,* S. Karger, Basel, 1975, 481.
15. **Toyokawa, H., Miyake, Y., and Maruchi, N.,** A statistical study on the structure of food consumption in Japan, *Proc. 10th Int. Congr. Nutr.,* S. Karger, Basel, 1975, 695.

Chapter 4

CARCINOGENIC PROPERTIES OF SOME PLANTS USED AS HUMAN FOODS OR HERBAL REMEDIES IN JAPAN

Iwao Hirono

TABLE OF CONTENTS

I. INTRODUCTION

The Japanese have long used the young buds and seeds of a variety of native wild plants as special seasonal foods. Certain wild plants have also been used as folk medicine. Some of these plants contain very toxic substances and can cause death when eaten. These plants are usually used as human foods only after these toxic principals have been removed by cooking processes. Recently, it was found that some of these wild plants were carcinogenic to experimental animals. These naturally occurring carcinogens of plant origin are so-called secondary metabolites of the plants and their physiological role is unknown. Only a few carcinogens of plant origin are known at present, because carcinogenicity tests on plant materials to detect environmental carcinogens were started only recently, but more carcinogens will probably be found in plants used as human foods or herbal remedies as these studies progress. This chapter deals with green plants used as human foods or folk medicines in Japan and found to be carcinogenic with their utilization, their carcinogenic activity, and epidemiology.

II. CYCAD

A. Cycad as a Food

Cycads are widely distributed in tropical and subtropical regions, and the species indigenous to Amami, Okinawa, and Yaeyama, the southwestern islands of Japan, is *Cycas revoluta* Thunb. (Figure 1). In these islands, the seeds and trunks of cycads were invaluable food when other food supplies were destroyed by typhoons before and during World War II. The cycad seeds (Figure 2) are still used as a source of starch and as a constituent of the bean paste "miso" in some parts of the islands. It is also known that the inhabitants of Guam use nuts of the cycad, *Cycas circinalis* L., as a source of food starch. A review of the literature of the utilization and toxicity of cycads has been compiled by Whiting.[1]

B. Carcinogenicity of Cycad

Laqueur et al.[2,3] found that crude meal prepared from dried and ground seeds of cycad induced tumors of the liver, kidney, and intestinal tract when fed to rats, and that the carcinogenic effect of the crude cycad material was mainly due to its content of cycasin (Figure 3), a toxic glycoside. This glycoside was first isolated from the seeds of *Cycas revoluta* Thunb. and identified in 1955 by Nishida et al.,[4] and later found by Riggs[5] in *C. circinalis* L. It has been reported that the carcinogenic effect of cycasin is so strong that a single dose of cycasin induces tumors in high incidence.[6] The carcinogenic effect of cycasin is not restricted to rats, but was also demonstrated in mice,[7-10] hamsters,[11] guinea pigs,[12] and rabbits.[13] Spatz et al.,[14,15] using germ-free rats, showed that cycasin is hydrolyzed to an aglycone (Figure 4) by the bacterial flora and that this aglycone is toxic and is a proximate carcinogen.

C. Cycasin in Foods and Cycasin-Intoxication

Cycasin occurs in the seeds, stems, and leaves of cycads. The amount of cycasin present in cycad nuts and dried ground nuts depends on the species of cycad and the method used for drying the nuts: 0.016% cycasin was found in ground and dried nuts of *C. circinalis* prepared in Guam (leached with water and then sun-dried),[16] whereas 2.3% cycasin was found in unwashed, vacuum-dried nuts.[17] To prepare cycad starch, cycad nuts are cut into small pieces, soaked in water in a container, or washed in running water, and dried. Since cycasin is readily soluble in water, cycad starch and parts of cycads that have been thoroughly washed with water are safe to eat.

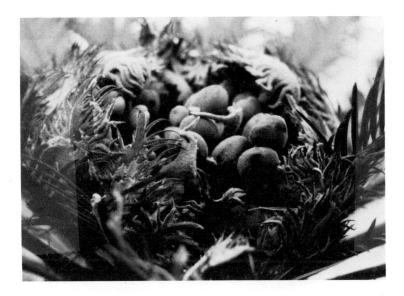

FIGURE 1. Cycad, *Cycas revoluta* Thunb.

7 8 9 20 1 2 3 4 5 6 7 8 9 30

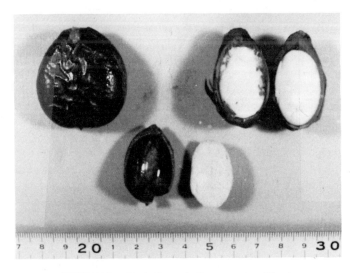

FIGURE 2. Seed of cycad, *Cycas revoluta* Thunb.

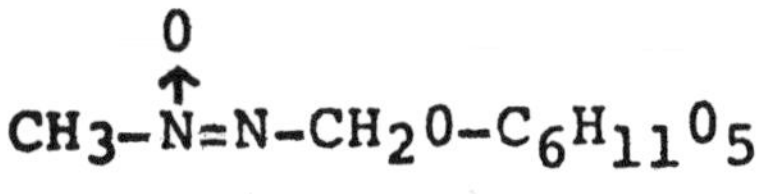
O
CH3-N=N-CH2O-C6H11O5

FIGURE 3. Cycasin.

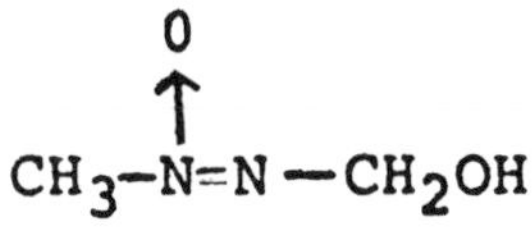
O
CH3-N=N—CH2OH

FIGURE 4. Aglycone of cycasin.

Toxicity to man has generally been attributed to improper washing of the cycad nuts or stem. Acute intoxication in humans caused by cycads has occasionally occurred accidentally in the Okinawa islands.[18] A total of 17 cases of cycad poisoning have been reported, all but one of them fatal. In most cases intoxication occurred after eating cycad "ojiya". The cycad ojiya, a kind of gruel boiled with bean paste or soy sauce, was prepared as follows: cycad stem was barked, cut into thin slices, dried in the sun for 7 to 10 days, and then immersed in water for about 2 days. Slices were taken out of water and wrapped in miscanthus until they became soft. Then they were washed several times with water and boiled with seasoning. The latent time from the ingestion of cycad ojiya to the appearance of symptoms was 12 to 24 hr in most cases. The acute toxicity of cycasin in experimental animals also appeared at least 12 hr after oral administration of cycasin, and it is thought that the symptoms appeared after a certain amount of aglycone has accumulated. In humans, the first sign of intoxication was the sudden development of nausea and vomiting. The patients then rapidly became unconscious and most of them died within 20 hr after the appearance of the first sign of acute intoxication. In most patients, swelling of the liver was observed and the one patient who regained consciousness developed jaundice.

As described above, cycasin was carcinogenic in several kinds of test animals, and swelling of the liver and jaundice, which are symptoms of liver damage due to the acute toxicity of cycasin, were observed in the surviving patient as well as in test animals. These findings strongly suggest that cycasin is carcinogenic to man.

In 1959, the Miyako Islands, Okinawa suffered from a succession of typhoons and the inhabitants lost all their crops and had to subsist largely on cycads. A statistical survey of the mortality from cancer was made in an attempt to assess the incidence of tumors in this community.[18] However, no appreciable increase in cancer mortality was observed. This negative result may be because the survey was made soon after the people had eaten cycads or because the cycad foods were well prepared.

Kobayashi[19] examined the amount of cycasin in cycad materials used as foods in Japan by polarography and gas chromatography. He tested for the presence of cycasin in five samples of homemade cycad bean paste, "sotetsumiso". Cycad bean paste is usually prepared as follows: cycad nuts are cut in half, the kernel is washed with water, and dried. The dry pieces are ground to a powder and mixed with rice or wheat to make "koji". Finally, beans and salt are added to koji and the mixture is left to ferment. The ratio of cycad flour in the paste amounts to about one fourth to one third of the total weight of the paste. He reported that none of the food materials from cycad that he tested, such as cycad bean paste and starch, contained any detectable cycasin.

III. BRACKEN

A. Bracken as a Human Food

Bracken, *Pteridium aquilinum*, is called "warabi" in Japanese. Young bracken fronds (Figure 5) in the fiddlehead or crosier stage of growth have long been used as human food in Japan, and most Japanese regard warabi as a special delicacy. The young shoots of bracken are used as a fresh vegetable in spring or they are salted, sun dried, or pickled for future use. Freshly picked bracken fronds are usually prepared for eating by immersing in plain boiling water or boiling water containing wood ash or sodium bicarbonate to remove the bitterness. Then they are boiled in plain water and served, flavored with fish powder and soy sauce. Salted bracken is boiled in water for a few minutes and then washed in running water to remove the salt. Dried bracken is usually soaked in water to make it soft before it is cooked.

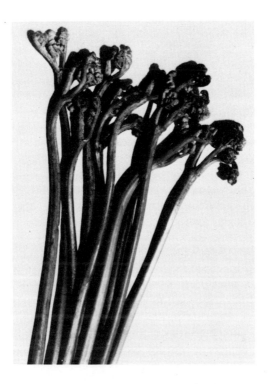

FIGURE 5.   Young bracken frond.

B. Carcinogenicity of Bracken

The carcinogenic activity of bracken was most clearly demonstrated in the experiments of Evans and Mason,[20,21] showing that rats fed bracken developed multiple intestinal adenocarcinomas. Pamukcu et al.[22-24] also found that bracken was carcinogenic to cows, rats, and mice. The young bracken fronds used as human food in Japan were also strongly carcinogenic, and rats fed diet containing unprocessed dry bracken powder in the proportion by weight of one part bracken to two parts basal diet for 4 months developed tumors of the ileum, cecum, and urinary bladder,[25] ileal tumors being induced in the highest incidence. Histologically, the intestinal tumors were epithelial tumors, such as adenomas and adenocarcinomas, and also sarcomas. The urinary bladder tumors were papillomas, transitional cell carcinomas, and squamous cell carcinomas. In Japan, bracken is usually used as a human food after its bitterness has been removed as described above. Experiments on rats suggested that the carcinogen contents of bracken treated with wood ash or sodium bicarbonate and of salt bracken were much less than that in unprocessed bracken. However, even after these treatments the bracken still retained carcinogenic activity.[26] Bracken was carcinogenic not only to rats[20,23,25] and cows,[22] but also to mice,[21,24,27] guinea pigs,[21,28] Japanese quails,[21] and hamsters.[21]

C. Nature of the Carcinogen in Bracken

The nature of the carcinogen in bracken has not yet been elucidated. Flavonoids,[29,30] indanones,[31,32] and pterolactam[33] have been isolated from bracken. However, there are no data to indicate that these chemicals are carcinogenic.[27,34] Evans and Osman[35] reported that shikimic acid is present in bracken and that it was carcinogenic in mice. They also suggested that another fraction of bracken contains a strong carcinogen, in addition to shikimic acid. However, in our experiments, rats fed diet containing shikimic acid did not develop tumors.[36] Thus, at least in rats, the carcinogenicity of bracken may be attributable to a substance(s) other than shikimic acid. Recently, Wang et al.[37] isolated carcinogenic tannin from bracken. The tannin induced bladder tumors when implanted intravesically into mice. However, neither intestinal nor bladder tumors were induced when a diet containing the tannin was fed to rats.[56] Thus, the nature of the carcinogenic substance in bracken is still uncertain. We studied the carcinogenicity to rats of a boiling water extract of bracken. All the rats fed the concentrated boiling water extract developed urinary bladder carcinomas and most of them also developed ileal tumors. These results show that the carcinogen in bracken can be extracted with boiling water and, thus, that it is probably water soluble.[38]

Young bracken is also used as folk medicine for asthma by a few people in Japan. For this purpose, a decoction of young dry bracken is usually drunk like tea. Since a boiling water extract of bracken is carcinogenic as mentioned above, the decoction of bracken probably contains carcinogen and, thus, use of this decoction probably represents a human hazard.

A comparative study on the carcinogenicities of various parts of bracken showed that the curled tops of young bracken fronds were more carcinogenic than the stalks.[39] It is interesting that people in some parts of Japan have a time-honored and peculiar custom of eating the stalks, but not the curled tops of young bracken.

D. Epidemiology of the Carcinogenicity of Bracken

Pamukcu and Price[23] suggested that the high incidence of human stomach cancer in Japan could be partially due to bracken, since this plant is eaten in considerable amounts in Japan. However, bracken is usually eaten after its bitterness has been removed by boiling water containing wood ash or sodium bicarbonate (processed bracken). Processed bracken contains much less carcinogen than unprocessed bracken. Therefore, it is difficult to evaluate the significance of bracken in relation to the high incidence of human stomach cancer in Japan. Kamon and Hirayama[40] made an epidemiological survey of cancer in a mountainous area of central Japan where the people eat much bracken, and they reported a significantly higher risk of esophageal cancer in people who ate hot tea gruel everyday and in those who ate bracken everyday; the risk was particularly high with a combination of both factors. Milk from cows that have eaten bracken contains a carcinogenic principle(s),[41] and may thus be a human hazard.

IV. PETASITES

A. Petasites as a Food and Folk Medicine

Petasites, *Petasites japonicus* Maxim., is a herb of the tribe Senecioneae in the family Compositae. Many species of this tribe commonly contain hepatotoxic pyrrolizidine alkaloids. Petasites is widely cultivated for use as a food in Japan. The mature terrestrial part of this plant is eaten either as a vegetable after being boiled and seasoned with soy sauce or as an addition to bean paste soup. Candied petasites is also eaten. Wild petasites is also used as a human food, especially in mountainous areas. The young flower stalks of wild petasites (Figure 6) are collected in early spring and used as food or a herbal remedy such as a cough cure, expectorant, or stomachic. They are usually used after their bitterness has been removed by boiling water. In some cases, fresh flower stalks are broiled and eaten with bean paste without removing the bitterness. Sometimes, fresh flower stalks are stored in salt.

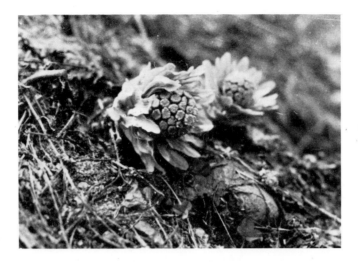

FIGURE 6.   Young flower stalks of *Petasites japonicus* Maxim.

B. Carcinogenicity of Flower Stalks of Petasites

Experiments showed that rats fed diet containing dry powder of the fresh flower stalks of wild petasites at a concentration of 4% or 8% develop hemangioendothelial sarcomas of the liver. Hepatocellular adenomas and hepatocellular carcinomas were also induced in a few animals.[27,42] The flower stalks of petasites were found to contain petasitenine (Figure 7) (fukinotoxin[43]), a new carcinogenic pyrrolizidine alkaloid, and a stereo-isomer of otosenine.[44,45] The flower stalks of cultivated petasites had much weaker hepatotoxicity than those of the wild type. The hepatotoxicity of the mature terrestrial part of cultivated petasites, which is one of the most popular vegetables in Japan, was very slight, and only proliferation of the bile ducts was observed in rats fed containing 32% petasites diet.[27] Since petasitenine is water soluble, it is possible to eliminate the carcinogenic activity to a certain extent by treatment with boiling water. However, it is conceivable that the flower stalks induce more liver damage in patients with liver diseases than in healthy persons, even when the amount of carcinogen is reduced by treatment with boiling water.[46]

V. COLTSFOOT

Like petasites, coltsfoot, *Tussilago farfara* L., is a member of the tribe Senecioneae, family Compositae. The leaves, Farfarae folium, are used in Europe as a cough medicine. A preparation of dried buds of the coltsfoot imported from China is called "Kan-tō-ka" in Japanese (Figure 8), and a decoction of this is used as a cough medicine. Rats given diet containing powdered buds of the coltsfoot developed hemangioendothelial sarcomas of the liver, hepatocellular adenomas, and carcinomas.[47] Chemical studies on the dried buds suggested that the carcinogenic effect was probably due to senkirkine, a hepatotoxic pyrrolizidine alkaloid.[48]

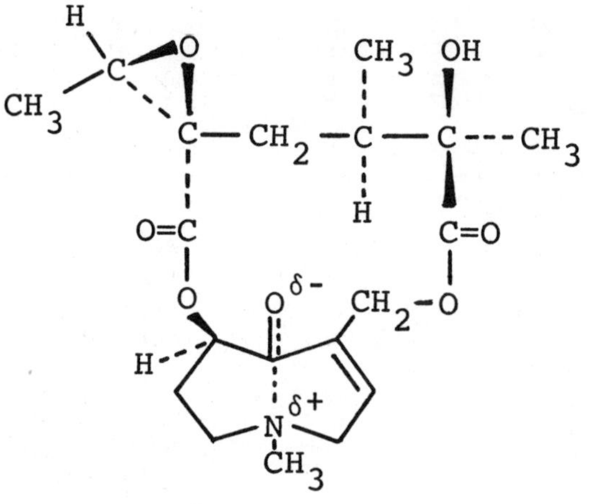

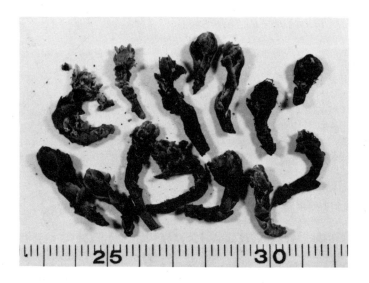

FIGURE 7.   Petasitenine.

FIGURE 8.   Dried buds of coltsfoot, *Tussilago farfara* L.

VI. *SYMPHYTUM OFFICINALE* L.

Symphytum officinale (Figure 9) is a herb of the family Boraginaceae, which includes the *Heliotropium* species that contain high levels of pyrrolizidine alkaloids. This plant is called comfrey or Russian comfrey and is cultivated for use in Japan as a green vegetable or tonic. The fresh leaves are used in salads and their juice is used as a drink. Sliced roots are also eaten. In Europe, comfrey is used as a demulcent in chronic catarrhs and certain disorders of the mucous membrane of the gastrointestinal tracts. Both the leaves and roots are hepatotoxic to rats, and rats fed diet containing powdered roots at high concentration showed centrolobular necrosis of the liver. Rats fed diet containing 8 to 33% comfrey leaves or 1 to 8% roots for long periods developed liver cell adenomas (Figure 10) and hemangioendothelial sarcomas of the liver. The roots had much higher

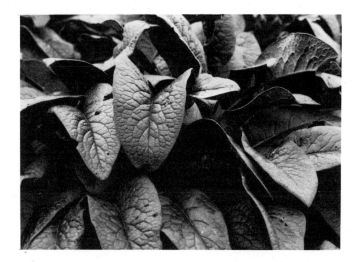

FIGURE 9.   Comfrey, *Symphytum officinale* L.

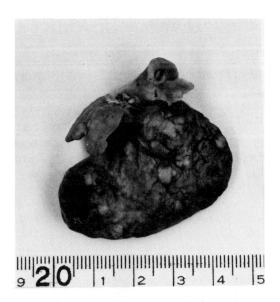

FIGURE 10.   Liver cell adenoma (grayish white nodules)
in a rat fed diet containing comfrey roots.

hepatoxicity and carcinogenicity than the leaves.[49] Histological changes in the liver, such as proliferation of the intrahepatic bile ducts, megalocytosis, formation of hyperplastic nodules, and liver cirrhosis, frequently developed in rats fed comfrey diet, even when the animals had no tumors. These histological changes of the liver are quite similar to those induced by some hepatotoxic pyrrolizidine alkaloids. It has been reported by Furuya and his co-worker[50,51] that symphytine and echimidine, which are pyrrolizidine alkaloids, are present in *Symphytum officinale*. The carcinogenic activity of comfrey is probably due to symphytine or some other hepatotoxic pyrrolizidine alkaloids.*

*Recently, it was proved that the carcinogenic activity of coltsfoot and comfrey is due to senkirkine and symphytine respectively.[57]

VII. FOOD HABITS RELEVANT TO A HIGH RISK OF CANCER OF THE STOMACH AND ESOPHAGUS IN JAPAN

Mortality from stomach cancer is higher in Japan than anywhere else in the world. A study of 220 Japanese patients with stomach cancer and 440 hospital controls in Hawaii by Haenszel et al.[52] showed that immigrants (Issei) from prefectures with the highest stomach cancer risks in Japan continued to display a high risk in Hawaii, but that their Nisei offspring had a normal risk. The associations of stomach cancer with the consumption of specific kinds of foods have been noted. High risks were found for Issei and Nisei who ate pickled vegetables and dried/salted fish, and those who ate most of these foods had the highest risks. Since the consumptions of raw fish and unprocessed vegetables were not associated with a high cancer risk, the methods for preparation of pickles and dried/salted fish may induce the high risk. Possible *N*-nitroso compounds are formed from secondary amines in dried fish and nitrites present in large amounts in pickled vegetables, and these *N*-nitroso compounds may cause a high incidence of stomach cancer. Low risks were suggested for several western vegetables such as tomatoes and celery, many of which are eaten raw.

The prefectures in Japan with the highest risk of stomach cancer are Akita, Yamagata, Niigata, and Toyama, bordering the Sea of Japan. In these prefectures, especially before World War II, rice, fish, and Japanese style salted pickled vegetables were the stable diet. The consumption of fresh raw vegetables was low all year round, and especially in the winter season, because of the heavy snow. However, life in these prefectures has changed much since World War II and meals have also become rather westernized. Probably these changes in the diet will decrease the risk of stomach cancer in Japan.

It is well known that the mortality rate from cancer of the esophagus is very high in Wakayama and Nara prefectures where the people have a time-honored custom of eating hot tea gruel. This custom is still preserved in these prefectures.[53] However, further studies are needed on whether the high risk of esophageal cancer is due to the temperature of the tea gruel or the tannin in the tea.

VIII. OTHER PLANTS TESTED

Various kinds of plants with a bitter or astringent taste are used as human foods in Japan. These plants are usually eaten after their bitterness has been removed by the treatment with boiling water. However, no carcinogenicity was observed when several of these untreated plants were fed to rats.[54,55] The plants examined were as follows: young leaves of artemisia (*Artemisia princeps* Pamp.), young horsetail (*Equisetum arvense* L.), young fronds of osmunda (*Osmunda japonica* Thunb.), ginkgo nuts (*Ginkgo biloba* L.), young terrestrial parts of cacalia (*Cacalia hastata* L.), rhizomes of dandelion (*Taraxacum platycarpum* Dahlst.), young furled fronds of ostrich-fern (*Matteuccia struthiopteris* (L.) Todaro), young terrestrial parts of aralia (*Aralia cordata* Thunb.), rhizomes of burdock (*Arctium-Lappa* L.), bamboo shoots (*Phyllostachys heterocycla* Matsum.), and rhizomes of the lotus (*Nelumbo nucifera* Gaertn.).

REFERENCES

1. **Whiting, M. G.,** Toxicity of cycads, *Econ. Bot.,* 17, 271, 1963.
2. **Laqueur, G. L., Mickelsen, O., Whiting, M. G., and Kurland, L. T.,** Carcinogenic properties of nuts from *Cycas circinalis* L. indigenous to Guam, *J. Natl. Cancer Inst.,* 31, 919, 1963.
3. **Laqueur, G. L.,** Carcinogenic effects of cycad meal and cycasin, methylazoxymethanol glycoside, in rats and effects of cycasin in germfree rats, *Fed. Proc. Fed. Am. Soc. Exp. Med.,* 23, 1386, 1964.
4. **Nishida, K., Kobayashi, A., and Nagahama, T.,** Cycasin, a new toxic glycoside of *Cycas revoluta* Thunb. I. Isolation and structure of cycasin, *Bull. Agric. Chem. Soc. Jpn.,* 19, 77, 1955.
5. **Riggs, N. V.,** Glucosyloxyazoxymethane, a constituent of the seeds of *Cycas circinalis* L., *Chem. Ind.,* 8, 926, 1956.
6. **Hirono, I., Laqueur, G. L., and Spatz, M.,** Tumor induction in Fischer and Osborne-Mendel rats by a single administration of cycasin, *J. Natl. Cancer Inst.,* 40, 1003, 1968.
7. **Hirono, I. and Shibuya, C.,** High incidence of pulmonary tumors in dd mice by a single injection of cycasin, *Gann,* 61, 403, 1970.
8. **Hirono, I., Shibuya, C., and Fushimi, K.,** Tumor induction in C57BL/6 mice by a single administration of cycasin, *Cancer Res.,* 29, 1658, 1969.
9. **O'Gara, R. W., Brown, J. M., and Whiting, M. G.,** Induction of hepatic and renal tumors by topical application of aqueous extract of cycad nut to artificial skin ulcers in mice, *Fed. Proc. Fed. Am. Soc. Exp. Med.,* 23, 1383, 1964.
10. **Shibuya, C. and Hirono, I.,** Relations between postnatal days of mice and carcinogenic effect of cycasin, *Gann,* 64, 109, 1973.
11. **Hirono, I., Hayashi, K., Mori, H., and Miwa, T.,** Carcinogenic effects of cycasin in Syrian golden hamsters and the transplantability of induced tumors, *Cancer Res.,* 31, 283, 1971.
12. **Spatz, M.,** Carcinogenic effect of cycad meal in guinea pigs, *Fed. Proc. Fed. Am. Soc. Exp. Med.,* 23, 1384, 1964.
13. **Watanabe, K., Iwashita, H., Muta, K., Hamada, Y., and Hamada, K.,** Hepatic tumors of rabbits induced by cycad extract, *Gann,* 66, 335, 1975.
14. **Spatz, M., McDaniel, E. G., and Laqueur, G. L.,** Cycasin excretion in conventional and germfree rats, *Proc. Soc. Exp. Biol. Med.,* 121, 417, 1966.
15. **Spatz, M., Smith, D. W. E., McDaniel, E. G., and Laqueur, G. L.,** Role of intestinal microorganisms in determining cycasin toxicity, *Proc. Soc. Exp. Biol. Med.,* 124, 691, 1967.
16. **Matsumoto, H. and Strong, F. M.,** The occurrence of methylazoxymethanol in *Cycas circinalis* L., *Arch. Biochem. Biophys.,* 101, 299, 1963.
17. **Campbell, M. E., Mickelsen, O., Yang, M. G., Laqueur, G. L., and Keresztesy, J. C.,** Effects of strain, age and diet on the response of rats to the ingestion of *Cycas circinalis, J. Nutr.,* 88, 115, 1966.
18. **Hirono, I., Kachi, H., and Kato, T.,** A survey of acute toxicity of cycads and mortality rate from cancer in the Miyako islands, Okinawa, *Acta Pathol. Jpn.,* 20, 327, 1970.
19. **Kobayashi, A.,** Cycasin in cycad materials used in Japan, *Fed. Proc. Fed. Am. Soc. Exp. Med.,* 31, 1476, 1972.
20. **Evans, I. A. and Mason, J.,** Carcinogenic activity of bracken, *Nature (London),* 208, 913, 1965.
21. **Evans, I. A.,** The radiomimetic nature of bracken toxin, *Cancer Res.,* 28, 2252, 1968.
22. **Pamukcu, A. M., Göksoy, S. K., and Price, J. M.,** Urinary bladder neoplasms induced by feeding bracken fern *(Pteris aquilina)* to cows, *Cancer Res.,* 27, 917, 1967.
23. **Pamukcu, A. M. and Price, J. M.,** Induction of intestinal and urinary bladder cancer in rats by feeding bracken fern *(Pteris aquilina), J. Natl. Cancer Inst.,* 43, 275, 1969.
24. **Pamukcu, A. M., Ertürk, E., Price, J. M., and Bryan, G. T.,** Lymphatic leukemia and pulmonary tumors in female swiss mice fed bracken fern *(Pteris aquilina), Cancer Res.,* 32, 1442, 1972.
25. **Hirono, I., Shibuya, C., Fushimi, K., and Haga, M.,** Studies on carcinogenic properties of bracken, *Pteridium aquilinum, J. Natl. Cancer Inst.,* 45, 179, 1970.
26. **Hirono, I., Shibuya, C., Shimizu, M., and Fushimi, K.,** Carcinogenic activity of processed bracken used as human food, *J. Natl. Cancer Inst.,* 48, 1245, 1972.
27. **Hirono, I., Sasaoka, I., Shibuya, C., Shimizu, M., Fushimi, K., Mori, H., Kato, K., and Haga, M.,** Natural carcinogenic products of plant origin, *GANN Monogr. Cancer Res.,* 17, 205, 1975.
28. **Ushijima, J., Matsukawa, K., and Yuasa, R.,** Oncogenic activity of bracken fern (transl.), *Jpn. J. Vet. Sci.,* 33, 129, 1971.
29. **Nakabayashi, T.,** Isolation of astragalin and isoquercitrin from bracken, *Pteridium aquilinum, Bull. Agric. Chem. Soc. Jpn.,* 19, 104, 1955.
30. **Wang, C. Y., Pamukeu, A. M., and Bryan, G. T.,** Isolation of fumaric acid, succinic acid, astragalin, isoquercitrin and tiliroside from *Pteridium aquilinum, Phytochemistry,* 12, 2298, 1973.
31. **Hikino, H., Takahashi, T., Arihara, S., and Takemoto, T.,** Structure of pteroside B, glycoside of *Pteridium aquilinum* var. *latiusculum, Chem. Pharm. Bull.,* 18, 1488, 1970.

32. **Fukuoka, M., Kuroyanagi, M., Toyama, M., Yoshihira, K., and Natori, S.,** Pterosins J, K, and L and six acylated pterosins from bracken, *Pteridium aquilinum* var. *latiusculum, Chem. Pharm. Bull.,* 20, 2282, 1972.

33. **Takatori, K., Nakano, S., Nagata, S., Okumura, K., Hirono, I., and Shimizu, M.,** Pterolactam, a new compound isolated from bracken, *Chem. Pharm. Bull.,* 20, 1087, 1972.

34. **Saito, M., Umeda, M., Enomoto, M., Hatanaka, Y., Natori, S., Yoshihira, K., Fukuoka, M., and Kuroyanagi, M.,** Cytotoxicity and carcinogenicity of pterosins and pterosides, 1-indanone derivatives from bracken *(Pteridium aquilinum), Experientia,* 31, 829, 1975.

35. **Evans, I. A. and Osman, M. A.,** Carcinogenicity of bracken and shikimic acid, *Nature (London),* 250, 348, 1974.

36. **Hirono, I., Fushimi, K., and Matsubara, N.,** Carcinogenicity test of shikimic acid in rats, *Toxicol. Lett.,* 1, 9, 1977.

37. **Wang, C. Y., Chiu, C. W., Pamukcu, A. M., and Bryan, G. T.,** Identification of carcinogenic tannin isolated from bracken fern *(Pteridium aquilinum), J. Natl. Cancer Inst.,* 56, 33, 1976.

38. **Hirono, I., Ushimaru, Y., Kato, K., Mori, H., and Sasaoka, I.,** Carcinogenicity of boiling water extract of bracken, *Pteridium aquilinum, Gann,* 69, 383, 1978.

39. **Hirono, I., Fushimi, K., Mori, H., Miwa, T., and Haga, M.,** Comparative study of carcinogenic activity in each part of bracken, *J. Natl. Cancer Inst.,* 50, 1367, 1973.

40. **Kamon, S. and Hirayama, T.,** Epidemiology of cancer of the oesophagus in Miye, Nara and Wakayama prefecture with special reference to the role of bracken fern, *Proc. Jpn. Cancer Assoc.,* 211, 1975.

41. **Pamukcu, A. M., Ertürk, E., Yalciner, S., Milli, U., and Bryan, G. T.,** Carcinogenic activity of milk from bracken fern fed cows, *Proc. AACR ASCO,* 17, 14, 1976.

42. **Hirono, I., Shimizu, M., Fushimi, K., Mori, H., and Kato, K.,** Carcinogenic activity of *Petasites japonicus* Maxim., a kind of coltsfoot, *Gann,* 64, 527, 1973.

43. **Furuya, T., Hikichi, M., and Iitaka, Y.,** Fukinotoxin, a new pyrrolizidine alkaloid from *Petasites japonicus, Chem. Pharm. Bull.,* 24, 1120, 1976.

44. **Yamada, K., Tatematsu, H., Suzuki, M., Hirata, Y., Haga, M., and Hirono, I.,** Isolation and the structures of two new alkaloids, petasitenine and neopetasitenine from *Petasites japonicus* Maxim, *Chem. Lett.,* 461, 1976.

45. **Hirono, I., Mori, H., Yamada, K., Hirata, Y., Haga, M., Tatematsu, H., and Kanie, S.,** Carcinogenic activity of petasitenine, a new pyrrolizidine alkaloid isolated from *Petasites japonicus* Maxim, *J. Natl. Cancer Inst.,* 58, 1155, 1977.

46. **Mori, H., Ushimaru, Y., Tanaka, T., and Hirono, I.,** Effect of carbon tetrachloride on carcinogenicity of *Petasites japonicus* and transplantability of induced tumors, *Gann,* 68, 841, 1977.

47. **Hirono, I., Mori, H., and Culvenor, C. C. J.,** Carcinogenic activity of coltsfoot, *Tussilago farfara* L., *Gann,* 67, 125, 1976.

48. **Culvenor, C. C. J., Edgar, J. A., Smith, L. W., and Hirono, I.,** The occurrence of senkirkine in *Tussilago farfara, Aust. J. Chem.,* 29, 229, 1976.

49. **Hirono, I., Mori, H., and Haga, M.,** Carcinogenic activity of *Symphytum officinale, J. Natl. Cancer Inst.,* 61, 865, 1978.

50. **Furuya, T. and Araki, K.,** Studies on constituents of crude drugs. I. Alkaloids of *Symphytum officinale* Linn., *Chem. Pharm. Bull.,* 16, 2512, 1968.

51. **Furuya, T. and Hikichi, M.,** Alkaloids and triterpenoids of *Symphytum officinale, Phytochemistry,* 10, 2217, 1971.

52. **Haenszel, W., Kurihara, M., Segi, M., and Lee, R. K. C.,** Stomach cancer among Japanese in Hawaii, *J. Natl. Cancer Inst.,* 49, 969, 1972.

53. **Segi, M.,** Tea-rice gruel as a possible factor of the esophageal cancer (transl.), *Proc. Jpn. Cancer Assoc.,* 32, 306, 1973.

54. **Hirono, I., Shibuya, C., Shimizu, M., Fushimi, K., Mori, H., and Miwa, T.,** Carcinogenicity examination of some edible plants, *Gann,* 63, 383, 1972.

55. **Hirono, I., Mori, H., Kato, K., Ushimaru, Y., Kato, T., and Haga, M.,** Safety examination of some edible plants. II, *J. Environ. Pathol. Toxicol.,* 1, 71, 1977.

56. **Wang, C. Y.,** personal communication.

57. **Hirono, I., Haga, M., Fujii, M., Matsuura, S., Matsubara, N., Nakayama, M., Furuya, T., Hikichi, M., Takanashi, H., Uchida, E., Hosaka, S., and Ueno, I.,** Induction of hepatic tumors in rats by senkirkine and symphytine, *J. Natl. Cancer Inst.,* 63, 469, 1979.

Chapter 5

THE CYCAD TOXIN

Gert L. Laqueur and Hiromu Matsumoto

TABLE OF CONTENTS

I. INTRODUCTION

Clinical observations made about 30 years ago brought to light an unusually high incidence of amyotrophic lateral sclerosis (ALS) among the Chamorros, native to the island of Guam.[1-3] Familial and sporadic forms were recognized, and it was also thought that an exogenous toxic factor might play a contributory role in individuals with a hereditary liability to the disease.[3]

Majorie Grant Whiting, experienced in ethnonutrition of the Pacific area, suggested that products or parts of cycad plants which were used for food on Guam might provide the exogenous toxic factor. The suggestion was based on published evidence that toxic properties of various parts of these plants produce an irreversible hind leg paralysis in cattle grazing on land where cycads grew. Observations of this nature had been recorded from such widely separated geographic areas as Australia and the Dominican Republic. Whiting gathered available information from the research literature of what was known about the uses of cycads as medicines, food, and fodder for man and animal, as well as their toxic effects. The results of her literature search, enlarged through personal experience on Guam and in Japan, were published and have remained an important reference source on the "toxicity of cycads".[4,5]

An exploration of the nature of the cycad plant toxins was started at the suggestion of Kurland and Whiting early in the 1960s at two places, the National Institutes of Health, Bethesda, Md. and the University of Hawaii. Post-mortem studies of laboratory animals in the initial experiments failed to demonstrate lesions in the brain and spinal cord resembling those seen in ALS. Osborne-Mendel and Holtzman strains of rats were used in these early studies and in subsequent experiments Sprague-Dawley and Fischer strains were employed, as well as mice, guinea pigs, and hamsters. The central nervous system was examined in all cases, but evidence of disease was not found. Loss of myelin and myelin degeneration in spinal cords were found in cycad-fed cattle, which exhibited signs of hindleg paralysis, by Hall and McGavin[6] in Australia, and by Mason and Whiting[7] in the Dominican Republic, in contrast to the negative results in small laboratory animals. Thus far, it is not possible to implicate definitively crude cycad material as the cause for the cattle disease, not to speak of the human disease, ALS. The toxic component in cycads in crystalline form would have to be available in quantities sufficiently large for testing it in cattle, in order to establish a causal relationship between consumption of cycads and the neurologic disease in cattle. The solution to this problem is further complicated, however, by our incomplete knowledge of the neuroanatomy of the central nervous system and spinal cord in cattle and the extent to which they are comparable to man. Although two interrelated toxic factors have been isolated from cycads, as will be described later, they are not only difficult to obtain but it has also not been established that they are the only toxic factors in cycads.[8] The toxins isolated and characterized thus far are the glucoside cycasin and its aglycone, methylazoxymethanol (MAM). The details of the isolation and action will be described later.

Clinical and pathological studies did not produce evidence for a neurologic disease in small laboratory animals after exposure to cycads, but the early experiments uncovered carcinogenic properties of crude cycad meal,[9] and of cycasin and its aglycone methylazoxymethanol.[10] These unexpected findings gave impetus to cancer-oriented research programs. Several conferences were held and the proceedings of two were published in the *Federation Proceedings* in 1964 and 1972.[11,12] Review papers concerning various aspects of cycad toxicity and carcinogenicity have appeared.[4,13-18]

A definite increase in cancer morbidity and mortality, which in some way could be related in cycads as a part of the diet, has not been observed in man. Mugera and Nderito from Kenya have suggested that the ingestion of cycad meal might play some contributory role in the etiology of liver cancer in parts of Africa where cycads are eaten.[19] Hirono et al.[20] searched for evidence of cycad toxicity and increases in cancer among the inhabitants of the Miyako Islands. It is known that the people had eaten cycads during the period of repeated strong typhoons in 1959, but no evidence of increase in cancer was found about 15 years later. The authors suggested that the cycad flour used by the islanders most likely had been properly prepared. There are experimental data which show properly prepared flour obtained from various families on Guam did not produce tumors in animals when fed to them in a concentration as high as 10%.[21]

II. DISTRIBUTION OF CYCADS

Cycads are ancient gymnosperms and are considered intermediate forms in the evolution from ferns to flowering plants. They were widely distributed throughout the world in the Mesozoic period. The cycads living today are limited to the tropical and subtropical zones around the globe, extending to the temperate regions such as in Florida, U.S., in Kagoshima Prefecture, Kyushu, Japan, and in parts of Australia. The family of cycads, referred to as Cycadaceae, today consists of nine living genera, each genus often having several species.

Cycas is most widely distributed and extends from East Africa across the Indian Ocean and Japan to the Mariana Islands. The important species are *Cycas circinalis* L. and *C. revoluta* Thunb. Much of the more recent work to be discussed later has been done with these two species. The seed from *C. circinalis* is a large single round to oval body, 6 to 8 cm in diameter, whereas the seed of *C. revoluta* is smaller. Both are covered by a husk, which is green and turns orange to red as the seeds mature. Masses of these seeds lie in the strobils and they can be seen from a great distance in the sunshine. At the time of the visit by one of the authors in 1970 (Laqueur), the people on Amami Oshima still added the starch of cycad seeds to make bean paste (miso).

Zamia is the second most widely distributed cycad. They grow on land bordering the Carribean Sea and the northern parts of South America. It was an important genus growing in southern Florida, where at the turn of the century a flour known as "koonti" or "sofkee" was commercially milled. Many of the cycad plants were cut in the course of this milling enterprise. The present day cycads in Florida are used only as ornamental plants in gardens. Two genera, *Macrozamia* and *Bowenia,* the latter of which grows mainly in Queensland, are found in Australia. The first isolation of toxic compounds in cycads was carried out with specimens of *Macrozamia. Encephalartos,* which grow in central and southern Africa, and *Stangeria* are the two African genera. *Microcycas* is found in Cuba and *Ceratozamia* in Mexico.[22,23]

The great age of this plant family, occasionally referred to as the living fossils in the literature, has attracted the interest of many botanists and naturalists. Examples of one or several genera and species are found in numerous botanical gardens either in greenhouses or out in the open, depending on the climatic condition. The Kew Gardens in London is an example of the first type, while the Fairchild Tropical Garden in Miami, Florida is an example of the second type. An extensive literature on cycads similarly reflects the widespread scholarly interest in this plant family, and several well-illustrated monographs are available with illustrations of representative members of the cycads.[24-27] Cycads now serve mainly as ornamental plants.

III. USES OF CYCADS

According to Whiting,[4] who covered in her review the nutritional uses of cycads, all parts of the plant depending on genus and species have been used for human consumption.

The native populations have been aware that without proper preparation the starchy component in seeds, stems, and roots is poisonous. The methods for detoxification used in widely separated parts of the world have been surprisingly similar. One can only assume that the detoxification methods originally were based on trial and error. The procedures empirically developed and used by the natives and their apparent success in detoxifying cycad material are readily understandable, in light of our present-day knowledge about cycad constituents and their chemical characteristics.

The method essentially consists of removing the outer husk and seed coat to obtain a firm kernel, which contains primarily starch. The kernel is cut into small pieces which are soaked in several changes of water. The glucoside in the kernel, because of its water solubility, is progressively removed with the repeated washings. The soaked kernel, with a reduced content of glucoside, is spread out in the sun to dry. It has been observed that a layer of foam, which is most likely the product of fermentation, forms on the surface during this drying process. The enzymes are partly provided by the cycad kernel, which contains a β-glucosidase capable of hydrolyzing the remaining glucosides, and partly provided by bacteria resulting from contamination in the hot and humid tropic environment. After further washing and drying, the starch is ground into a fine flour and used for cooking or stored for emergency, such as after a typhoon.

The critical step in the preparation of cycad flour for human consumption is the washing, which progressively removes the toxin. It has been said that the starch is free of poison when chickens survive drinking the last wash water. If true, a primitive but remarkably effective test in safety is used. The preparation of the flour takes several days or close to a week. It is possible that shortcuts in this process may have resulted in incomplete removal of the toxin in emergency situations, and illness or death of individuals or several members of a family, as in the Miyako Islands cases, may have occurred in the past, as reported by Hirono and co-workers.[20] The cases of cycad poisoning collected by Whiting[4] (Table 3 of reference 4) as well as those of Hirono and Mugera and Nderito from Kenya are similar. They indicate early involvement of the gastrointestinal tract beginning about 12 hr after ingestion of a meal and ending after 34 to 48 hr with signs of generalized intoxication with or without jaundice, depending apparently on the length of survival.[19,20] The appearance of jaundice in lethally poisoned humans is significant because dose-dependent hepatic injury with bile-stained fluid in the serosal cavities has been a consistent and early evidence of cycad toxicity in the experimental studies described below.

It would seem that one of the reasons why increases in cancers in general and cancers of the liver in particular have not been observed until now in man is that death occurs within 24 to 48 hr after ingestion of poisonous cycads. This observed time is reasonable for a poison which requires liberation of the toxin by enzymatic hydrolysis in the lower intestinal tract. The enzyme is of bacterial origin. No records are available which will allow projection of possible effects of many repeated but nonlethal, noninjurious amounts of cycads consumed over a period of years. If the observations in animals can be cautiously applied to man, a search for an increase in incidence of primary hepatomas might be carried out in the future. However, in the absence of detailed clinical studies and autopsy reports in instances of assumed cycad poisoning in man, there is no proof but only suspicion that death was the result of severe generalized intoxication, including massive liver injury.

IV. ACUTE TOXIC EFFECTS

The acute toxic effects in animals of crude cycad meal prepared from seeds of *Cycas circinalis* collected on Guam have been described.[9] The degree of toxic manifestations roughly paralleled the concentration of the meal in the diet and in turn depended on the concentration of cycasin in the crude meal. The concentration of cycasin varied from 1.2 to 3% in the meals used and depended in part on the stage of ripeness of the seeds, green seeds being more toxic than brown mature seeds. Boiling cycad slices has been observed by Dastur and Palekar,[28] to result in higher yields of cycasin. This effect has been explained by these authors to have resulted from inactivation of the enzyme β-glucosidase by the boiling, and thus prevented hydrolysis of cycasin to MAM and glucose. According to these authors a wide range in cycasin content of seeds was found varying from 0.55% to 3.6% in different batches.[29] The widespread variations in values obviously were unsatisfactory for comparative studies. The situation became greatly improved after the crude cycad meal was replaced by the glucoside cycasin and its aglycone, MAM. Short-term experiments, lasting only 5 to 10 days, first established that the toxic manifestations of cycasin and MAM were identical to those which had been observed with crude cycad meal. The toxicity of cycasin and MAM will now be briefly described as they were observed in rats in the early experiments. In addition to the similarity of the early changes induced in tissues with crude cycad meal, cycasin, and MAM, there was also no difference in the acute response between strains of rats which had been used in different laboratories.

V. STRUCTURAL CHANGES

The first experiments, in which crude cycad meal containing 1.2 and 3% cycasin was fed, used several hundred weanling Osborne-Mendel male rats. The cycad meal contained in the diets varied in concentrations from 0.25 to 10%. Rats receiving a diet containing 5% or more of cycad meal died within 2 weeks, whereas concentrations of 0.25 and 0.5% of the less toxic cycad meal (1.2% cycasin) in the basal diet did not produce any sign of toxicity nor mortality up to 5 months after the beginning of feeding when they were killed. No significant lesions were found in them on histopathologic examination.

The earliest changes were noted in the liver within 24 hr when the diet contained 2.3% cycasin. The changes consisted of loss of glycogen and cytoplasmic basophilia first from isolated liver cells around the central vein and subsequently from all liver cells in the centrilobular zones. Cytoplasmic eosinophilia with shrunken nuclei indicating cellular necrosis was noted in nearly all of the centrilobular cells, and the changes which had first been seen in scattered areas rapidly involved the entire liver by the 5th day. This process of liver cell necrosis was accompanied by hemorrhage in most lobules. Rats which had died or were moribund and killed at this stage frequently had free fluid in their body cavities and striking edema of the pancreas. Punctate hemorrhages were noticeable on serosal and mucosal surfaces occasionally accompanied by free blood in the lumen of the gut. It was noted that those rats which were developing liver cell necrosis became progressively more aggressive and sensitive to noise and motion.

Connective tissue repair or regeneration of liver cells occurred in rats with less severe injury or with hepatic damage absent, and after several weeks resulted in varying degree of cirrhotic livers or in essentially normal livers. Phagocytes laden with iron-containing pigment granules were often found in the scars as well as in the periportal fields in such livers.

Ultrastructural studies of liver cells during the early stages of cycasin poisoning have been published by Ganote and Rosenthal,[30] who gave MAM-acetate by stomach tube, and by Zedeck et al.,[31] who administered MAM-acetate intravenously to rats. The observations of both groups were supportive of each other. The earliest changes in liver cells became apparent as early as 15 min after the intravenous administration,[31] whereas 2 hr were required after intragastric instillation.[30] The changes showed loss of free ribosomes, membrane associated polysomes, and nucleolar alterations, indicating altered ribonucleic acid synthesis. Marked hypertrophy of smooth endoplasmic reticulum suggested increases in the activities of drug-metabolizing enzymes.

VI. ONCOGENIC EFFECTS

Survivors of the original experiment,[9] in which cycad meal containing 2.3% cycasin had been added in various concentrations, developed signs of neoplastic disease beginning after about 5 months. Swelling of the abdomen, apparently resulting from free fluid and a greatly enlarged nodular liver, palpable by external examination, pale eyes and pate, cold paws, and difficulties in breathing, suggested malignant disease associated with internal hemorrhage. When such animals were killed or spontaneously died, the most important autopsy findings consisted of massive intraperitoneal hemorrhage which usually could be traced to a point of rupture of the hepatic capsule to which blood clots were attached. The liver was replaced by one or several large nodular tumor masses with central umbilication and occasionally nearly filled the abdominal cavity. The liver parenchyma between tumor nodules was firm, indicating fibrosis. In few rats, solitary tumors were found surrounded by liver tissue without evidence of preexisting disease. The great majority of rats had single or multiple white and firm tumor nodules in one or both kidneys. Intestinal intussusception had resulted from growth of mucosal polypoid tumors in cecum in two instances. Details of the pathologic findings in the original experiment establishing the presence of carcinogen in crude cycad meal can be seen in Table 2 of Reference 9.[9] As the evidence accumulated for the presence of a carcinogen in crude cycad meal, the identification of the carcinogen became of paramount importance.

There were two types of carcinogens which were considered foremost in 1961 when the toxicity of cycad materials was explored. They were the aflatoxins and the *N*-nitroso compounds. The presence of a widespread fungal toxin produced by certain species of *Aspergillus flavus* and capable of inducing cancer in animals had just been reported from Great Britain by Lancaster et al.[32] Several of the seeds shipped to the laboratory from Guam for study were noted to be covered in places on the surface by a mold. The possibility existed, therefore, that the carcinogenic effects of crude cycad meal may also be due to an aflatoxin, as the toxin of *A. flavus* became to be known. The possibility was explored by Forgacs and Carll,[33] who reported on toxic fungi on seeds of *C. circinalis* in 1964 including a strain of *A. flavus* Link, which produced a high titer of aflatoxin. These authors reported only on the toxicity of the fungi in short-term experiments in mice. Long-term studies were not undertaken to test for carcinogenicity.

Matsumoto and Strong[10] produced confirmative evidence for a glucoside in crude cycad meal, which had previously been isolated by Nishida et al.[34] in Japan and by Riggs[35] in Australia. A possible relationship to the *N*-nitroso compounds was entertained because of similarities in the nature of the acute toxic hepatic injury and the late neoplastic response in liver and kidneys with both compounds.[36-38] The aglycone is isomeric with methylhydroxymethylnitrosamine. Over the years, additional information has been uncovered indicating further similarities in the metabolism of both compounds which most likely have the same ultimate carcinogen.[39-42]

VII. ONCOGENIC EFFECTS IN VARIOUS SPECIES

It was found that cycasin and MAM were the toxic and oncogenic factors in crude cycad meal and, when fed to young rats as part of the diet, induced tumors in liver, kidneys, and colon after long-term feeding, whereas the frequency of tumor sites was kidneys, colon, and liver in short-term experiments.[9,43] The difference in principal tumor sites, depending on the length of exposure, was similar to that reported for dimethyl-nitrosamine.[44] The oncogenicity of MAM, originally suggested by the findings of Matsumoto and Strong,[10] was subsequently confirmed and extended to include the synthetic MAM-acetate.

The oncogenic effects will be cited in the ensuing descriptions independent of the compound used, in view of the similarity in the histologic composition of the tumors induced with crude cycad meal, the isolated crystalline cycasin, its aglycone MAM, and the synthetic MAM-acetate. Comments will be offered if sex, age at the start of the experiments, duration of treatment, or route of administration to contribute to the outcome of the observed results. The tumors which have most frequently been seen will be described briefly under the heading of each species, i.e. rats, mice, guinea pigs, and hamsters, as they were found.

A. Rats

Rats, among the small laboratory animals, have most frequently been used for studies in carcinogenesis with cycad materials, and tumor inductions has been successful in all strains in which it was attempted. The most commonly involved organ sites included liver, kidneys, and colon; less frequently and more dependent on experimental arrangements were tumors in lung, brain, small intestines, ear canals, renal pelvis and urinary bladder, and peripheral nerves.

Hepatocellular carcinomas of the liver generally resulted after long-term feeding of crude cycad meal or of cycasin mixed with the diet. They occurred either as large often solitary carcinomas which were surrounded by normal appearing liver parenchyma, or as multiple primary hepatic carcinomas growing in a liver exhibiting evidence of old severe injury. In retrospect it appears likely that the kind of liver found in association with the carcinomas largely was related to the severity of the acute injury and that in turn depended on the amount of cycasin consumed. The majority of the animals with hepatic carcinomas showed evidence of intraabdominal malignancy 5 to 6 months after the onset. The carcinomas were large as a rule and could be palpated in many instances. Fatal intraperitoneal hemorrhage after rupture of Glisson's capsule was relatively common and, when present, was the cause of death. The tumor cells freely invaded the surrounding parenchyma and branches of the hepatic veins. Multiple, usually bilateral, metastatic tumor nodules with hemorrhagic components were seen in the lungs. A few of the hemorrhagic tumor nodules in the liver were composed of angiomatous structures in which the cells lining the vascular spaces were made up of anaplastic endothelial tumor cells. Foci of extramedullary erythropoiesis were noted within the carcinomas and sarcomas as well as in the uninvolved liver in several tumor-bearing rats. In addition to the malignant neoplasms, cystic and papillary cystadenomas, often multiple and of considerable size such as illustrated in reference 45, were thought to have arisen from the intrahepatic biliary system.[45] They were more frequently seen after intraperitoneal administration of MAM or the synthetic MAM-acetate than after feeding cycad meal or a cycasin-containing diet.

Although liver tumors have most readily been induced in long-term feeding experiments with cycasin or crude cycad meal, they have also developed after single intragastric instillation of cycasin or following subcutaneous injection of cycasin into newborn rats,[46] subcutaneous and intraperitoneal administration of cycasin to preweanling rats,[47] and after single or repeated doses of MAM or MAM-acetate given to conventional and germ-free rats.[48,49] The hepatocellular response to MAM was perhaps most directly illustrated in the study described by Borenfreund et al.[50] These authors reported that successfully made cultures of liver cells, when treated with MAM, developed about 6 to 8 weeks after exposure morphologic abnormalities including chromosomal aberrations, heteroploidy, and shortening of replication time. Furthermore, MAM-treated cells, when inoculated into cheek pouches of cortisone-treated hamsters or into nude mice, formed tumor nodules within 2 to 3 weeks. Microscopic study of the tumors showed them to be composed of spindle cells with many abnormal mitotic figures, and they retained the ability to secrete albumin.

Tumors of the kidney were most frequently encountered in rats exposed for short periods of time to either cycasin or crude cycad meal as part of the diet. They were found also, though less frequently, after administration of MAM or MAM-acetate. The cycasin-induced tumors usually developed mutliply and bilaterally, and histologically different types were observed in the kidneys of the same rat. The tumors were derived either from epithelial cells lining the tubules, or from mesenchymal cells giving rise to adenomas and adenocarcinomas, or to mesenchymal tumors with a low degree of aggressiveness, and sarcomas on occasion with pulmonary metastases. A few lipomatous tumors in cycasin-treated rats and even fewer such tumors were found in kidneys serving as controls. Among the renal tumors, those now referred to as mesenchymal tumors have been variously interpreted as to their histogenesis. The tumors originally were designated by us as undifferentiated proliferative lesions or interstitial tumors. The cycasin-induced tumors resembled those found in rats fed a diet containing dimethylnitrosamine, which were originally described by Magee and Barnes.[44] Hard and Butler have restudied the DMN-induced tumors of the rat kidney and have particularly contributed to the understanding of the mesenchymal tumors.[51,52] Hard has recently summarized these studies.[53] Two aspects of the cycasin-induced tumors perhaps have been noteworthy: (1) the frequency with which the mesenchymal tumors showed areas of sclerosis in the center, foci of sclerotic vascular changes occasionally remaining the only suggestive indication of a prior presence of such a tumor nodule; and (2) the limitation of smooth muscle cells as part of the mesenchymal tumor to female rats. Leiomyomas also were found in females. Similar observations were reported by Reuber,[54] who described a greater susceptibility for the development of leiomyomas and leiomyosarcomas of the kidney in 4-day-old female than in 4-day-old male BUF rats receiving intraperitoneally MAM-acetate at a dose of 20 mg/kg bodyweight, once weekly for 9 weeks. Light and electron microscopic studies of cycasin-induced renal tumors have been published by Gusek et al.[55-58] and Buss and Gusek,[59] and they cover both the epithelial and mesenchymal types of tumors. A valuable general review on experimental kidney tumors has been presented by Guerin et al.[60]

Tumors of the colon were the third most frequently observed neoplasm in the early studies in which crude cycad meal or cycasin mixed with the basal diet was fed to rats.[9,61] The tumors were situated principally in the proximal half of the colon and several in the cecum. Small intestines and lower colon and rectum were free of neoplasms. This situation drastically changed in subsequent experiments in which the aglycone of cycasin, MAM, the synthetic MAM-acetate and MAM-glucuronide were used. The proximate carcinogen used in either its natural or synthetic form resulted in a considerable increase in the number of tumors and a much wider involvement of the intestinal tract in the neoplastic process. MAM and MAM-acetate administered either in a single or in multiple intraperitoneal doses induced tumors in the small intestine, particularly carcinomas in the duodenum in addition to large bowel tumors,[45,48] but intrarectal instillation of MAM-acetate for 2 to 26 days into Donryu rats induced a very high incidence of carcinomas extending from cecum to rectum.[62]

The intestinal tumors were sessile or polypoid, benign or malignant. Broadly sessile carcinomas often growing through the serosa were predominantly seen in the duodenum and rectum infiltrating the bowel wall to various depths. They produced a carcinomatous peritonitis secondarily involving pancreas, spleen, and liver in the case of the duodenal cancer, and the pelvic organs when the primary site was in the rectum. At both locations, mucus production was common, and calcific deposits as well as foci of osseous metaplasia were noted in primary tumors. Sessile carcinomas accounted for some of the colonic carcinomas, but polypoid adenocarcinomas were more common. They frequently led in the advanced stages to intussusception with hemorrhagic infarction of the dependent part of the polypoid growth. Bloody feces or fresh blood around the anal opening often indicated the presence of a colonic neoplasm.

The uncovering of the oncogenic effects of cycad materials in various organ sites, including the colon, took place at a time when Matsumoto et al.[63] developed a method for the synthesis of the aglycone part, MAM, of the glucoside cycasin. The method, described in detail below, started from 1,2-dimethylhydrazine and proceeded through azomethane to azoxymethane methylazoxymethanol. At this time, Druckrey[64] and his co-workers were extending their investigations of carcinogenic N-nitroso compounds to the symmetrical 1,2-dialkylhydrazines and to the azo- and azoxyalkanes. The first report describing the successful induction of colon cancer with 1,2-dimethylhydrazine was published in 1967. A more extensive review of this subject appeared in 1970.[68]

Druckrey proposed a scheme for the metabolic activation of dimethylhydrazine.[66] The dimethylhydrazine is first oxidized to azomethane, a gas, which is converted to azoxymethane probably by a microsomal N-oxygenase.[67] The azoxymethane is further oxidized to MAM. Miller suggested that azoxymethane may be hydroxylated by the monooxygenase system in the liver or perhaps in the colon mucosa.[68] This scheme is the same as that for the chemical synthesis of MAM-acetate, except that the free MAM is generated in vivo instead of the ester. Fiala used ^{14}C-labeled dimethylhydrazine to demonstrate that the in vivo oxidation does follow the proposed metabolic scheme.[69,70] The major metabolite of injected ^{14}C-dimethylhydrazine was azomethane, which was exhaled with air.[71] Trace amounts of azoxymethane and MAM were detected in the urine of rats injected with ^{14}C-dimethylhydrazine.[72]

The availability of the chemicals provided the means for many investigators to experimentally explore the many problems of intestinal cancer, particularly that of the carcinoma of the colon which had assumed an important place in morbidity and mortality among cancers in man. It is not within the scope of this paper to review the numerous studies with 1,2-dimethylhydrazine and related compounds which were carried out in the attempts to create animal models for exploring the many factors contributing to human colon cancer. A selection of several more recent articles is given in the references.[73-77]

Cancer of lung and brain occurred with few exceptions in rats which had been exposed to the carcinogenic activity of cycads either during late fetal life or immediately after birth.[78-80] Although no definite explanation can be offered for the increased incidence in lung and brain tumors, the metabolic situation around the day of birth probably was unusually suitable for an interaction between the ultimate carcinogen of MAM and the cellular constituents in these two organ sites. The pulmonary tumors frequently developed multiply and usually involved both lungs. Histologically they resembled alveolar cell adenomas or carcinomas. They were visible as gray, subpleurally situated nodules. The brain neoplasms were not localized in a particular site and none had developed in the cerebellum. Histologically, the majority resembled oligodendrogliomas identical to those seen in man. A few were mixed with astrocytic elements or resembled astrocytomas.

According to Hoch-Legeti et al.[81] who examined ground fresh and dried cycad seed husks for oncogenic effect, malignant tumors of liver and kidneys were induced in nearly all rats. Yang et al.[82] came to the same conclusions. These observations are important because the juice of cycad husks is used by the Guamanians to relieve thirst, and dried husks are used in the place of sweets, as originally observed by Whiting.[4] The acute toxic effects of cycad husks in rats have also been described.[83] Although the studies thus far discussed have been principally conducted with cycasin, the glucoside obtained from either *Cycas revoluta* or *C. circinalis,* tumor induction has also been successful with seeds of *Encephalartos hildenbrandtii* from Kenya.[84] The azoxyglycoside in this cycad is macrozamin, according to Dossaji and Herbin.[85] The tumors induced in liver, kidney, and lungs were similar to those described with cycasin. Another member of the cycad family, Zamia, was examined on specimen of *Zamia floridana* tubers from Florida. Two percent of ground *Zamia* tubers added to the basal diet induced tumors in only 12% of the rats, but the tumor incidence increased to 60% when 3% ground tubers were mixed into the basal diet. Seven of the induced tumors were in the kidney, six in the liver, three in the colon, and one was an undifferentiated sarcoma in the omentum.[86]

B. Mice

Oncogenic effects of cycads in mice were first described by O'Gara et al.,[87] who observed tumors in liver and kidney in male C57 BL mice after repeated topical application of an aqueous emulsion of seeds of *C. circinalis* to skin ulcers artificially induced with 10% croton oil in mineral oil. The experiment was designed to simulate situations in life where cycad juices have reportedly been used as treatment of skin wounds and ulcers.[4] Tumors were found in 3 of 11 mice surviving the acute toxic effects. One had a hepatocellular carcinoma, adenomas within kidneys, and a subcutaneous hemangioma at the site of injection. A second mouse had a large adenoma in one kidney and multiple cystic lesions in the liver, while a third mouse had a large hemangiosarcoma of the liver. The hemangioma developing at the site of administration has remained the only example of a local neoplastic response. These studies, exploratory in nature, unfortunately could not be continued by the late Dr. O'Gara. They are of special interest, however, because the results displayed local as well as distant tumor development. The simultaneous presence of cycasin and MAM and of β-glucosidase in the seeds of cycads provides the chemicals necessary for tumor induction both at the site of application and at distant sites.

Oncogenic effects in mice after a single subcutaneous injection of cycasin into C57 BL/6 mice were described by Hirono et al.[88] They noted a marked difference in relative tumor incidence between newborn mice, in which 6% later developed liver and reticulum cell neoplasms, and mature mice, in which the tumor incidence was only 12% and liver, kidney, and lung were the principal tumor sites. They also noted that liver tumors had developed and metastasized more frequently in mice treated as newborns then as adults. A subsequent study further emphasized the importance of age in the immediate postnatal period when a single subcutaneous administration of cycasin produced a 100% tumor incidence in the newborn, but only 16% in 14-day-old mice at comparable doses.[89] Newborn mice of the dd strain received single subcutaneous injections of cycasin at two-dose levels in a third experiment. Lung tumors developed in 88% of mice surviving beyond 150 days and 64 had liver tumors with the smaller dose, but the larger dose produced 83% lung tumors and 37% liver tumors in the mice. Early mortality was high in this group amounting to 50% by the 16th day.[90] Many of the mice of the second group had various degrees of ataxia due to a maldevelopment of the cerebellar cortex, which will be discussed later in greater detail.

C. Hamsters

Observations on tumor induction in hamsters with cycasin have been made by Hirono et al.,[91,92] and with MAM by Spatz,[93,94] and by Laqueur and Spatz.[95] The intrahepatic bile ducts showed the most extensive changes, and 21 intrahepatic bile duct carcinomas were recorded among 151 hamsters when cycasin was given subcutaneously to newborn hamsters or by stomach tube to adult hamsters. Several of them were subsequently established as transplantable tumor lines.[91] The same authors observed a carcinoma of the gall bladder, hepatocellular carcinomas, and hemangioendothelial sarcomas of the liver in hamsters treated as newborns, whereas such tumors were rarely seen in hamsters which had received cycasin as adults by stomach tube. A few colonic tumors, pulmonary adenomas and an occasional renal tumor, were also observed.[91] Spatz reported in 1970 on the successful induction of hepatic and colonic carcinomas and of two carcinomas of the gall bladder in hamsters with MAM. It was administered either in a single intravenous dose, 20 mg/kg body weight, or in multiple intravenously given injections in which the dose varied from 10 to 20 mg/kg body weight.[93] Many adenomas and adenocarcinomas were found in the colon in addition to benign and malignant hepatic lesions involving liver cells and bile duct epithelium. The incidence of colonic neoplasms after a single intravenous administration of MAM amounted to 42%, and after multiple intraperitoneal doses reached 100%. Metastases from colonic carcinomas were found in 25% of the hamsters receiving multiple doses. Gall bladder carcinomas were found in two hamsters 32 and 37 weeks after they had received three intraperitoneal injections of MAM, the total doses of MAM being 5.06 and 6.16 mg of MAM respectively. There were no tumors in kidneys, lungs, or small intestines.[93,94]

D. Guinea Pigs

It was desirable to have available in the course of metabolic studies in guinea pigs, originally unrelated to the cycad investigation, a hepatoxic agent which would alter liver function. Observations which had just been made indicated that crude cycad meal contained a toxic factor which would bring about liver injury, its degree and severity being dependent on the concentration of the toxic factor added to the basal diet. The experience gained with the rats was used and meal varying in concentration from 5 to 10% was mixed into a guinea pig ration and fed to the pigs for one or two 5-day periods. The acute changes in the liver of the pigs were identical to those previously seen in rats and alterations were dose-dependent, although the pigs were twice as tolerant to the cycad poison than rats. Among 27 survivors which were killed between 11 and 22 months after first exposure to cycad meal, nine guinea pigs had liver tumors of which four were hepatocellular and five biliary in type. There were no metastases, but several pigs had focal hyperplastic lesions in the mucosa of gall bladder and esophagus.[93,94] The rather unexpected finding of hepatocellular neoplasms led to studies using a standard guinea pig diet and known doses of MAM or MAM-acetate instead of crude cycad meal.[95] Hepatocellular carcinomas were found in 30 of 45 guinea pigs surviving 6 months or longer, and 23 of them had metastasized. Bile duct carcinomas were found in two. Several additional mostly malignant tumors, among which one jejunal adenocarcinoma, three squamous cell carcinomas of the anterior nasal cavity, and one hemangiosarcoma of the nose, were observed.

E. Fishes

Only one report is available that describes the development of tumors in the liver of an aquarium fish, *Brachydanio rerio,* after initial subtotal destruction of the parenchyma by cycasin.[96]

VIII. TRANSPLACENTAL PASSAGE OF CYCAD TOXIN

When the work with cycads began in 1961, the scientific world was startled by reports that infants were born with severe malformations to mothers who, as was subsequently shown, had taken a drug called thalidomide (Contergan) during early pregnancy, usually for sedation. The epidemic outbreak ceased after withdrawal of the drug from the market. References to the original reports are to be found in Warkany's book.[97]

Because we were working with a highly toxic water-soluble substance in a natural product, cycad starch, which was consumed by people, it seemed highly appropriate to inquire into its transplacental passage. Preparations were made to test for both transplacental tumor induction and malformation once it had become apparent that the cycad toxin was also a carcinogen.

Transplacental passage was strongly suggested when acute liver lesions were found in pups of rats fed crude cycad meal during pregnancy. Similar observations were made with a litter of shoats, indicating transmammary passage, because the pigs had at no time access to cycad meal except through the milk from the sow.[98] Subsequent to the identification and isolation of the cycad toxins, cycasin, and its aglycone MAM,[10] it was shown that both chemicals passed through the placenta into fetal rats, and MAM was also demonstrated to be present in fetal hamster tissue when MAM had been intravenously given to pregnant hamsters.[99] It was shown, in addition, that after passage through the placenta MAM reacted by methylation with constituents of rat liver[100] with fetal rat brain after intraperitoneal administration of ^{3}H-MAM-acetate into pregnant rats,[101] as well as with nucleic acid in vitro.[102] A detailed summary of the observations on transplacental effects as of 1972 has been published.[79]

IX. TRANSPLACENTAL ONCOGENESIS

Transplacental tumor induction with cycad material was first accomplished with crude cycad meal containing 3% cycasin when fed to impregnated rats of the Sprague-Dawley strain during the 1st, 2nd, or 3rd week or throughout the entire period of gestation. The concentration of the meal in the diet varied from 1.3 to 5%. Of 81 long term survivors, 15 or 18.5% had tumors at various sites. Among them were 5 gliomas, and 7 jejunal tumors occurring in 4 to 7 litter mates.[78]

MAM and MAM-acetate were used in a subsequent series and given to pregnant Fischer rats in one intraperitoneal or intravenous administration of 20 mg/kg body weight. Details of this study, in which 42 or 12% out of 340 rats examined after transplacental exposure to the compounds had tumors, have been described.[94] A few rats had multiple primaries raising the total number of primary tumors to 50. The majority of the tumor-bearing rats had received the carcinogen within the 3rd week of intrauterine life or at the 21st day of gestation. This was particularly impressive with respect to the pulmonary and cerebral tumors, suggesting that this was the most sensitive day for later tumor development, and simultaneously indicating a metabolic situation favorable to a chemical interaction between carcinogen and the cellular constituents at these two sites. This period most likely extends for 1 or 2 days after birth as shown by the frequency of pulmonary and cerebral tumors in rats receiving injection of cycasin on day 1 of life.[46]

X. MALFORMATIONS

The teratogenic activity of MAM was first demonstrated in hamsters by intravenous injection of MAM into golden hamsters at day 8 of pregnancy and killing the animals at day 12 for examination under a dissecting microscope of the fetuses for malformation. The method was originally devised by Ferm for screening compounds for teratogenic activity.[103] It was found that with proper dosing, living hamster fetuses were obtainable on day-12 gestation with malformation of the brain and spinal cord, eyes, and extremities. The effective dose range was extremely narrow and 20 to 23 mg MAM/kg body weight were found optimal. Larger doses strikingly increased fetal death and resorption, whereas smaller doses failed to induce malformation. Illustrations of the malformation induced with MAM were included in the original report.[104]

A. Cerebellar Malformations

The first experimental production of a neurological disorder with cycasin was induced in mice and reported by Hirono and Shibuya.[105] The disorder consisted of various degrees of gait disturbances, and in the most severely affected mice, of hind leg paralysis. It was established in a subsequent paper that the disease was not strain-limited and that the same disorder could be induced in hamsters. The report described, furthermore, the pathologic process which found its explanation in extensive necrosis of the cells forming the external granular layer from which the cerebellar cortex, with exception of the layer of Purkinje cells, postnatally forms. Consequently, only scattered cells were found in the molecular and granule cell layers between which Purkinje cells were noted in apparently normal numbers but without their proper alignment. The changes persisted and were seen as late as 260 days after birth. Prerequisite for a successful induction of the cerebellar cortical alteration was the administration of cycasin on the day of birth.[106] These observations were confirmed using MAM-acetate, which was given to newborn hamsters 2 to 4 days postnatally.[107] The necrosis of cells in the external granular layer was more severe in the anterior than in the posterior lobes, when MAM-acetate was administered from the 4th to 6th day of postnatal life. Rows of cells, resembling those of the granule cell layer, occupied a zone midway through the molecular layer in the anterior lobes. They suggested regeneration from remnants of the external granular layer but incomplete migration of cells, when the cerebella were examined 20 days postnatally.[107] Similar observations were also made in rats treated postnatally with MAM-acetate.[108] Jones et al.[109] confirmed the changes in mice as did Sanger et al.,[110] who additionally described focal accumulations of granular cells in the molecular layer of pups treated with MAM-acetate within 24 hr after birth. Haddad et al.,[111] who systematically investigated the response of the brain to cycasin and MAM, confirmed the reported alterations in mice and hamsters. They observed dose-dependent changes in size and architecture of the cerebellum of rats, but fairly large dosing such as 50 mg/kg body weight subcutaneously of MAM-acetate at day of birth was required. Particularly striking effects both clinically and anatomically were observed in ferrets, a carnivore. Even with a relatively small dose of 10 mg/kg body weight at birth, pronounced permanent motor deficits were exhibited.[111] Fine structural alterations of cerebella in mice which were treated with cycasin within 24 hr after birth and examined 25 days later showed marked reduction in the number of granule cells and their processes including presynaptic terminals. Purkinje cells were present and were essentially normal.[112,113] Golgi-stained sections of cerebellum of 4-month-old rats, however, showed abnormal cells with reduced and abnormally oriented dendritic arborization.[114] As a reflection of the rapid postnatal growth of the cerebellar cortex, high thymidine incorporation into DNA and RNA were obtained in the cerebellum of treated rats when compared with untreated rat cerebral cortex.[115] Subcutaneous administration of MAM-acetate to rats at various days postnatally reduced the DNA content by 50% and with partial recovery during subsequent days resulted in a DNA deficit of 20% in the adult.[116]

B. Cerebral Malformations

Four litters of Fischer rats, 13 to 14 months old, were found to have on examination unusually small brains. The rats were part of an investigation which was searching for evidence of transplacental tumor induction discussed above.[78] The mothers of these litters had received on days 14, 15, and 16 of gestation intraperitoneal injections of MAM totalling 20 mg/kg body weight. The pregnancies ran their normal course. A slightly depressed area over the frontal lobe, revealing a gray translucent area, was found in one of the offsprings. Sectioning of the lobe suggested a brain tumor which was confirmed later by microscopic study.[117] Reproducibility, strain dependency, optimal dose, and time required for successful induction of the observed malformations were examined in subsequent experiments. Sister to brother matings of rats from microcephalic litters were carried out, and a long term project was started to look for intellectual deficits in microcephalic rats. The malformation was readily reproducible not only in Fischer rats but also in Osborne-Mendel rats. Fischer et al.[118] confirmed the induction of microencephaly with MAM in Long-Evans rats, and an identical effect was also obtained in Sprague-Dawley rats.[119] A single administration of 20 mg/kg body weight of MAM on day 15 of gestation was determined to be optimal. Matings between microcephalic sisters and brothers produced, as expected, normal offsprings.

Histologic examination of the brain 48 hr after the administration of MAM showed extensive necrosis among the cells of the subependymal matrix zone, which provides the cells for the developing cerebral cortex under normal situations.[117] One of the astounding observations was the great uniformity within each litter in the reduction in weight of the cerebrum, although differences were noted between litters. Except for variable degrees of ventricular dilation and accumulation of fluid, no other malformations were found in the brains. An estimate of the cellular loss from the hemispheres of MAM-treated rats was obtained by comparing the quantitative changes with age in the DNA content of microcephalic brain with those of controls. The difference amounted to about 25% at birth, which persisted into maturity. The hemispheres of a 7-day-old MAM-treated rat contained about one half of the DNA content of the same parts of the brain in controls, when the hemispheres and remainder of the brain were analyzed separately. There was no difference in the remaining brain.[120] The reduction in the number of cells in the hemispheres was accompanied by cellular changes in the organization of the cerebral cortices in the MAM-treated brains. The cortical laminae were indistinct — in places even absent — and scattered foci of ectopic islands of small undifferentiated cells were found in the narrow rim of cortex overlying dilated ventricles. The high degree of reproducibility should make this type of microcephaly useful for studies of the neurons and cells which are involved at different days of fetal life in the development of the cerebral cortex.[121] A study of this nature has recently described an abnormally dense noradrenergic innervation of the thin neocrotex following the destruction of many of its intrinsic neurons on day 15 of fetal life by MAM.[119]

A different type of structural disorganization in microcephalic brains was detected by Singh in postnatal hooded rats which had been exposed to MAM acetate once or three times during the 3rd week of fetal life.[122] Although the hippocampus was normal at birth, foci or ectopic neurons were detectable opposite gaps in the continuity of the pyramidal layer of Ammon's horn starting at the 5th day of life. The number of gaps and ectopic neuronal foci increased within the ensuing 2 to 3 weeks. Necrosis of cells which preceeded the development of the other central nervous system lesions were not observed by the author, and the mechanism responsible for the evolution of these lesions has remained uncertain.

The rats were active and unrestricted in their spontaneous activities in spite of their rather severe brain alterations. There remained the possibility, however, that microcephalic rats might differ from their controls when properly tested for behavioral and intellectual performance. Such rats were tested in a Hebb-Williams maze devised for testing intellectual functions of the rat. The performance of the microcephalic rats was substantially and significantly inferior to that of normal rats.[123] The error rate was considerably greater for females than males in the group of microcephalic rats, but this difference was absent among the controls. On repeating the test the microcephalic rats decreased their error rate in a manner similar to the controls. The method to induce microencephaly was subsequently confirmed in rats of the Long-Evans strain. A dose-dependent microencephaly was demonstrated that also correlated well with the deficits in intellectual performance. A summary of these experiments indicated that various aspects of behavior were not uniformly affected in the rats. Deficiencies in solving tasks in maze problems existed, but none was observed in operant conditioning schedules nor in discrimination learning set. Interestingly, the authors also found that an enriched environmental condition during rearing considerably improved the performance of microencephalic-impaired rats in problem-solving tasks.[124]

A study of representative animals of rodents, lagomorphs, and carnivores revealed that among all animals tested (mouse, rat, hamster, rabbit, ferret, cat, dog, and pig), the ferret was perhaps most responsive to the effects of MAM and yielded the greatest amount of information at both the prenatal and postnatal age.[111-114,125] The cerebellar effects in ferrets treated with MAM-acetate from the gestational age of 38 days until immediately after birth (42 days) have been cited above. Injections of MAM-acetate into pregnant ferrets on days 27 to 32 of gestation resulted in young with severe degrees of microencephaly and lissencephaly. Such ferrets were maintained for about 1 year, in spite of an associated hydrocephaly severe enough to flatten the anterior cerebellar surface.[11,125] Both malformations, cerebellar hypoplasia and microencephaly, were induced in ferrets administered MAM-acetate on the 38th day of gestation, whereas two doses were necessary when given on the 15th day of gestation and on day of birth, to produce both malformations in the rat.[111]

C. Retinal Malformations

Severe retinal hypoplasia was noted in hamsters which received injections of MAM-acetate between the 4th and 6th days of life and examined on the 20th postnatal day. The thinning was most conspicuous in the prospective unclear layer of the retina and was accompanied by formation of rosettes.[107] Similar observations were made in mice and rats treated with cycasin on the 1st day of life.[92] Goerttler et al.[126] induced and described the same lesions in rats after intraperitoneal administration of MAM-acetate at a dose of only 10 mg/kg body weight. The retina, histologically examined shortly after a dose of MAM had been given, showed multiple, closely spaced foci of unclear debris. During attempted regeneration rosettes were formed in the nuclear layer.[92] The detailed description of the development of the retina in normal rats during fetal and postnatal life should be consulted for comparison.[127]

D. Comments on Induced Malformations

Looking at these three examples of malformations involving the cerebrum, cerebellum, and the retina of rats, the initial recognizable process was identical in all except possibly for the changes in the hippocampus. It started with death of cells of selected parts of the brain, which at specific times during fetal development were growing in numbers through cell division and excessively sensitive to the action of cycad toxin. The toxin was shown to cross the placenta and was capable of chemically reacting with cellular components of fetal tissues. It would seem likely that the reactions between the ultimate carcinogen of MAM and nucleic acids and proteins of the fetal cells which eventually result in tumors also occurred simultaneously in cells adjacent to those which at that stage of development were highly sensitive to the toxin and disintergrated. Otherwise, it would be difficult to visualize the development of a glioma in an area contributing to the microencephalic portion of the cerebral cortex with a single dose of MAM. Excretory studies of the cycasin in crude cycad materials, as well as of crystalline cycasin, have shown that the greater portion was excreted in the first 24 hr after its administnation, but only small amounts were excreted during the second period of 24 hr. With any lengthy storage of this low molecular weight, water soluble toxin seems unlikely and no evidence has been found to suggest it.

XI. OTHER NEUROTOXIC FACTORS

A new basic amino acid, α-amino-β-methylaminopropionic acid, was isolated in 1967 by Vega and Bell[128] from seeds of *Cycas circinalis.* The compound was synthesized and reported to be markedly neurotoxic to chicks and rats. It was found in seeds and leaves of the genus *Cycas* but not in the seeds of the other genera. However, leaf extracts of *Dioon, Zamia, Bowenia, Macrozamia, Lepidozamia,* and *Encephalartos* contained a compound similar to α-amino β-methylaminopropionic acid.[129,130] Although the significance of this compound in terms of the human disease, ALS, and the disease in cattle is uncertain, chronic toxicity studies are indicated before a final decision is made with respect to the importance of this compound for the diseases of cattle and man.

XII. CYCASIN, MACROZAMIN, AND OTHER AZOXYGLYCOSIDES

Cooper,[131] in 1941, isolated a toxic crystalline compound from *Macrozamia spiralis* and named it macrozamin. Eight years later, the sugar moiety of macrozamin was identified as primeverose, 6-(β-D-xylopyranosyl)-D-glucopyranose.[132] The aglycone of the glycoside, although not isolated, was demonstrated to be an aliphatic azoxy compound, hydroxyazoxymethane. The aglycone was believed to be incapable of independent existence.[133] Later, when the aglycone was prepared from the glucoside isolated from *C. circinalis,* it was named methylazoxymethanol (MAM) to indicate that it was the alcohol portion of the glucoside.[10]

Nishida et al.,[34] in 1955, isolated a glycoside from *C. revoluta* and showed that it was related to macrozamin. The MAM moiety was attached to glucose instead of the disaccharide primeverose as in the case of macrozamin. The compound was named cycasin.[34] Riggs showed that the same compound was present in *C. circinalis.*[35] Proton magnetic resonance spectroscopy evidence indicated that the unsubstituted methyl group of cycasin is attached to the quaternary nitrogen atom[134] and the chemical structure is as shown in Figure 1. Cycasin is soluble in water and aqueous ethanol, but only sparingly soluble in alcohol and insoluble in most organic solvents. It has an optical rotation of $[\alpha]_D^{28}$ = 41.3 and melts at 144 to 145°C with decomposition.[34]

Both glycosides, macrozamin and cycasin, are hydrolyzed by 0.1 N hydrochloric acid at 100°C. The free aglycone rapidly decomposes stoichiometrically as follows:

$$CH_3\text{-}\overset{\overset{\displaystyle O}{\uparrow}}{N}=N\text{-}CH_2\text{-}O\text{-sugar} \xrightarrow{H^+} HCHO + CH_3OH + N_2 + \text{sugar}$$

The reaction of alkaline hydrolysis is complex, and among the products identified are cyanide ion (ca. 0.5 mol), formic acid (ca. 0.5 mol), and traces of methylamine and ammonia.[33] The generation of cyanide ion by alkaline hydrolysis has been used as a qualitative test for the presence of azoxyglycosides.[34]

Nishida and co-workers have shown that there are seven other azoxyglycosides in minute quantities in *Cycas revoluta.*[135,136] These compounds are thought to be products of transglycosylation and could be considered as β-glucosylcycasin, and thus have been named neo-cycasins. All parts of *C. revoluta,* the leaf, stem, male strobil, and seed, have

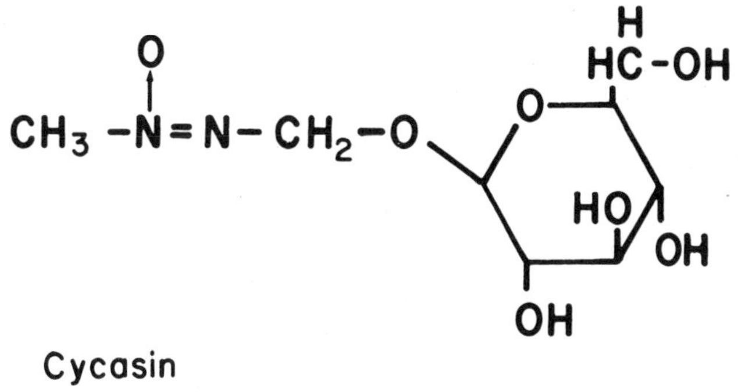

Cycasin

FIGURE 1. Structure of cycasin, β-D-glucopyranosyloxyazoxyme-
thane or methylazoxymethyl-β-D-glucopyranoside.

been analyzed for the presence of cycasin.[136] The azoxyglycosides appear to exist in all the cycad genera and cycasin and macrozamin seem to be the major azoxyglycosides present.

A. Hydrolysis of Azoxyglycosides In Vivo

Early in the experimental work with crude cycad starch and later with crystalline cycasin, the question arose as to the fate of the ingested azoxyglycosides in the animals. Cooper[131] reported as early as 1941 that macrozamin required passage through the gastrointestinal tract to produce toxicity. Nishida et al.[137] found the same to be true in the case of cycasin. These investigators also noted that a period of 12 to 24 hr was required for toxic effects to become evident, and they suspected some enzymatic activity, perhaps of bacterial origin, within the intestinal tract as the cause of the delay in toxicity. This situation was clarified by Kobayashi and Matsumoto,[138] who showed in quantitative studies that parenterally administered cycasin was nearly quantitatively excreted in the urine, whereas only a portion of the cycasin given by stomach tube was excreted in the urine, and the remainder, varying between 23 and 70% of the intake, was metabolized in the gut.

The importance of the intestinal tract for the metabolism of cycasin was also supported by the observation that, in long term studies of the carcinogenicity of cycasin, a small but recurring percentage of animals did not develop tumors with total dosages of cycasin well within the tumor-inducing range.[9] Although excretory studies were not done at that time, it was noted that liver damage usually seen with dosages at the levels used was also absent. The cycasin fed with the diet apparently had passed unchanged through the intestinal tract. Evidently rats differed in their ability to hydrolyze cycasin.

To elucidate the possible cause for this variability, germ-free rats appeared useful to evaluate the general importance of the intestinal flora for cycasin hydrolysis. Excessive amounts of cycasin were fed (200 mg/100 g feed) to conventional and germ-free Sprague-Dawley rats for 20 days. All germ-free rats gained weight and were alive and well after 20 days, whereas the majority of the conventional rats had died or were moribund. A group of germ-free rats identically treated were set aside and maintained for two additional years. They were found free of those tumors commonly induced with cycasin.[43,46] Further studies in which cycasin intake and excretion were measured showed that germ-free rats excreted about 97% of the intake, whereas only 20% of the intake was recovered from the urine of conventional rats; the remainder was hydrolyzed.[139] It appeared, therefore, that the enzyme necessary for cycasin hydrolysis was of bacterial origin, and monocontamination of germ-free rats with bacteria known to produce β-glucosidase promptly restored to the intestinal tract the ability to hydrolyze cycasin. On the other hand, monocontamination with organisms that do not produce β-glucosidase failed to hydrolyze cycasin.[140] In retrospect, it would seem possible that variations in the intestinal bacterial flora could explain those cases in which rats exposed to tumor-inducing amounts of cycasin by the enteric route failed to develop evidence of hepatotoxicity and neoplasm. It is regrettable that fecal cultures were not done routinely when the experiments were performed to determine the nature of the bacterial flora.

A somewhat different situation exists when rats and mice are administered a single injection of cycasin into the subcutis in the neck region during the neonatal and early postnatal periods. These animals developed tumors in later life.[46,88] Of 55 rats, 46 (or 84%) developed tumors at various sites but not locally. Cycasin had apparently been hydrolyzed in the subcutis as the observations of Spatz[141] would indicate, and freed the aglycone for resorption and tumor induction at a distant site. A more extensive study was reported by Matsumoto et al.,[47] who investigated the activity of β-glucosidase in tissues of various organs of preweanling rats. The tumor incidence in a parallel study was determined in groups of rats into which cycasin had been parenterally injected on postnatal days corresponding to those at which the determinations for β-glucosidase activity were conducted. The greatest activity was found in the small intestine at about the 15th postnatal day. Persistently low levels of activity were found in skin, pancreas, liver, muscle, and stomach. Enzyme activity in kidney tissue remained low but slightly increased after weaning. There was good correlation between levels of activity in the small intestine and the tumor yield when the two experiments were compared.

B. Methylazoxymethanol and its Acetate

Early attempts at separation of the glucoside cycasin into its components, alcohol and glucose, resulted in the decomposition of the aglycone.[34] Subsequently Kobayashi[142] hydrolyzed cycasin with purified cycad β-glucosidase and obtained evidence that as long as heat is not applied to the reaction mixture the free aglycone could exist, but he did not attempt to isolate it. Matsumoto and Strong[10] first obtained the aglycone, methylazoxymethanol (MAM), from the lipid fraction *C. circinalis* seeds, which had been extracted with ethyl ether. MAM, free of water, was found to be reasonably stable. The ultraviolet spectrum of MAM was the same as that of cycasin, but the purified material was free of glucose. Kobayashi and Matsumoto[138] used a commercially available β-glucosidase, almond emulsion, to hydrolyze cycasin, and extracted the free aglycone with ether in a continuous liquid extractor. A system in which 5% cycasin dissolved in 0.03 M phosphate buffer at pH 5.2 and incubated at 35° for 5 hr with 0.2% emulsin was established to be satisfactory for large-scale hydrolysis of cycasin. The algycone was purified by repeated vacuum fractional distillation. The compound is a colorless liquid boiling at 51°C (0.6 mm) and crystallizes at 1 to 3°C. It is completely miscible with water and alcohol, soluble in chloroform but less soluble in ether, and in aqueous solution slowly decomposes even at room temperature. The ultraviolet spectrum is the same and infrared spectrum is similar to that of cycasin.[138]

The isolation of cycasin is too time-consuming and difficult and thus a synthetic compound was needed, as interest in experimental use of cycasin and MAM increased. The ideal compound to synthesize would have been MAM, but because of its relative instability, the acetate ester of the compound was synthesized. The synthesis started with the symmetrical 1,2-dimethylhydrazine which was oxidized to azomethane with mercuric oxide. The azoxymethane was brominated in the allylic position by the Wohl-Ziegler reaction. The bromoazoxymethane was converted with silver acetate, in a two-phase reaction, to MAM-acetate. The compound was purified by vacuum distillation.[63] MAM-acetate is now commercially available. The synthesis also made possible the preparation of radioisotope-labeled MAM-acetate. The preparation of the starting compound was modified and radioisotope-labeled methyl group was incorporated into the 1,2-dimethylhydrazine.[143]

MAM-acetate has been shown to be deacetylated by serum esterase, and thus free MAM is generated in experimental animals parenterally administered with the ester.[144]

The qualitative identification of cycasin by the detection of the cyanide formed when the compound is treated with alkali has already been mentioned. A cycasin containing solution is made alkaline with a few drops of 2N sodium hydroxide and heated to boiling. The solution is acidified with sulfuric acid and the evolution of hydrocyanic acid is detected by a blue coloration of a copper-benzidine test paper placed at the mouth of the test tube, which is gently heated if necessary.[34]

Separation of cycasin from other compounds can be carried out with either paper or thin layer chromatography. The developing solvent in n-butanol/acetic acid/water, (4/1/1), and visualization is with aniline hydrogen phthalate in butanol or with a 1% ethanolic resorcinol solution and 2N hydrochloric acid (1:9). The sprays detect glucose of cycasin.[34] A specific reaction for the azoxy group of cycasin is obtained by spraying the compounds separated on a thin layer plate with 0.2% chromotropic acid in 2M sulfuric acid and heating the plate at 100 to 110°C for 5 to 10 min. The reactions involved are: the hydrolysis of cycasin to release free MAM, the decomposition of the MAM to yield formaldehyde, the reaction of formaldehyde with chromotropic acid to produce a blue color.[10]

Cycasin in cycad seeds or in prepared cycad meal can be determined quantitatively by utilizing the chromotropic acid color reaction. The intensity of the color developed is determined colorimetrically at 570 nm and the quantity of cycasin is read off a standard curve. The standard curve can be prepared with a standardized formaldehyde solution if pure cycasin is not available.[10] The chromotropic acid reaction does not distinguish between the various azoxyglycosides. A gas chromatographic method has been used for the specific quantitation of cycasin. The dried residue of a cycasin containing extract is trimethylsilylated and the cycasin derivative is separated in a gas chromatograph.[145] This method can be used to determine macrozamin as well as cycasin, but macrozamin is barely detectable. A more satisfactory method for the estimation of a mixture of cycasin and macrozamin is to dissolve the residue in 1% ethanol and determine the azoxyglycosides by liquid chromatography using an ODS reversed–phase column. This method separates cycasin and macrozamin, and for equimolar amounts of the two compounds the peak heights are essentially equal, but larger quantities are needed than for gas chromatography.

The determination of minute quantities of cycasin and macrozamin in animal tissue is more difficult. The tissue is extracted with 70% ethanol and the ethanol is removed by vacuum distillation. The resulting water-soluble extract is further purified. Interfering materials are removed and the glycosides concentrated. The method of Kobayashi and Matsumoto which absorbs the glycosides on Darco® G-60-celite column works well. A thorough washing of the column with water removes most of the interfering impurities and the absorbed glycosides can be eluted with 20% ethanol. The eluate is dried and the azoxyglycosides in the dry residue are derivatized with Tri-Sil® reagent and quantitated by gas chromatography.[146]

XIII. BIOCHEMICAL CHANGES

The reaction of MAM with cellular constituents and the effect on some enzyme activities have been studied in attempts to understand the mechanism of carcinogenic action of the compound. Methylation is the primary reaction which occurs and its effects range from what appears to be cell membrane destruction to inhibition or inactivation of nucleic acid and protein synthesizing enzymes.

Progressive loss of up to around 30% of the total rat liver RNA was produced by cycasin fed in increasing levels. The loss of liver phospholipids paralleled that of RNA[147,148] and correlated with the disintegration of cytoplasmic basophilia as observed with the light microscope. The changes suggested that the primary effect of cycasin could be on the lipo-protein-rich endoplastic reticulum membrane. MAM inhibited the incorporation of thymidine into rat liver small intestine and kidney DNA.[30] Uridine triphosphate (UTP) incorporation was inhibited in nuclei isolated from MAM treated rat liver.[149] An "aggregate" enzyme system containing chromatin and RNA polymerase, a nuclear preparation devoid of membrane, also showed that there was inhibition of UTP incorporation into RNA.[150] Orotic acid was incorporated into nucleolar RNA but cytidine was significantly less incorporated.[149] The monomer-plus dimer of rat liver RNA was approximately 35% in the control, but in cycasin-treated liver the monomer-dimer increased to 52% and 67% in MAM-acetate treated liver. Cycasin deaggregates poly-ribosomes, but MAM-acetate was more effective. This difference was attributed to the less efficient release of MAM from cycasin by the bacterial enzymes of the intestinal microflora.[100] Single strand breaks in liver DNA induced by MAM was demonstrated by alkaline sucrose gradient centrifugation. Maximum damage occurred a few hours after MAM administration but the repair process took longer than 14 days.[151] The product of MAM methylation of nucleic acid has been identified as 7-methylguanine. Liver RNA was methylated to a greater extent than either the kidney or small intestine.[100] Small amounts of 7-methylguanine was detected in the DNA isolated from the descending colon of rats treated with MAM-acetate.[152] MAM injected into pregnant rats methylated guanine in the seven position of both DNA and RNA of fetuses, indicating that the compound is transported across the placenta.[101] MAM can also methylate DNA and RNA in vitro to produce 7-methylguanine.[102]

Cycasin inhibited protein synthesis in the liver but not in the kidney, spleen, or ileum.[100] This inhibition was not evident for 5 hr, but once established it persisted for 20 hr. Similar inhibition was observed after MAM-acetate as well as an aqueous extract of *Macrozamia communis*[30,153] were administered to rats. Microsomal protein synthesis in rat liver was inhibited 50% below control levels in 1 hr and to a maximum of 70% in 2 hr. Circular dichroism analysis of the "aggregate" enzyme preparation from MAM-treated rat liver indicated a conformational change of the nuclear protein component, suggesting a MAM-nuclear proteins interaction.[150]

MAM is an excellent methylating agent which decomposes spontaneously. Organic acids and phenols, as well as the guanine of DNA and RNA, have been shown to be methylated when mixed with MAM and Kept at 37°C for several hours.[102] The biochemical action of MAM is strikingly similar to that of dimethylnitrosamine (DMNA).[100] MAM and methylhydroxymethylnitrosamine are isomeric, and thus it has been speculated that both compounds may produce the same transient intermediate. Two intermediates, diazomethane[68] and methyldiazonium hydroxide,[65] have been suggested. Proton magnetic resonance studies on the decomposition of MAM in D_2O eliminated the possibility of formation of diazomethane.[155] Methyldiazonium hydroxide, as proposed by Druckrey,[65] is suggested as the transient methyl donor. Methyldiazonium hydroxide can arise either directly from MAM or indirectly from a cyclic intermediate through the azene and the diazo-hydroxide.[155] The spontaneous decomposition of methyl-hydroxymethylnitrosamine probably follows a parallel course and could explain the similarities of the biochemical action of MAM and DMNA.

More recently, there have been attempts to relate the mechanism of action with the organ specificity of MAM in the induction of tumors. Schoental[39] first suggested that

MAM might be activated through oxidation to methylazoxyformaldehyde by alcohol dehydrogenase (ADH). Grab and Zedeck[156] have demonstrated that MAM can serve as a substrate for ADH. They found that NAD^+ dependent ADH activity was present in those tissues, such as liver and colon, which are sensitive to acute and carcinogenic effects of MAM. There was no NAD^+ dependent ADH activity in the kidney but with $NADP^+$ ADH was more active with MAM than with ethanol. Pyrazole, an ADH inhibitor, blocked the oxidation of MAM, and when given to rats 2 hr prior to the administration of MAM reduced its lethality. Thus, the authors suggest that ADH activity in the metabolism of MAM may provide the mechanism for the organ specificity of MAM tumor induction.[156]

Injected MAM induces tumors in the colon and the route it takes to get to the colon lumen to react with colon tissue has been investigated. It was suggested that MAM is conjugated with glucuronic acid in the liver and secreted with bile.[157] The conjugate, MAM-glucosiduronic acid (MAM-GlcUA), is carried down to the colon with the bile where bacterial β-glucuronidase hydrolyzes the compound and releases free MAM, which induces neoplastic growth. This hypothesis was tested with MAM-GlcUA which was synthesized by oxidation of the primary alcohol of the glucose moiety of cycasin to a carboxylic acid.[158] The bile collected from male Wistar rats with cannulated bile ducts and injected with varying quantities of MAM-GlcUA (20 to 160 mg/kg body weight) was analyzed for the compound. The compound was not found in the bile. All the compound was found excreted in the urine at all levels administered. There was no indication that MAM-GlcUA was formed when MAM was injected into cannulated rats.[159] Zedeck et al.[160] concluded that a relationship exists between the segments of intestine acutely affected by MAM-acetate, as indicated by inhibition of DNA synthesis, and the sites of eventual tumor formation. They found that injected MAM-acetate inhibits DNA synthesis in the duodenum and colon of rats with cannulated bile ducts, which suggested to them that the carcinogen can exert its biological effects upon the epithelium via the circulation rather than via the intestinal lumen. Hirono and co-workers[161] subjected rats to single-barreled colostomies, which cut off fecal flow to the distal two thirds of the colon. Rats were given ten consecutive once a week i.v. injections of MAM-acetate. These animals developed a high incidence of tumors in the anal two thirds section of the colon where the mucosa did not have contact with the fecal stream and no passage of bile had occurred. The oral stump of the section distal to the colostomy also had a high incidence of tumors, which they explained might be due to increased vascularization and increased contact with the carcinogen. The three experiments[159-161] described above can be interpreted that the carcinogen MAM, when injected, reaches the colon mucosa via the circulatory system.

MAM-GlcUA and cycasin have a common aglycone, MAM, and thus it would be expected that MAM-GlcUA, when administered orally, would induce tumors at the same sites as those induced by cycasin. However, the largest number of neoplasms induced by a single oral administration of MAM-GlcUA was located in the intestinal tract and predominantly in the colon. The intestinal tumors in the small and large intestines were sessile or polypoid adenomas or carcinomas. Neoplasms of the liver were only few in number and consisted either of liver cell nodules or of single or multiple cystadenomas of bile duct origin. There was no evidence of malignancy. Renal tumors were few in number. There is β-glucuronidase activity in both the small and large intestine, but MAM-GlcUA was not carcinogenic to germ-free rats.[162] Bacterial enzyme must hydrolyze MAM-GlcUA orally administered to rats, as in the case with cycasin. It could be concluded that the conversion of the primary alcohol group of cycasin to a carboxylic acid group changed the compound from a predominantly kidney tumor inducer to an intestinal tumor inducer.

XIV. RADIOMIMETIC AND MUTAGENIC EFFECTS

Cycasin induced chromosomal aberrations in root-tip cells of *Allium cepa* comparable to those found after exposure to 200 R of gamma irradiation.[163] The chromosomal changes included dot deletions, rod deletions, and chromosome bridges. The observations on *A. cepa* were extended to include a representative member of the cycad family, *Zamia integrifolia*. Cycasin and emulsin (β-glucosidase) are not radiomimetically active in the intact *Zamia*. However, cycasin and emulsin as well as MAM produced significant damage in intact root cells.

Root tips of both plants *Allium* and *Zamia* were treated with cycasin, emulsin, a mixture of cycasin and emulsin, and X-rays. The incidence of anaphase bridges was used for comparison. Cycasin and emulsin given separately to *Zamia* roots produced chromosomal damage which was more severe than when cycasin and emulsin had been incubated first to produce MAM. *Allium* roots, when placed in a cycasin solution for several hours, produced a low level of β-glucosidase activity, and chromosome damage was greater in *Allium* than in *Zamia* under these conditions.[164] It was suggested that some protective mechanism, either compartmentalization or chemical inhibition, was operative in the intact cycad plant under normal conditions.

In this context, the observations that larvae of the arctiid moth, *Seiractia echo,* fed on cycad plants without ill effects are of interest. They suggested a different system in which protection through detoxification could be demonstrated. Extracts of larvae feeding on cycad leaves, when analyzed, had relatively large amounts of cycasin. The cycasin was carried over into the pupa, adult, and egg.[165] It was also observed that all stages of *Seiractia* except the egg contained an emulsin-like enzyme, although free MAM was not detected in undamaged insects or in the plant tissues. Teas, in a subsequent study, reported that larvae of *S. echo* fed MAM in an artificial diet for 24 hr had the largest amount of cycasin in the hemolymph followed by the Malpighian tubules. Only relatively small amounts were detected in other tissues, including the gut. However, enzymatic activity measured as β-glucosidase was greatest in the gut and absent from the other sites. Apparently, the MAM fed to the larvae had been glycosylated to cycasin and retained in part in the hemolymph, and excreted in part by the Malpighian tubules, thus protecting the larvae from the potentially hazardous effects of MAM.[166]

Tests for mutagenicity have shown that cycasin was not mutagenic, but MAM was found to be a good mutagen.[167] The effect was first demonstrated by measuring the frequency of reversion to histidine independence of several histidine requiring mutants of *Salmonella typhimurium*. These observations were confirmed and extended to include the synthetic conjugates of MAM.[168] The acetate ester of MAM was slightly mutagenic but preincubation with bacterial cells markedly increased the number of revertants. Pretreatment with β-glucuronidase was required in the case of the glucuronide of MAM before mutagenicity was demonstrable. Gabridge, Denunzio, and Legator,[169] using the host-mediated assay, injected intraperitoneally histidine auxotrophs of *S. typhimurium* 2 hr after MAM and cycasin were orally given. Two hours were allowed for the hydrolysis of cycasin to proceed to its maximum. Mutation frequency was increased over control many fold more with MAM than with cycasin. Cycasin administered parenterally did not increase the mutation frequency above the spontaneous level. It has recently been reported that the mutagenicity of MAM-acetate could be inhibited with lithocholic acid when it is included in the preincubation mix. Similarly, mutagenicity was not observed when pyrazole, which inhibits alcohol dehydrogenase, was added to the preincubation mix.[170] Alcohol dehydrogenase is thought to convert MAM to its reactive derivative.

Mutagenesis was also tested in *Drosophila melanogaster* by Teas and Dyson.[171] The feeding test used MAM and MAM-acetate to induce sex-linked recessive lethals in males. Cycasin was not mutagenic but MAM and MAM-acetate were significantly mutagenic. Homogenates of *Drosophila* and the yeast strain used in the medium showed substantial esterase activity to explain the mutagenic activity of the MAM-acetate. No β-glucosidase activity was observed in the medium and mutagenicity of cycasin was not demonstrable. Cycasin was found to be mutagenic in those plants which contain emulsin capable of hydrolyzing glycosides to their respective aglycones. A high mutation frequency was found when the common bean (*Phaseolus vulgaris, L.*), which possesses β-glucosidase activity, was treated with cycasin.[172]

XV. RESUME

The uncovering of oncogenic properties of cycad starch, used in the past by scattered groups of people living in the tropics and subtropics to prepare food, was incidental to a search for a neurotoxin to explain the high incidence of amyotrophic lateral sclerosis among the natives of Guam, who used cycad starch. Atlhough the posionous nature of crude cycad starch was known and similar methods were developed for the removal of the toxic substance, whether on Guam, in Kenya, or on Kyushu, Japan, and its neighboring islands, its tumor-producing capabilities had not been recognized. The likely explanation for this apparent incongruity might be the severeness of the acute toxicity which caused death within a few days following consumption of improperly detoxified starch. A few reports describing lethal effects have been published, but many more may have possibly occurred without a causal connection being suspected between death and eating of cycad starch.

The studies concerned with the elucidation of the nature of the cycad toxins have shown that they are glycosides with a common aglycone, methylazoxymethanol, but with different sugar components. Cycasin, the most extensively studied compound, has glucose attached to the aglycone in a β-linkage. The successful synthesis of the aglycone as the acetate ester has not only made the carcinogen available for general experimental use, but has also independently led to the discovery of carcinogens, such as 1,2-dimethylhydrazine and azoxymethane, which are intermediate compounds in the synthesis of the aglycone of cycasin.

Investigations into the fate of cycasin in the animal body have shown that it was innocuous when administered parenterally and carcinogenic when given enterically, and only a small fraction of unmetabolized cycasin was found in the urine. The aglycone was effective independent of the route of administration, and thus was the proximate carcinogen and toxin of cycasin.

The importance of the intestinal passage of cycasin for the development of toxic and carcinogenic properties to become apparent required further studies to clarify what specific role the intestines played in the changing of the glucoside to the aglycone. The upper small intestinal tract provided the necessary hydrolytic enzyme, a β-glucosidase, during the early postnatal period, and a comparable enzymatic activity resided in the subcutis of newborn and early postnatal conventional and germ-free rats. This activity disappeared after weaning. Cycasin given enterically to mature germ-free rats was excreted, indicating that the intestinal bacterial floral provided the hydrolytic enzyme and not the mucosa of the gut. Monocontamination of germ-free rats with proper bacterial strains restored to the intestinal tract the ability to hydrolyze cycasin.

These studies provided a model that a naturally occurring and locally used food can be altered in the intestinal tract through the activity of bacteria-derived enzyme to produce a toxin and carcinogen. The story of the cycad toxin reviewed here supports the notion that some cancers may be caused by environmental factors, including things man eats.

There has been a renewed interest in the relationship between cancer and diet and, as part of this general problem, in the intestinal bacterial flora of animals, particularly of man. The observation that cycasin is carcinogenic when hydrolyzed by bacterial enzyme has stimulated an interest in examining the microflora of people living in areas with grossly different incidences of colon cancer. The aim is to demonstrate that populations with high risks are characterized by bacteria which have the potential to convert to carcinogens certain constituents of food ingested by humans. These time-consuming investigations, it is hoped, will ultimately contribute to our still developing knowledge of the physiology and pathophysiology of the gastrointestinal tract and its bacterial flora as they relate to diet and cancer.

REFERENCES*

1. **Kurland, L. T. and Mulder, D. W.,** Epidemiologic investigations of amyotrophic lateral sclerosis. 1. Preliminary report on geographic distribution, with special reference to the Mariana Islands, including clinical and pathologic observations, *Neurology,* 4, 355, 1954.
2. **Hirano, A., Malamud, N., Elizan, T. S., and Kurland, L. T.,** Amyotrophic lateral sclerosis and Parkinsonism-dementia complex on Guam, *Arch. Neurology,* 15, 35, 1966.
3. **Kurland, L. T., Mulder, O. W., and Westlund, K. B.,** Multiple sclerosis and amyotrophic lateral sclerosis, *N. Eng. J. Med.,* 252, 649, 1955.
4. **Whiting, M. G.,** Toxicity of cycads, *Econ. Bot.,* 17, 270, 1963.
5. **Whiting, M. G.,** Food practices in ALS foci in Japan, the Marianas, and New Guinea, *Fed. Proc. Fed. Am. Soc. Exp. Med.,* 23, 1343, 1964.
6. **Hall, W. T. and McGavin, M. D.,** Clinical and neuropathological changes in cattle eating the leaves of *Macrozamia lucida* or *Bowenia serrulata* (family Zamiaceae), *Pathol. Vet.,* 5, 26, 1968.
7. **Mason, M. M. and Whiting, M. G.,** Caudal motor weakness and ataxia in cattle in the carribean area following ingestion of cycads, *Cornell Vet.,* 58, 541, 1968.
8. **Louw, W. R. A. and Oelofsen, W.,** Carcinogenic and neurotoxic components in the cycad *Encephalartos altensteinii* Lehm. (family Zamiaceae), *Toxicon,* 13, 447, 1975.
9. **Laqueur, G. L., Mickelsen, O., Whiting, M. G., and Kurland, L. T.,** Carcinogenic properties of nuts from *Cycas circinalis* L. indigenous to Guam, *J. Natl. Cancer Inst.,* 21, 919, 1963.
10. **Matsumoto, H. and Strong, F. M.,** The occurrence of methylazoxymethanol in *Cycas circinalis* L., *Arch. Biochem. Biophys.,* 101, 299, 1963.
11. **Kurland, L. T.,** Introductory remarks, *Fed. Proc. Fed. Am. Soc. Exp. Med.,* 23, 1337, 1964.
12. **Mickelsen, O.,** Introductory remarks, *Fed. Proc., Fed. Am. Soc. Exp. Med.,* 31, 1465, 1972.
13. **Laqueur, G. L. and Spatz, M.,** Toxicology of cycasin, *Cancer Res.,* 28, 2262, 1968.
14. **Yang, M. G. and Mickelsen, O.,** Cycads, in *Toxic Constituents of Plant Foodstuffs,* Liener, I. E., Ed., Academic Press, New York, 1969, 159.
15. **Spatz, M.,** Toxic and carcinogenic alkylating agents from cycads, *Ann. N. Y. Acad. Sci.,* 163, 848, 1969.
16. **Jones, M., Mickelsen, O. and Yang, M.,** Methylazoxymethanol neurotoxicity, in *Progress in Neuropathology, II,* Zimmerman, H. M., Ed., Grune & Stratton, New York, 1973, 91.
17. **Laqueur, G. L.,** Oncogenicity of cycads and its implications, in *Advances in Modern Toxicology,* Vol. 3, Kraybill, H. F. and Mehlman, M. A., Eds., Hemisphere Publishing Corp. Washington, D.C., 1977, 231.
18. **Matsumoto, H.,** Naturally occurring food toxicants: cycasin, in *CRC Handbook Series in Nutrition and Food,* Rechcigl, M., Ed., CRC Press, Boca Raton, Fla., in press.
19. **Mugera, G. M. and Nderito, P.,** Cycad as hepatic carcinogens in Kenya, in *Cancer in Africa,* Clifford, P., Linsell, C. A., and Timmor, G. L., Eds., Intl. Publ. Serv., New York, 1968.
20. **Hirono, I., Kachi, H., and Kato, T.,** A survey of acute toxicity of cycads and mortality rate from cancer in the Miyako islands, Okinawa, *Acta Pathol. (Jpn.),* 20, 327, 1970.

*   After submitting the review on the Cycad Toxin, the authors have become aware of two important references which are appended: (a) Haddad, R., Rabe, A., and Dumas, R., Neuroteratogenicity of methylazoxymethanol acetate: behavioral deficits of ferrets with transplacentally induced lissencephaly, *Neurotoxicology,* 1, 171, 1979; and (b) Haddad, R. and Rabe, A., Use of the ferret in experimental neuroteratology: cerebral, cerebellar, and retinal dysplasias induced by methylazoxymethanol acetate, *Adv. Study Birth Defects,* 4, 45, 1980.

21. **Yang, M. G., Mickelsen, O., Campbell, M. E., Laqueur, G. L. and Keresztesy, F. C.,** Cycad flour used by Guamanians: effects produced in rats by long-term feeding, *J. Nutr.,* 90, 153, 1966.
22. **Fosberg, F. R.,** Resume of the cycadaceae, *Fed. Proc. Fed. Am. Soc. Exp. Med.,* 23, 1340, 1964.
23. **Birdsey, M. R.,** A brief description of the cycads, *Fed. Proc. Fed. Am. Soc. Exp. Med.,* 31, 1467, 1972.
24. **Hertrich, W.,** *Palms and Cycads, Huntington Botanical Gardens,* The Henry F. Huntington Library and Gallery, C. F. Brown & Co., Alhambra, Calif., 1951.
25. **Sporne, K. R.,** *The Morphology of Gymnospermus,* Hutchinson & Co., London, 1965.
26. **Tryon, R. M.,** Ancient seeds plants: the cycads, *Bull. Mo. Bot. Garden,* 1955, 43.
27. **Smiley, N.,** Around the world in search of cycads, *Bull. Fairchild Trop. Garden,* Miami, Fla., April 1965.
28. **Dastur, D. K. and Palekar, R. S.,** Effect of boiling and storing on cycasin content of *Cycas circinalis* L., *Nature (London),* 210, 841, 1966.
29. **Palekar, R. S. and Dastur, D. K.,** Cycasin content of *Cycas circinalis, Nature (London),* 206, 1363, 1965.
30. **Ganote, C. E. and Rosenthal, A. S.,** Characteristic lesions of methylazoxymethanol-induced liver damage, *Lab. Invest.,* 19, 382, 1968.
31. **Zedeck, M. S., Sternberg, S. S., Pynter, R. W., and Gowan, F.,** Biochemical and pathological effects of methylazoxymethanol acetate, a potent carcinogen, *Cancer Res.,* 30, 801, 1970.
32. **Lancaster, M. C., Jenkins, F. P., and Phillip, F. M.,** Toxicity associated with certain samples of groundnuts, *Nature (London),* 192, 1095, 1961.
33. **Forgacs, J. and Carll, W. T.,** Toxic fungi from the seeds of *Cycas circinalis* L., *Fed. Proc. Fed. Am. Soc. Exp. Med.,* 23, 1370, 1964.
34. **Nishida, K., Kobayashi, A., and Nagaham, T.,** Cycasin a new toxic glycoside of *Cycas revoluta* Thumb., I. Isolation and structure of cycasin, *Bull. Agric. Chem. Soc. Jpn.,* 19, 77, 1955.
35. **Riggs, N. W.,** Glycosyloxyazoxymethane, a constituent of the seeds of *Cycas circinalis* L., *Chem. Ind. (London),* 926, 1956.
36. **Barnes, F. M. and Magee, P. N.,** Some toxic properties of dimethylnitrosamine, *Br. J. Ind. Med.,* 11, 167, 1954.
37. **Magee, P. N. and Barnes, J. M.,** The production of malignant primary hepatic tumours in the rat by feeding dimethylnitrosamine, *Br. J. Cancer,* 10, 114, 1956.
38. **Magee, P. M. and Barnes, J. M.,** The experimental production of tumours in the rat by dimethylnitrosamine (*N*-nitro dimethylamine), *Acta Unio. Int. Contra Cancrum,* 15, 187, 1959.
39. **Schoental, R.,** The mechanisms of action of the carcinogen nitroso and related compounds, *Br. J. Cancer,* 28, 436, 1973.
40. **Magee, P. M. and Barnes, F. M.,** Carcinogenic nitroso compounds, *Adv. Cancer Res.,* 10, 163, 1967.
41. **Miller, J. A.,** Carcinogenesis by chemicals: an overview — G. H. A. Clowes memorial lecture, *Cancer Res.,* 30, 559, 1970.
42. **Druckrey, H.,** Specific carcinogenic and teratogenic effects of "indirect" alkylating methyl and ethyl compounds, and their dependency on stages of ontogenic developments, *Xenobiotica,* 3, 271, 1973.
43. **Laqueur, G. L.,** Carcinogenic effects of cycad meal and cycasin, methylazoxymethanol glycoside, in rats and effects of cycasin in germfree rats, *Fed. Proc. Fed. Am. Soc. Exp. Med.,* 23, 1386, 1964.
44. **Magee, P. M. and Barnes, J. M.,** Induction of kidney tumours in the rat with dimethylnitrosamine (*N*-nitrosodimethylamine), *J. Pathol. Bacteriol.,* 84, 19, 1962.
45. **Laqueur, G. L. and Matsumoto, H.,** Neoplasms in female Fischer rats following intraperitoneal injection of methylazoxymethanol, *J. Natl. Cancer Inst.,* 37, 217, 1966.
46. **Hirono, I., Laqueur, G. L., and Spatz, M.,** Tumor induction in Fischer and Osborne-Mendel rats by a single administration of cycasin, *J. Natl. Cancer Inst.,* 40, 1003, 1968.
47. **Matsumoto, H., Nagata, Y., Nishimura, E. T., Bristol, R., and Haber, M.,** β-glucosidase modulation in preweanling rats and its association with tumor induction by cycasin, *J. Natl. Cancer Inst.,* 49, 423, 1972.
48. **Laqueur, G. L., McDaniel, E. G., and Matsumoto, H.,** Tumor induction in germfree rats with methylazoxymethanol (MAM) and synthetic MAM acetate, *J. Natl. Cancer Inst.,* 39, 355, 1967.
49. **Zedeck, M. S. and Sternberg, S. S.,** Tumor induction in intact and regenerating liver of adult rats by a single treatment with methylazoxymethanol acetate, *Chem.-Biol. Interactions,* 17, 291, 1977.
50. **Borenfreund, E., Higgin, P. J., Steinglass, J., and Bendick, A.,** Properties and malignant transformation of established rat liver parenchymal cells in culture, *J. Natl. Cancer Inst.,* 55, 375, 1975.
51. **Hard, G. C. and Butler, W. H.,** Cellular analysis of renal neoplasia. Light microscope study of the development of interstitial lesions induced in the rat kidney by a single, carcinogenic dose of dimethylnitrosamine, *Cancer Res.,* 30, 2806, 1970.
52. **Hard, G. C. and Butler, W. H.,** Ultrastructural study of the development of insterstitial lesions leading to mesenchymal neoplasia induced in the rat renal cortex by dimethylnitrosamine, *Cancer Res.,* 31, 337, 1971.
53. **Hard., G. C.,** Tumours of the kidney, renal pelvis and ureter, in *Pathology of Tumours in Laboratory Animals* Vol. 1, Tumours of the Rat, Part II, Turnsov, V. S., Ed., IARC Scientific Publication No. 6, Lyon, 1976.

54. **Reuber, M. D.,** Leiomyomas and leiomyosarcomas of the kidney in 4-day old BUF rats given methyl-azoxymethanol acetate intraperitoneally, *J. Natl. Cancer Inst.,* 56, 405, 1976.
55. **Gusek, W., Buss, H., and Kruger, C. H.,** Morphologische and histochemische Befunde an experimentellen Nierentumoren der ratte, *Verh. Dtsch. Ges. Path.,* 50, 337, 1966.
56. **Gusek, W., Buss, H., and Laqueur, G. L.,** Histologische-histochemische Untersuchungen am "Intersti-tiellen cycasin-tumor" der Ratteniere, *Beitr. Path. Anat.,* 135, 53, 1967.
57. **Gusek, W. and Mestwerdt, W.,** Cycasin-induzierte Nierentumoren bei der Wistarratte unter besonderer Beruchsichtigung der Adenome, *Beitr. Path. Anat.,* 139, 199, 1969.
58. **Gusek, W.,** Die Ultrastructur cycasin-induzierter Nierenadenome, *Virchows Arch. Path. Anat. Histol.,* 365, 221, 1975.
59. **Buss, H. and Gusek, W.,** Untersuehungen uber die interstitiellen Zellen der Nierenrinde, *Virchows Arch. Abt. B Zellenpath.,* 1, 251, 1968.
60. **Guerin, M., Chouroulinkov, I., and Riviere, M. R.,** Experimental kidney tumors, in *The Kidney. Mor-phology, Biochemistry, Physiology,* Vol. 2, Rouiller, C. and Muller, A. F., Eds., Academic Press, New York, 1969.
61. **Laqueur, G. L.,** The induction of intestinal neoplasms in rats with the glycoside cycasin and its aglycone, *Virchows Arch. Path. Anat. Physiol.,* 340, 151, 1965.
62. **Narisawa, T. and Nakano, H.,** Carcinoma of the large intestine of rats induced by rectal infusion of methylazoxymethanol, *Gann,* 64, 93, 1973.
63. **Matsumoto, H., Nagaham, T., and Larson, H. O.,** Studies on methylazoxymethanol, the aglycone of cycasin: a synthesis of methylazoxymethyl acetate, *Biochem. J.,* 95, 13C, 1965.
64. **Druckrey, H., Preussman, R., Matzkies, F., and Ivankovic, S.,** Selective Erzeugung von Darmkrebs bei Ratten durch 1,2-Dimethyl-hydrazin, *Naturwissenschaften,* 54, 557, 1966.
65. **Druckrey, H.,** Production of colonic carcinomas by 1,2-dialkyl-hydrazines and azoxyalkanes, in Burdett, W. J., Ed., *Carcinoma of the Colon and Antecedent Epithelium,* Burdett, W. J., Ed., Charles C Thomas, Springfield, Ill., 1970, 267.
66. **Druckrey, H.,** Organospecific carcinogenesis in the digestive tract, in *Topics in Chemical Carcinogenesis,* Nakahara, W., Takayama, S., Sugimura, T., and Odashima, S., Eds., University Park Press, Baltimore, 1972, 73.
67. **Ziegler, D. M., Mitchell, C. H., and Jollow, D.,** Microsomes and Drug Oxidations, Gillette, J. R., Conney, A. H., Cosmides, G. J., Esterbrook, R. W., Fouts, J. R., and Mannering, G. J., Eds., Academic Press, New York, 1969, 173.
68. **Miller, J. A.,** Comments on chemistry of cycads, *Fed. Proc. Fed. Am. Soc. Exp. Med.,* 23, 1361, 1964.
69. **Fiala, E. S.,** Investigations into the metabolism and mode of action of the colon carcinogen 1,2-dime-thylhydrazine, *Cancer,* 36, 2407, 1975.
70. **Fiala, E. S.,** Investigations into the metabolism and mode of action of the colon carcinogens 1,2-dime-thylhydrazine and azoxymethane, *Cancer,* 40, 2436, 1977.
71. **Fiala, E. S., Kulakis, C., Bobotas, G., and Weisburger, J. H.,** Detection and estimation of azomethane in expired air of 1,2-dimethylhydrazine-treated rats, *J. Natl. Cancer Inst.,* 56, 1271, 1976.
72. **Fiala, E. S., Bobotas, G., Kulakis, C., and Weisburger, J. H.,** Separation of 1,2-dimethylhydrazine me-tabolites by high-pressure liquid chromatography, *J. Chromatogr.,* 117, 181, 1976.
73. **Wiebecke, B., Krey, U., Loehrs, U., and Eder, M.,** Morphological and autoradiographical investigations on experimental carcinogenesis and polyp development in the intestinal tract of rats and mice, *Virchows Arch. Abt. A Path. Anat.,* 360, 179, 1973.
74. **Ward, J. M.,** Morphogenesis of chemically induced neoplasms of the colon and small intestine in rats, *Lab. Invest.,* 30, 505, 1974.
75. **Ward, J. M., Yamamoto, R. S., and Brown, C. A.,** Pathology of intestinal neoplasms and other lesions in rats exposed to azoxymethane, *J. Natl. Cancer Inst.,* 51, 1029, 1973.
76. **Pozharisski, K. M.,** Morphology and morphogenesis of experimental epithelial tumors of the intestine, *J. Natl. Cancer Inst.,* 54, 1115, 1975.
77. **Nigro, N. O., Bhadrachari, N., and Chochai, C.,** A rat model for studying colonic cancer: effect of cholestyramine on induced tumors, *Dis. Colon Rectum,* 16, 438, 1973.
78. **Spatz, M. and Laqueur, G. L.,** Transplacental induction of tumors in Sprague-Dawley rats with crude cycad material, *J. Natl. Cancer Inst.,* 38, 233, 1967.
79. **Laqueur, G. L. and Spatz, M.,** Transplacental induction of tumours and malformations in rats with cycasin and methylazoxymethanol, in *Transplacental Carcinogenesis,* Tonatis, L. and Mohr, U., Eds., IARC Scientific Publication No. 4, Lyon, 1973, 59.
80. **Laqueur, G. L.,** Multiple primary tumors induced with the glucoside cycasin and its aglycone, in *Multiple Primary Malignant Tumours,* Severi, L., Ed., 5th Perugia University, Perugia, Italy, 1975, 99.
81. **Hoch-Ligeti, C., Stutzman, E., and Arvin, J. M.,** Cellular composition during tumor induction in rats by cycad husk, *J. Natl. Cancer Inst.,* 41, 605, 1968.

82. **Yang, M. G., Sanger, V. L., Michelsen, O., and Laqueur, G. L.,** Carcinogenicity of long-term feeding of cycad husk to rats, *Proc. Soc. Exp. Biol. Med.,* 127, 1171, 1968.

83. **Yang, M. G. and Mickelsen, O.,** Cycad husk from Guam: its toxicity to rats, *Econ. Bot.,* 22, 149, 1968.

84. **Mugera, G. M. and Nderito, P.,** Tumours of the liver, kidney and lungs in rats fed *Encephalartos Hildebrandtii, Br. J. Cancer,* 22, 563, 1968.

85. **Dossaji, S. F. and Herbin, G. A.,** Occurrence of macrozamin in the seeds of *Encephalartos Hildebrandtii, Fed. Proc. Fed. Am. Soc. Exp. Med.,* 31, 1470, 1972.

86. **Laqueur, G. L.,** unpublished data, 1964.

87. **O'Gara, R. W., Brown, J. M., and Whiting, M. G.,** Induction of hepatic and renal tumors by topical application of aqueous extract of cycad nut to artificial skin ulcers in mice, *Fed. Proc. Fed. Am. Soc. Exp. Med.,* 23, 1383, 1964.

88. **Hirono, I., Shibuya, C., and Fushimi, K.,** Tumor induction in C 57 BL/6 mice by a single administration of cycasin, *Cancer Res.,* 29, 1658, 1969.

89. **Shibuya, C. and Hirono, I.,** Relation between postnatal days of mice and carcinogenic effects of cycasin, *Gann,* 64, 109,1973.

90. **Hirono, I. and Shibuya, C.,** High incidence of pulmonary tumors in dd mice by a single injection of cycasin, *Gann,* 61, 403, 1970.

91. **Hirno, I., Hayashi, K., Mori, H., and Miwa, T.,** Carcinogenic effects of cycasin in Syrian golden hamsters and the transplantability of induced tumors, *Cancer Res.,* 31, 283, 1971.

92. **Hirono, I.,** Carcinogenicity and neurotoxicity of cycasin with special reference to species differences, *Fed. Proc. Fed. Am. Soc. Exp. Med.,* 31, 1493, 1972.

93. **Spatz, M.,** Carcinogenicity of methylazoxymethanol (MAM) in guinea pigs and hamsters, *Abstr. 10th Int. Cancer Congr.,* Medical Arts Publ., Houston, 1970, 24.

94. **Spatz, M.,** Carcinogenic effect of cycad meal in guinea pigs, *Fed. Proc. Fed. Am. Soc. Exp. Med.,* 23, 1384, 1964.

95. **Laqueur, G. L. and Spatz, M.,** Oncogenicity of cycasin and methylazoxymethanol, in *Recent Topics in Chemical Carcinogenesis,* Odashima, S., Sato, H., and Takayama, S., Eds., Gann Monograph on University of Tokyo Press, Tokyo, 1975, 189.

96. **Stanton, M. E.,** Hepatic neoplasms of aquarium fish to *Cycas circinalis, Fed. Proc. Fed. Am. Soc. Exp. Med.,* 25, 661, 1966.

97. **Warkany, J.,** *Congenital Malformations,* Year Book Medical Publ., Chicago, 1971, chap. 11.

98. **Mickelsen, O., Campbell, E., Yang, M. G., Mugera, G., and Whitehair, C. K.,** Studies with cycad, *Fed. Proc. Fed. Am. Soc. Exp. Med.,* 23, 1363, 1964.

99. **Spatz, M. and Laqueur, G. L.,** Evidence of transplacental passage of the natural carcinogen cycasin and its aglycone, *Proc. Soc. Exp. Biol. Med.,* 127, 281, 1968.

100. **Shank, R. C. and Magee, P. N.,** Similarities between biochemical actions of cycasin and dimethylnitrosamine, *Biochem. J.,* 105, 521, 1967.

101. **Nagata, Y. and Matsumoto, H.,** Studies on methylazoxymethanol: methylation of nucleic acids in the fetal rat brain, *Proc. Soc. Exp. Biol. Med.,* 132, 383, 1969.

102. **Matsumoto, H. and Higa, H. H.,** Studies on methylazoxymethanol, the aglycone of cycasin: methylation of nucleic acids in vitro, *Biochem. J.,* 98, 20C, 1966.

103. **Ferm, V. H.,** The rapid detection of teratogenic activity, *Lab. Invest.,* 14, 1500, 1965.

104. **Spatz, M., Daugherty, W. J., and Smith, D. W. E.,** Teratogenic effects of methylazoxymethanol, *Proc. Soc. Exp. Biol. Med.,* 124, 476, 1967.

105. **Hirono, I. and Shibuya, C.,** Induction of a neurological disorder by cycasin in mice, *Nature (London),* 216, 1311, 1967.

106. **Hirono, I., Shibuya, C., and Hayashi, K.,** Induction of a cerebellar disorder with cycasin in newborn mice and hamsters, *Proc. Soc. Exp. Biol. Med.,* 131, 593, 1969.

107. **Shimada, M. and Langman, J.,** Repair of the external granular layer of the hamster cerebellum after prenatal and postnatal administration of methylazoxymethanol, *Teratology,* 3, 119, 1970.

108. **Laqueur, G. L.,** unpublished observation, 1969.

109. **Jones, M., Yang, M., and Mickelsen, O.,** Effects of methylazoxymethanol glucoside and methylazoxymethanol acetate on the cerebellum of the postnatal Swiss albino mouse, *Fed. Proc. Fed. Am. Soc. Exp. Med.,* 31, 1508, 1972.

110. **Sanger, V. L., Yang, M., and Mickelsen, O.,** Cycasin-induced central nervous system lesion in postnatal mice, *Fed. Proc. Fed. Am. Soc. Exp. Med.,* 31, 1524, 1972.

111. **Haddad, R. K., Rabe, A., and Dumas, R.,** Comparison of effects of methylazoxymethanol acetate on brain development in different species, *Fed. Proc. Fed. Am. Soc. Exp. Med.,* 31, 1520, 1972.

112. **Hirano, A. and Jones, M.,** Fine structure of cycasin-induced cerebellar alterations, *Fed. Proc. Fed. Am. Soc. Exp. Med.,* 31, 1517, 1972.

113. **Hirano, A., Dembitzer, H. M., and Jones, M.,** An electron microscopic study of cycasin-induced cerebellar alterations, *J. Neuropathol. Exp. Neurology,* 31, 113, 1972.

114. **Haddad, R. K., Rabe, A., Shek, J., Donahue, S., and Dumas, R.,** Primary and secondary alterations in cerebellar morphology in carnivore (ferret) and rodent (rat) after exposure to methylazoxymethanol acetate, in *Neurotoxicology,* Roizin, L., Shiraki, H., and Grcevic, N., Eds., Raven Press, New York, 1977, 603.
115. **Sung, S. C.,** DNA synthesis in the developing rat brain, *Can. J. Biochem.,* 47, 47, 1969.
116. **Chanda, R., Woodward, D. J., and Griffin, S.,** Cerebellar development in the rat after early postnatal damage by methylazoxymethanol: DNA, RNA and protein during recovery, *J. Neurochem.,* 21, 547, 1973.
117. **Spatz, M. and Laqueur, G. L.,** Transplacental chemical induction of microencephaly in two strains of rats. I., *Proc. Soc. Exp. Biol. Med.,* 129, 705, 1960.
118. **Fischer, M. H., Welber, C., and Waisman, H. A.,** Generalized growth retardation in rats induced by prenatal exposure to methylazoxymethyl acetate, *Teratology,* 5, 223, 1972.
119. **Johnston, M. V., Grzanna, R., and Coyle, J. T.,** Methylazoxymethanol treatment of fetal rats results in abnormally dense noradrenergic inervation of neocortex, *Science,* 203, 369, 1979.
120. **Matsumoto, H., Spatz, M., and Laqueur, G L.,** Quantitative changes with age in the DNA content of methylazoxymethanol-induced microencephalic rat brain, *J. Neurochem.,* 19, 297, 1972.
121. **Szumanska, G. and Spatz, M.,** Histochemical investigation of experimental microencephaly induced by methylazoxymethanol acetate (MAMA), *Neuropathol. Pol.,* 15, 17, 1977.
122. **Singh, S. C.,** Ectopic neuronoes in the hippocampus of the postnatal rat exposed to methylazoxymethanol during foetal development, *Acta Neuropathol. (Berlin),* 40, 111, 1977.
123. **Haddad, R. K., Rabe, A., Laqueur, G. L., Spatz, M., and Valsamis, M. P.,** Intellecural deficit associated with transplacentally induced microencephaly in the rat, *Science,* 162, 88, 1969.
124. **Rabe, A. and Haddad, R. K.,** Methylazoxymethanol-induced microencephaly in rats: behavioral studies, *Fed. Proc. Fed. Am. Soc. Exp. Med.,* 31, 1536, 1972.
125. **Haddad, R. K., Rabe, A., and Dumas, R.,** CNS birth defects in animal models, *Comp. Pathol. Bull.,* 7, 2, 1975.
126. **Goerttler, K., Arnold, H. P., and Michalk, D. V.,** Uber carcinogeninduzierte diaplacentare Wirkungen bei Ratten, *Z. Krebsforsch.,* 74, 396, 1970.
127. **Braekevelt, C. R. and Hollenberg, M. J.,** The development of the retina of the albino rat, *Am. J. Anat.,* 127, 281, 1970.
128. **Vega, A. and Bell, E. A.,** γ-amino-δ-methylaminopropionic acid, a new amino acid from seeds of *Cycas circinalis, Phytochemistry,* 6, 759, 1967.
129. **Polsky, F. T., Nunn, P. B., and Bell, E. A.,** Distribution and toxicity of γ-amino-δ-methylaminopropionic acid, *Fed. Proc. Fed. Am. Soc. Exp. Biol.,* 31, 1473, 1972.
130. **Dossaji, S. F. and Bell, E. A.,** Distribution of γ-amino-δ-methylaminopropionic acid in *Cycas, Phytochemistry,* 12, 143, 1973.
131. **Cooper, J. M.,** Isolation of a toxic principle from the seeds of *Macrozamia spiralis, J. Proc. R. Soc. N. S. Wales,* 74, 450, 1941.
132. **Lythgoe, B. and Riggs, N. V.,** Marcozamin, part I. The identity of the carbohydrate component, *J. Chem. Soc. (London),* 2716, 1949.
133. **Langley, B. W., Lythgoe, B., and Riggs, N. V.,** Macrozamin, part II. The aliphatic azoxy structure of the aglycone part, *J. Chem. Soc. (London),* 2309, 1951.
134. **Korsch, B. H. and Riggs, N. V.,** Proton magnetic resonance spectra of aliphatic azoxy compounds and the structure of cycasin, *Tetrahedron Lett.,* 10, 523, 1964.
135. **Nishida, K., Kobayashi, A., Nagahama, T., and Numata, T.,** Studies on some new azoxy glycosides of *Cycas revoluta* Thunb. Part I. On neocycasin A., δ-laminaribosyloxyazoxymethane, *Bull. Agric. Soc. Jpn.,* 23, 460, 1959.
136. **Nagahama, T.,** Studies on neocycasins, new glycosides of cycads, *Bull. Fac. Agric. Kagoshima Univ.,* 14, 1, 1964.
137. **Nishida, K., Kobayashi, A., Nagahama, T., Kojima, K., and Yamane, M.,** Studies on cycasin. A new toxic glycoside of *Cycas revoluta* Thunb., part IV. Pharmacological study of cycasin, *Seikagaku,* 28, 218, 1956.
138. **Kobayashi, A. and Matsumoto, H.,** Studies on methylazoxymethanol, the aglycone of cycasin: isolation, biological and chemical properties, *Arch. Biochem. Biophys.,* 110, 373, 1965.
139. **Spatz, M., McDaniel, E. G., and Laqueur, G. L.,** Cycasin excretion in conventional and germfree rats, *Proc. Soc. Exp. Biol. Med.,* 121, 417, 1966.
140. **Spatz, M., Smith, D. W. E., McDaniel, E. G., and Laqueur, G. L.,** Role of intestinal microorganisms in determining cycasin toxicity, *Proc. Soc. Exp. Biol. Med.,* 124, 691, 1967.
141. **Spatz, M.,** Hydrolysis of cycasin by δ-glucosidase in skin of newborn rats, *Proc. Soc. Exp. Biol. Med.,* 128, 1005, 1968.
142. **Kobayashi, A.,** Biochemical studies on cycasin, part II. Existence of free aglycone of cycasin in its enzymatic hydrolysis, *Agric. Biol. Chem. Jpn.,* 26, 208, 1962.

143. **Horisberger, M. and Matsumoto, H.,** Studies on methylazoxymethanol, synthesis of ^{14}C and ^{3}H labelled methylazoxymethanol acetate, *J. Labelled Compd.,* 4, 164, 1968.
144. **Poynter, R. W., Ball, C. R., Goodban, J., and Thackrah, T.,** The influence of physostigmine on the activation of methylazoxymethanol acetate, a potent carcinogen, by a serum factor in vitro, *Chem.-Biol. Interactions,* 4, 139, 1972.
145. **Wells, W. W., Yang, M. G., Bolzer, W., and Mickelsen, O.,** Gas-liquid chromatographic analysis of cycasin in cycad flour, *Anal. Biochem.,* 25, 325, 1968.
146. **Hasegawa, Y. and Matsumoto, H.,** unpublished data.
147. **Williams, J. N.,** Effect of cycad and cycasin feeding on liver RNA, DNA, succinic oxidase, and lipids in the rat, *Fed. Proc. Fed. Am. Soc. Exp. Med.,* 23, 1374, 1964.
148. **Williams, J. N. and Laqueur, G. L.,** Response of liver nucleic acids and lipids in rats fed *Cycas circinalis,* L. endosperm of cycasin, *Proc. Soc. Exp. Biol. Med.,* 118, 1, 1965.
149. **Zedeck, M. S., Sternberg, S. S., McGowan, J., and Poynter, R. W.,** Methylazoxymethanol acetate: induction of tumors and early effects on RNA synthesis, *Fed. Proc. Fed. Am. Soc. Exp. Med.,* 31, 1485, 1972.
150. **Grab, D. J., Zedeck, M. S., Swislocki, N. I., and Sonneberg, M.,** In vitro synthesis of RNA with "aggregate" enzyme, chromatin, and DNA from liver of methylazoxymethanol acetate-treated rats, *Chem.-Biol. Interactions,* 6, 259, 1973.
151. **Damjonov, I., Cox, R., Sarma, D. S. R., and Farber, E.,** Patterns of damage and repair of liver DNA induced by carcinogenic methylating agents in vivo, *Cancer Res.,* 33, 2122, 1973.
152. **Zedeck, M. S. and Brown, G. B.,** Methylation of intestinal and hepatic DNA in rats treated with methylazoxymethanol acetate, *Cancer,* 40, 2580, 1977.
153. **Healy, P. J.,** Studies on poisoning by *Macrozamia communis* — I. Biochemical disturbances in the liver, *Biochem. Pharmacol.,* 18, 85, 1969.
154. **Lundeen, P. B., Banks, G. S., and Ruddon, R. W.,** Effects of the carcinogen methylazoxymethanol acetate on protein synthesis and drug metabolism, *Biochem. Pharmacol.,* 20, 2522, 1971.
155. **Nagasawa, H. T., Shirota, F. M., and Matsumoto, H.,** Decomposition of methylazoxymethanol, the aglycone of cycasin, in D$_2$O, *Nature, (London),* 236, 324, 1972.
156. **Grab, D. and Zedeck, M. S.,** Organ-specific effects of the carcinogen methylazoxymethanol related to metabolism nicotinamide adenine dinucleotide-dependent dehydrogenases, *Cancer Res.,* 37, 4182, 1977.
157. **Weisburger, J. H.,** Colon carcinogens: their metabolism and mode of action, *Cancer,* 28, 60, 1971.
158. **Matsumoto, H., Takata, R. H., and Komeiji, D. Y.,** Synthesis of the glucuronic acid conjugate of methylazoxymethanol, *Cancer Res.,* 39, 3070, 1979.
159. **Matsumoto, H. and Takata, R. H.,** Metabolic fate of methylazoxymethanolglucosiduronic acid injected into rats, unpublished data.
160. **Zedeck, M. S., Grab, J. J., and Sternberg, S. S.,** Differences in the acute response of the various segments of rat intestine to treatment with the intestinal carcinogen, methylazoxymethanol acetate, *Cancer Res.,* 37, 32, 1977.
161. **Matsubara, N., Mori, H., and Hirono, I.,** Effect of colostomy on intestinal carcinogenesis by methylazoxymethanol acetate in rats, *J. Natl. Cancer Inst.,* 61, 1161, 1978.
162. **Laqueur, G. L., Matsumoto, H., and Yamamoto, R. S.,** Carcinogenicity of MAM-glucuronide, unpublished data.
163. **Teas, J. J., Sax, H. J., and Sax, K.,** Cycasin: radiomimetic effect, *Science,* 149, 541, 1965.
164. **Porter, E. D. and Teas, H. J.,** Comparative radiomimetic effect of emulsin, cycasin, methylazoxymethanol and X-ray in *Zamia integrifolia, Radiat. Bot.,* 11, 21, 1971.
165. **Teas, H. J., Dyson, J. G., and Whisenant, B. R.,** Cycasin metabolism in *Seirarctia echo* Abbot and Smith (Lepidoptera:arctiidae), *J. Ga. Entomol. Soc.,* 1, 21, 1966.
166. **Teas, H. J.,** Cycasin synthesis in *Seirarctia echo* (Lepidoptera) larvae fed methylazoxymethanol, *Biochem. Biophys. Res. Commun.,* 26, 686, 1967.
167. **Smith, D. W. E.,** Mutagenicity of cycasin aglycone (methylazoxymethanol), a naturally occurring carcinogen, *Science,* 152, 1273, 1966.
168. **Matsushima, T., Matsumoto, H., Shirai, A., Sawamura, M., and Sugimura, T.,** Mutagenicity of the naturally occurring carcinogen cycasin and synthetic methylazoxymethanol-conjugates on *Salmonella typhimurium, Cancer Res.,* 39, 3780, 1979.
169. **Gabridge, M. G. A., Denunzio, A., and Legator, M. S.,** *Cycasin:* detection of associated mutagenic activity in vivo, *Science,* 163, 689, 1969.
170. **Kanagalingam, K. and Andrews, A. W.,** Inhibition of the mutagenicity of methylazoxymethanol acetate (MAMOAc) by lithocholic acid (LA), *Am. Assoc. Cancer Res. Proc.,* Abst. 519, 1979.
171. **Teas, H. J. and Dyson, J. G.,** Mutation in *Drosophila* by methylazoxymethanol, the aglycone of cycasin, *Proc. Soc. Exp. Biol. Med.,* 125, 988. 1967.
172. **Moh, C. C.,** Mutagenic effect of cycasin in beans (*Phaseolus vulgaris* L.), *Mutation Res.,* 10, 251, 1970.

Chapter 6

DIET AND CANCER

Leo Kinlen

TABLE OF CONTENTS

I. INTRODUCTION

The wide acceptance that most cancers in man are caused by environmental factors has brought much attention to the role of tobacco smoke and modern industry in the etiology of cancer in Western countries, perhaps to the neglect of other factors. And yet cancer mortality (except for lung cancer) has changed little this century in Western countries, suggesting that some longstanding aspects of life are important in the etiology of many of the cancers that are more common in the West than in certain other parts of the world. One obvious candidate is diet. It is rather surprising therefore that widespread interest in the role of human diet in cancer etiology has developed only recently, particularly since ingestion is such an obvious route for carcinogens or their precursors to enter the body. There would seem to be no single explanation for the increasing interest. It has been known for some time that dietary manipulation can alter the yield of tumors in certain experimental animals. More recently, several workers have drawn attention to the striking correlations that exist in man between death rates from certain cancers and the per capita consumption of particular dietary items in different countries. The problems of interpreting such correlations are well–known but encouragement for the view that they indicate real effects of diet comes from migrant groups such as the Japanese in the U.S. who have shown changes in their cancer risks following their adoption of a more Western diet.

Unfortunately it is difficult to apply the usual epidemiological methods of inquiry to the question of diet and cancer. Thus the case-control approach, first used in this field by Stocks and Karn in 1933,[1] is complicated by the fact that it is difficult for people to summarize what they eat now, let alone many years previously which may be more relevant. Similarly, the prospective approach has limited application since it is difficult to identify groups of people within a country who have markedly different diets. Nevertheless in spite of these problems Bjelke has profitably applied both these methods and his findings suggest that vegetables may be protective against the development of certain cancers, perhaps due to their content of β-carotene, the precursor of vitamin A. Further stimulus to work on diet and cancer has come with the realization that diet affects the intestinal flora and might thereby influence the risk of large bowel cancer. In addition, Burkitt with his development of the fiber hypothesis has drawn attention to the possible adverse effects of a low fiber intake on the risk of a variety of diseases.

But research — as well as speculation — on the role of diet in the causation of cancer in man has undoubtedly been influenced by appreciation of the great variety of mechanisms by which diet may affect carcinogenisis in experimental animals. Such mechanisms that may be relevant to cancer in man, have recently been classified as follows:[2]

1. Ingestion of carcinogens or carcinogen precursors.
2. Dietary effects on the production, activation, or inactivation of carcinogens by the intestinal flora.
3. Dietary effects on the endogenous production, activation, or inactivation of carcinogens.
4. Dietary effects on tissues to alter their susceptibility to carcinogenesis.

Many examples could be proposed of dietary constituents that might influence human carcinogenesis simply because they do so in animals. Thus, substances such as nitrosamines have been detected in human food, as have others that can *oppose* the development of certain cancers. Examples of this last group include vitamins A and C, tannins, antioxidants and substances that induce microsomal enzyme activity. But clearly additional evidence is required before such constituents can be regarded as relevant to cancer in *man*. The following review of the evidence for dietary factors in the etiology of human cancer has been restricted to studies of cancer in man.

II. ESOPHAGUS CANCER

A. Alcohol

A dietary factor in the etiology of esophagus cancer has been suspected for 50 years or more since the Registrar General first analyzed causes of death in England in relation to the occupations stated on death certificates and showed that innkeepers, barmen, and waiters had an increased risk of this disease.[3] A link with alcohol is again apparent in the high correlation that exists between the per capita consumption of alcohol and esophageal cancer mortality rates in males (but not in females) in different countries.[4] And even though personally reported drinking habits are often inaccurate, the relationship is also evident when individuals are studied. Workers in the U.S.,[5] Puerto Rico,[6] Europe,[7] and China[8] have found that patients with esophagus cancer more often drink alcohol than do the controls — and also more of them drink it in large amounts.

The relationship is not simple, however, and several workers have confirmed the observation by Wynder and Bross[5] that there is a multiplicative interaction between alcohol and tobacco smoking such that alcohol has greater effects on the risk of esophagus cancer in heavy smokers than in nonsmokers. Another factor is the type of alcohol. France has the highest mortality rate in males in Europe largely due to the high rates prevailing in Normandy and Brittany where the sex ration for this disease is 25 to 1. Tuyns and his colleagues have investigated the question there for the International Agency for Research on Cancer (I.A.R.C.) and have focused attention on the relationship between esophagus cancer and the consumption of the homemade ciders and apple brandies for which these areas are noted. As in other areas, a multiplicative effect of drinking alcohol and smoking has been found, but attempts to implicate specific constituents of the popular local drinks have not been successful.[10] Nitrosamines have been detected, but only in the small amounts found in many other foods.[9]

In some of the high incidence areas for the disease in Africa, Cook[11] has adduced evidence for a relationship with the consumption of beer made from maize. This would explain much of its distribution within Africa, the male preponderance and the apparent recent increase in incidence.

Alcohol consumption in the first half of this century declined in Britain and so also did mortality from esophagus cancer. Recently however, following the marked increases in alcohol intake in recent decades, esophagus cancer has increased. The precise role of alcohol in relation to esophagus cancer is not clear but it may not be carcinogenic itself since in animals it can both increase the susceptibility of tissues to carcinogens and facilitate their cellular absorption.

B. Other Factors

Alcohol cannot explain why northern Iran should have for both males and females the highest incidence of esophageal cancer in the world; the people are observant Moslems. In this region a long-continued investigation by the I.A.R.C. and the Institute of Public Health Research of Teheran University has recently reported its findings.[12] Compared to adjoining lower incidence areas, the high incidence areas are characterized by a higher intake of sheep's milk, yogurt, "majoveh" (made with seeds, pepper, and raisins), a special kind of bread, and also by a lower intake of protein, vitamins A and C, and riboflavin. A high prevalence of opium use was also noted in the high incidence areas. However in more sensitive studies in which affected patients were compared to controls, it seemed that their lower intake of fruit and raw vegetables was important rather than most of the other area differences, though it was not possible to investigate opium use by individuals. However, the recent demonstration of mutagenic activity in residues from opium pipes in this region[13] suggests that the use of opium may be important perhaps in conjunction with nutritional deficiency for which there is well-established evidence in the high incidence areas.

Dietary factors in the etiology of esophageal cancer are also implied by the evidence that nutritional deficiencies are involved in the Plummer-Vinson syndrome. This disorder which is associated with an increased risk of cancers of the hypopharynx and the upper esophagus characteristically occurs in women with chronic iron deficiency. In addition, its former frequency in women in northern Sweden (where cancer of the hypopharynx is still relatively common) has been attributed to their low intake of meat, fruit, and fresh vegetables.[14] Bracken fern has been found to be carcinogenic in several animal species, and in Japan, where the young fronds are often eaten, patients with esophagus cancer reported eating bracken significantly more often than did control patients.[15]

III. MOUTH AND PHARYNX CANCER

Cancers of the oral cavity and pharynx appear to share some of the dietary risk factors for esophagus cancer and evidence from several studies indicates that alcohol has a multiplicative effect with tobacco.[6] Thus heavy drinkers who smoke a given amount of tobacco, experience a much higher incidence of these cancers than do nondrinkers who smoke a similar amount. In addition, studies of patients with oral cancer in India and Pakistan[16,17] have found lower blood levels of retinol and β-carotene than in controls, suggesting that dietary sources of these substances are protective.

IV. STOMACH CANCER

Stomach cancer has a strong claim for attention in this review since its marked international variation, its decline in many countries in which nutrition is considered to have improved this century, and the intimacy of contact between any carcinogens in food and the gastric mucosa encourage speculation about dietary factors in its etiology. Similarly the marked socioeconomic gradient shown by this cancer may reflect the better food that is available to those who are well off.

Correlations of stomach cancer mortality in different countries with a wide range of dietary variables have indicated a negative association with fat consumption and a positive association with fish consumption. However, the relationship with fish is entirely dependent upon the extreme values for Japan and Iceland, indicating that fish consumption makes only a small contribution to the international variation in stomach cancer mortality rates.[18]

Several studies have compared the diet reported by patients with stomach cancer to that of controls.[19-23] The principal findings in these studies have been summarized in Table 1, and although the findings are not consistent, the observation in several studies of a negative relationship with vegetable intake is striking. Bjelke[31,34] has commented on the low intake of vegetables by stomach cancer patients both in his Minnesota and Norwegian studies and he has pointed out supportive evidence collected by other workers. Several studies have also suggested associations between stomach cancer and a low intake of fruits, or with a high intake of salty foods. Haenszel and his colleagues[33] found in Japan that of the six foods that showed appreciable differences between cases and controls, five were vegetables or fruits and all of these had been eaten less often by patients with cancer. In a recent study in Israel, Modan and his colleagues[32] were impressed by the greater intake of starch-containing foods by stomach cancer patients

Table 1
CASE-CONTROL STUDIES OF DIETARY FACTORS IN STOMACH CANCER

Location	Numbers (Approx.)		Association		Ref.
	Patients	Controls	Positive	Negative	
Japan	2000	4000	Rice as staple	—	19
Liverpool, N. Wales	200	9000	Fried foods	—	20
Japan, U.S.A., Iceland, Yugoslavia	521	653	—	—	21
Netherlands	340	1060	Bacon	Citrus fruits	22
England	100	200	—	—	23
Kansas	93	279	Fried foods, animal fats	Fresh fruit, dairy produce	24
New York	276	2221	Potatoes, cabbage	Lettuce	25
Japan	454	454	Salted foods	Milk	26
Bombay	162	131	—	Strict Vegetarian diet with dairy produce	27
Japan	1524	3792	Highly salted pickles	Milk, meat, green and yellow vegetables	28
Hawaii	220	440	Pickles (dried)/Salted fish	Raw "western" vegetables	29
New York	228	228		Raw vegetables	30
Minnesota	83	1657	Cooked cereals, smoked fish, canned fruits	Lettuce, tomatoes, vegetables, vitamin C	31
Norway	228	1394	Salted fish	Vegetables, fruit, vitamin C	31
Israel	166	471	Starches	Squash, egg plant	32
Japan	783	1566	—	Lettuce, celery	33

but noted that the intake of eggplant and squash was less than in their three control groups. There have been few prospective studies in which groups of people included in dietary surveys have been followed to determine their mortality pattern. Bjelke used this method and although relatively few cases of stomach cancer have occurred so far his findings with regard to vegetables are consistent with those in the case control studies. It is tempting to speculate that the apparent protective effect of vegetables is due to their carotene content since this is a precursor of vitamin A, a substance which inhibits carcinogenesis in certain experimental situations, but it may be more prudent at this stage to keep in mind that vegetables also contain many other substances.

Hirayama has reported that in Japan milk drinkers have a low risk of stomach cancer[15] and this was also found in Hawaii by Haenszel for those born in Japan, though not for their offspring.[29] However, data from other parts of the world are somewhat conflicting and it is difficult to evaluate the significance of these observations.

Differences in the extent of adoption of a Western diet among the Japanese in Hawaii provide a valuable opportunity for epidemiological study. Haenszel and his colleagues[29] compared the diet in Hawaii of 220 Japanese patients with stomach cancer with that of 440 hospital controls. Those born in Japan who had adopted a Western diet did not show the lower risk found in their offspring suggesting that diet in early life is important in this disease. Associations were found between stomach cancer and the consumption of pickled vegetables and dried or salted fish. In keeping with this observation is the report that salted fish consumption is high in certain areas of Japan notable for their high incidence of stomach cancer. Bjelke also found that frequent use of salted fish in Norway was associated with an increased risk of stomach cancer.[31]

Nitrosamines are such potent carcinogens in several animal species that they have attracted much attention as possible causes of cancer in man, particularly since it is easy to envisage their formation from the amines and the nitrate (or nitrite) that are common dietary constituents. Mortality from stomach cancer has been related to nitrate levels in water but a definite relationship has not been firmly established. Thus an area of Colombia is noted both for its high incidence of stomach cancer and high nitrate levels in its well water but more detailed field studies have so far not confirmed the relationship.[35] In England mortality from stomach cancer was reported to be higher in a Nottinghamshire town with a high water-nitrate level than in certain other towns in the region,[36] but a later analysis showed that this difference in fact disappeared when account was taken of certain demographic features.[37]

Bracken fern is carcinogenic in certain animals but seems an unlikely human carcinogen. However in Japan where the young fronds are eaten, an association with stomach cancer has been suggested. In addition the fact that some constituents of the fern might reach man in produce from animals that graze on bracken and in water has prompted speculation that it may play some part in the high incidence of stomach cancer in North Wales where bracken abounds. However a recent study of cancer mortality in rural areas of Scotland in relation to data on bracken coverage failed to yield any support for this suggestion.[38]

The widespread decline of stomach cancer in many parts of the world encourages speculation about the possible effects of improved methods of food preservation and storage but firm evidence on this question is lacking.

V. COLORECTAL CANCER

Cancers of the colon and rectum are here considered together since they share many epidemiological features. Thus, countries with a high incidence of colon cancer usually have a high rate of rectum cancer, though the fact that the former usually predominates in women and the latter in men indicates that they are not similar in all respects. Evidence from several sources points to dietary factors in the etiology of these cancers. There is a strong correlation between the incidence of colon cancer in different countries and the corresponding average consumption of animal protein, fat, or meat.[18] Also, the incidence of colorectal cancer is much higher in blacks in the U.S. than in Africa, while mortality from colon cancer is higher in Japanese migrants to the U.S. than in Japan.[39,40] Moreover, even in Japan, the diet of colon cancer patients was found to be more often of western type than that of controls.[41] Similar changes towards the western pattern of colon cancer have been noted in migrants from Poland and Norway to the U.S.[42,43] and from Poland to Australia.[44]

With such claims for attention it is not surprising that work on dietary factors in colon cancer has followed several different lines. Bjelke[31] and others have investigated the question by case control and prospective studies while Burkitt[45] and others have stressed the contrast in dietary fiber intake between countries with a marked difference in colon cancer incidence. Other workers such as Hill have incorporated epidemiological elements into their laboratory work on bacterial and chemical constituents of feces.

The possible importance of fats in relation to this disease was apparently first indicated by Wynder and Shigematsu[46] who pointed out that in Japan, where the disease is relatively rare, a much smaller proportion of the caloric intake comes from fats than in the U.S. where large bowel cancer is common. They also suggested that long-chain fatty acids present in feces might be relevant carcinogens since related substances are carcinogenic in experimental animals. A role for fats also appeared to be implied when, in 1971, Hill and his colleagues[48] reported that people in countries with a low incidence of this cancer had a fecal concentration of neutral and acid steroids derived from cholesterol and bile salts than did people in high incidence countries such as Britain and the U.S. In addition, western peoples had fewer aerobic bacteria in their feces but more anaerobic bacteria particularly those which metabolize bile salts. These bacteria produce 7 alpha dehydrogenase which can convert cholic acid to desoxycholate, a carcinogen at least in animals. The same workers have also reported that, compared to controls, the feces of colon cancer patients contained more nuclear dehydrogenating clostridia and higher concentrations of bile acids.[49] Other workers have not found such bacteriological and chemical differences between bowel cancer patients and controls, or between groups with different risks of colon cancer within the same country.[50-55] Moreover, a study organized by the International Agency for Research on Cancer[56] found no difference in the concentration of fecal bile acids or in stool carriage rates of dehydrogenating clostridia between people living in Kuopio in rural Finland and those in Copenhagen where the incidence of colon cancer is four times higher than Kuopio. However, certain differences were noted including a greater consumption of meat, lower intakes of dietary fiber and milk, and lower stool weights in the high than in the low incidence area. Although there are many inconsistencies in the observations relating to the bacteriological and chemical constituents of feces in relation to colon cancer, it is still possible that certain dietary factors in the etiology of colon cancer are mediated by their effects on the intestinal microflora. Moreover, there is the striking observation that animals can be protected from the intestinal tumors produced by cycasin by rendering them bacteriologically sterile.

Also, the fat hypothesis has not generally been supported by studies of meat consumption which, in fact, shows an even closer international correlation with colon cancer than is shown by total fat intake. A link with meat was encouraged by the report that Californian Seventh Day Adventists, many of whom are vegetarians, had an unusually low incidence of colorectal cancer.[47] However in all other studies that have compared the diet of patients with colorectal cancer with that of controls only one suggested that a high meat intake markedly increased the risk of the tumor. Haenszel and his col-leagues[57] found among Japanese migrants to Hawaii, where an unusual degree of dietary heterogeneity exists, that bowel cancer patients ate meat and string beans more often than did the controls. These workers stressed the difference in beef consumption, but in fact the younger patients showed increases in risk in association with all major meat items. But the initial interpretation of the low risk reported in the largely vegetarian Adventists, has been affected by the finding that Mormons in Utah, who eat *more* beef than the United States average, have just as low a risk. More recently Kinlen[59] has reported that mortality from colorectal cancer in women belonging to strict religious orders who abstained from meat was similar to that in the general population.

The most striking fact about studies of the diet reported by patients with colorectal cancer (listed in Table 2) is that in spite of many differences in design and method of selecting controls, several suggest a protective effect of vegetables. Stocks[1,20] was the first to make such an observation though he did not stress the finding. Modan and his col-leagues[60] found that the diets reported by patients with colon cancer included fruits and a variety of vegetables less often than did the controls. They also found that a low fiber consumption was reported more often by the colon cancer patients than by the controls. Bjelke[31] found that both in Norway and in Minnesota colorectal cancer patients reported a lower intake of certain vegetables than did controls. Somewhat lower intakes than for the controls were also reported for cereal products, milk, coffee, and fish products but no differences were detected with respect to total meat consumption. The findings by the same worker in his prospective studies in Norway and the U.S. with respect to vegetable intake support the observations made in the case-control studies.[34]

But what constituent of vegetables is responsible for their apparent protective effect? Burkitt has for some years been stressing that the low fiber content of western diets may be the cause of several different diseases that are common in the West — including colon cancer. He has also pointed out that the longer intestinal transit time and low stool weight associated with low residue diets would tend to increase both the concentrations of any fecal carcinogens and the contact with colonic mucosa. Since dietary fiber in the form of bran has been shown to reduce the degradation of bile salts,[62] perhaps by decreasing their contact with colonic bacteria, this hypothesis may not necessarily conflict with the theory about intestinal bacteria and fatty breakdown products. The fiber hy-pothesis was initially thought to be weakend by the poor correlation that was found when the average intake of crude fiber in different countries was compared with the corresponding mortality rates from colon cancer. However, crude fiber is far from being equivalent to fiber in the sense used by Burkitt and Trowell which concerns the fraction of vegetable matter not digested by human enzymes. Of great interest, therefore, is the recent report[63] of a significant negative correlation between colon cancer in different British regions and the average intake of the pentose fraction of total dietary fiber, since this fraction appears to be particularly important in increasing fecal bulk.

Another constituent of vegetables that may be relevant is carotene since this is a precursor of vitamin A which has been shown to inhibit carcinogenesis in animals in recent experimental situations. Few studies have been analysed so that the effect of carotene might be distinguished from other substances. Modan and his colleagues[64] recently did so, however, in their analysis of data from Israel and found that the pro-tection appeared to come from constitutents other than carotene. Vegetables such as cabbage, turnips and broccoli also contain indoles which reduce the yield of tumors in animals in certain experimental situations, perhaps through their capacity to induce benzopyrene hydroxylase activity in the gut.

A marked association between beer drinking and colorectal cancer emerged when Breslow and Enstrom[65] correlated cancer mortality and the per capita consumption of

Table 2
CASE-CONTROL STUDIES OF DIETARY FACTORS IN COLORECTAL CANCER

Location	Numbers		Association		Ref.
	Patients	Controls	Positive	Negative	
England-Wales	300	9000	Beer	—	20
U.S.A.	340	1020	—	—	24
New York	791	409	Beer	—	46
Bombay	1636	1314	—	Vegetarian diet high in dairy products	27
Japan	157	307	Fruit and milk	Rice	41
Hawaii	179	357	Meat, string beans, Starches		57
Norway	278	1394	Processed meats	Vegetables, vitamin A, coffee	31
Minnesota	373	1657	Meat (rectum only)	Vegetables, fruit, coffee, crude fiber	31
California	41	123	Meat, fish, Dairy Products (except milk) in the past	—	47
Israel	275	550	—	Vegetables	60
New York	982	2392	—	Vegetables	61

cigarettes, spirits, wine, and beer in different U.S. areas. This relationship persisted when similar data were examined for 24 other countries. Enstrom[66] followed up this work by a more sensitive analysis in which he found that among eight major sites of cancer examined in males, rectum produced the strongest correlation between changes in the per capita beer consumption in different U.S. states since World War II and later changes in cancer mortality. Furthermore, the male to female ratio of rectum cancer mortality rates correlated strongly with per capita beer consumption in different areas of the U.S. in a cautious review of other relevant evidence. Nevertheless, it is interesting to note that Stocks[20] found a significant relationship in Liverpool and the North Wales area between intestinal cancer and beer drinking, while Bjelke found in a prospective study of 12,000 men that heavy beer drinkers developed colorectal cancer more often than light or nondrinkers of beer.

The International Agency for Research on Cancer has attempted to take further the question of a relationship between beer and large bowel cancer by sponsoring two cohort studies among brewery workers in Copenhagen and Dublin who are allowed a free quota of the brewery product. But although a significant excess of death from rectum cancer was observed among the Dublin workers,[67] this was not seen in Copenhagen.[68] There are of course chemical and other differences between the stout brewed in Dublin and the lagers brewed in Denmark. It may also be relevant that the national consumption of beer, and also mortality from rectal cancer, is higher in Denmark than in Ireland. It is clear that more work is needed to clarify this subject.

VI. LIVER CANCER

The outbreak of an epidemic of mycotoxicosis among turkeys in 1960 was a stimulus to research the aflatoxins which are produced by the *Aspergillus* group of molds,[69] and led to their recognition as potent carcinogens in several species of animals.[70] Later a similarity was noted between the geographical distribution of populations with a high incidence of liver cancer and those with dietary staples often contaminated by *Aspergillus* molds. Since then, many attempts have been made to investigate this possible relationship. In Swaziland, a close correlation was found between the incidence of liver cancer in three areas and the frequency of contamination of ground nuts with aflatoxin.[71] In Uganda there was a positive correlation between the levels of contamination in several foods and the incidence of this tumor in different tribes.[72] Further confirmation has come from studies in Mozambique,[73] Thailand,[74] and Kenya[70] that related the aflatoxin levels in food ready for ingestion to local incidence rates for this cancer. But in view of the problems involved, it is not surprising that the risk of liver cancer has not been studied in relation to aflatoxin exposure on an individual basis.

It is well known that there is a high incidence of primary liver cancer in patients with hepatic cirrhosis whether caused by alcohol or other factors. However it is not established whether alcohol has any role in the etiology of this cancer independently of cirrhosis. The poor nutritional status of many alcoholics who develop hepatoma may be relevant and this is supported by the significant negative correlation between the incidence of this cancer in different countries and the consumption of calories, protein, and fat.[18]

VII. BREAST CANCER

Several workers have confirmed the strikingly close correlation first noted by Lea[75] in 1966 between the mortality from breast cancer and the per capita consumption of fat in different countries. Indeed, Armstrong and Doll[18] found in a detailed examination of international data for a variety of cancers and for many different dietary and economic

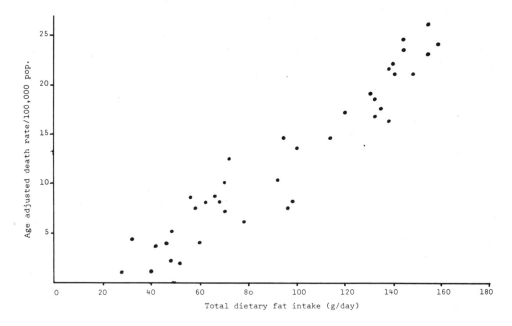

FIGURE 1. Correlation between per capita consumption of dietary fat and age-adjusted mortality from breast cancer in different countries.

variables, that no correlation was more striking than that between breast cancer mortality and average fat intake (Figure 1). Moreover these observations appear to have a corollary in the marked effects of fat intake on mammary carcinogenesis in mice and rats.

Recent evidence from Japan where the incidence of breast cancer is exceptionally low encourages the view that diet exerts a role in this disease. Whereas in most countries the incidence of this cancer continues to increase after the menopause, this does not happen in Japan. In recent years, both mortality and incidence rates in Japan have been increasing particularly at ages 45 to 59 and it may be relevant that since World War II there has been a marked increase in the consumption of saturated fat. Futhermore, Japanese migrants to the U.S. who in general have adopted a western type of diet have also shown an increase in breast cancer mortality rates compared with those in Japan, although it is noteworthy that this increase is first evident in children of migrants (Nisei) and in the third generation.[76,77,40]

Recently Nomura and his colleagues[78] reported that of 6860 Japanese males included in a prospective study of colon cancer and diet, 86 reported that their wives had developed breast cancer. If it is assumed that dietary patterns of spouses are likely to be similar, it is relevant that these 86 men consumed more meat, butter, margarine, cheese, and corn than did other men in the study (who also ate more Japanese foods).

Since much of the fat consumed in western countries comes from meat, the incidence of breast cancer in vegetarians is of relevance. Phillips reported that Seventh Day Adventists living in California, many of whom eat little meat, had a lower breast cancer mortality than that of the general U.S. population.[47] More recently, however, it has been reported that the reduction in breast cancer is less marked than previously thought.[79] Also, there is evidence that Adventists have a high intake of animal fats such as butter and milk so that their intake of animal fats may not be unusual for the United States.

Recently Kinlen[59] has completed a study of cancer mortality in members of religious orders who abstain from meat. No appreciable reduction of breast cancer mortality was detected in religious sisters who do not eat meat as compared with the general population.

In view of the high correlation between breast cancer mortality and fat consumption in the international studies, the failure to find a reduced incidence of the disease in this study might seem inconsistent. However, this study concerned women who altered their diet in adult life and the findings may point towards the importance of diet in the years of childhood and adolescence. This might explain why the daughters of Japanese immigrants to the U.S. show a higher risk than their parents.[40] Indeed, the fact that age at menarche which is influenced by nutritional factors is also a risk factor for breast cancer makes this possibility more plausible.

Few studies have attempted to compare the diet of breast cancer patients with that of controls. Recently, Choi, Miller, and their colleagues[80,81] have reported the results of such a study conducted in four areas of Canada in which 400 patients with breast cancer and a similar number of neighborhood controls matched for age and marital status were studied by means of a dietary questionnaire, a 24-hr dietary recall, and a 4-day dietary record. The patients with breast cancer reported a greater intake of all nutrients and particularly of total fat than did the controls. Unfortunately, this study largely focused on diet *after* diagnosis of breast cancer, so it is difficult to evaluate the findings and there is a need for further comparisons of the previous diet of affected patients with that of controls.

The only study to link dietary information collected from women with their subsequent experience of breast cancer is that reported by Hirayama in Japan.[15] A high incidence was found in women who were obese and who had a high intake of eggs and meat, particularly pork. The same worker has also reported that breast cancer shows independent relationships with height and weight both of which are related to nutrition. Similar, if less marked, findings on weight and height have also been reported from the Netherlands.[82] A relationship with height supports the view that nutrition early in life is important but the data concerning obesity implies that later dietary effects may also be relevant. Moreover since there is evidence that estrone plays a part in the etiology of breast cancer, the conversion of androtenedione to estrone in fat depots of postmenopausal women suggests a mechanism through which dietary factors in adult life might operate.[83]

VIII. LUNG CANCER

A relationship between lung cancer and vitamin A was suggested in 1975 by Bjelke[84] who followed up 11,038 men aged 65 years or over whose dietary habits had been surveyed some 5 years previously. He found a negative association between lung cancer and a "vitamin A index" (which in fact largely comprised its precursor carotene). This finding could not be explained by some relationship between smoking and vitamin A intake, for the protective effects were evident within each of the cigarette smoking categories examined. Overall, a 2.5-fold increase in the relative risk of lung cancer was associated with a low intake compared to a high intake of vitamin A. These observations are more interesting in view of laboratory work on animals which has shown that vitamin A can reduce the yield of tumors in several experimental systems.

Confirmatory findings for this relationship have emerged from another prospective study and from two case-control comparisons. In Japan, a lower relative risk for lung cancer was found among people who ate vegetables daily that were high in carotene, and this relationship persisted after controlling for smoking habits. In Singapore,[85] a twofold excess of lung cancer was found in females in association with a low intake of vegetables rich in β-carotene, after controlling for smoking and socioeconomic status while in New York[86] a relative risk of more than twofold was found for this cancer among patients with a low intake of vitamin A. Moreover, Wald and his colleagues have recently reported that in a prospective study, those patients who later developed lung cancer had lower serum retinol levels at the start of the study than did controls and that this effect was independent of smoking.[87] A similar finding has been reported by Kark.[88]

IX. LARYNX CANCER

Case-control studies of larynx cancer have indicated relationships both with alcohol and smoking.[88] It is well–known that heavy drinkers smoke more than the average but smoking cannot explain the observed relationship with alcohol. Thus Wynder and his colleagues[89] found that after controlling for smoking, alcohol (and particularly heavy whiskey) consumption was associated with a tenfold elevation of the risk of larynx cancer as compared to that in moderate or nondrinkers.

X. BLADDER CANCER

Coffee has mutagenic activity and at least three case-control studies in the U.S. have found an association between bladder cancer and coffee consumption.[90-92] No clear dose-response relationship has been found however and a causal relationship is not established. Recently, Mettlin and Graham[93] have reported from New York that patients with bladder cancer have a lower intake of vitamin A than controls. They also raised the possibility that the previously reported association with coffee consumption may result from a tendency observed in their study for heavy coffee drinkers to have a relatively low intake of vitamin A. In veiw of this suggestion of a protective effect of vitamin A in bladder carcinogenesis, it is of interest that changing the vitamin A intake of animals has been shown to alter the yield of bladder tumors in response to carcinogens.

Bracken has been shown to cause bladder cancer in cattle.[94] Although it is possible that the unidentified consitituent in question might reach man in milk or meat from animals that graze on bracken, no evidence has emerged to link bracken with bladder cancer in man.

But the suggested dietary factor in bladder cancer that has received most attention is undoubtedly saccharin. This began with the report that rats receiving large amounts of saccharin in their diet developed bladder tumors. In man most studies of the question gave no indication of a hazard although a Canadian study claimed to detect a positive relationship. So much concern was aroused in the United States, where a great deal of saccharin is consumed, that the Food and Drug Administration commissioned, through the National Cancer Institute, what may be the largest case-control study ever carried out in one country;[95] it failed to find any evidence that artificial sweeteners had a marked relationship with bladder cancer.

XI. ENDOMETRIAL CANCER

Endometrial cancer like breast and colon cancer shows a high correlation with fat when its incidence or mortality in different countries is correlated with the corresponding average per capita fat consumption. Other evidence for the role of diet in the etiology of endometrial cancer, including its relationship to obesity, has been summarized by Armstrong.[2] As with breast cancer the conversation of androstenedione to estrone in the fat depots of postmenopausal women suggests a mechanism whereby diet might influence the incidence of the disease. Moreover the recent evidence that exogenous estrogens as hormone replacement therapy can cause endometrial cancer is a further indication of the importance of estrogens in its etiology.

XII. OTHER CANCERS

Correlations have been noted between dietary variables and mortality in different countries from other cancers including cancers of the prostate, testis, and kidney though these are less marked than those previously discussed for colon and breast cancers.[18] Thus prostate and testis cancers are positively correlated with fat consumption, and kidney cancer with both animal protein and coffee consumption. However, a case-control study failed to confirm these associations with renal cancer[96] while more sensitive studies of prostate and testis cancers are still awaited.

XIII. SUMMARY

There is much evidence for the role of diet in human cancer although few causative links have been firmly established. Indeed of specific dietary items studied in individuals, only alcohol is well-established as an etiological factor in human cancer and even here it seems likely that alcohol is not itself carcinogenic but acts indirectly. This lack of certainty about dietary factors in human cancer is partly however, a reflection of the problems implicit in their study. We do not eat basic dietary ingredients or chemicals as such; our diet is mixed and complex and difficult to define and summarize. Nevertheless there is much to suggest that diet is important in the etiology of human cancer. In particular, there are encouraging signs that certain dietary constituents such as vegetables, vitamin A and its precursor, carotene, may be protective but more work is required both to confirm these effects and to determine whether they are independent.

REFERENCES

1. **Stocks, P. and Karn, M. K.,** A co-operative study of the habits, home life, dietary and family histories of 450 cancer patients and of an equal number of control patients, *Ann. Eugen. (London),* 5, 237, 1933.
2. **Armstrong, B. K.,** The role of diet in human carcinogenesis with special reference to endometrial cancer, in *Origins of Human Cancer,* Hiatt, H. H., Watson, J. A., and Winsten, J. A., Eds., Cold Spring Harbor Laboratory, Cold Spring Harbor, N.Y., 1977, 557.
3. **Anon.,** Registrar General's Decennial Supplement, Part 2, England and Wales 1921, His Majesty's Stationery Office, London, 1927.
4. **Chilvers, C., Fraser, P., and Beral, V.,** Alcohol and oesophageal cancer and assessment of the evidence from routinely collected data, *Epidemiol. Commun. Health,* 33, 127, 1979.
5. **Wynder, E. L. and Bross, I. J.,** A study of etiological factors in cancer of esophagus, *Cancer,* 14, 389, 1961.
6. **Martinez, I.,** Factors associated with cancer of the esophagus, mouth, and pharynx in Puerto Rico, *J. Natl. Cancer Inst.,* 42, 1069, 1969.
7. **Schwartz, D., Lasserre, O., Flament, R., and Lellouch, J.,** Alcool et cancer. Etude de pathologie geographique portant sur 19 pays, *Eur, J. Cancer,* 2, 367, 1966.
8. **Wu, Y. K., and Loucks, H. H.,** Cancer of the esophagus or cardia of the stomach, *Ann. Surg.,* 134 946, 1951.
9. **Tuyns, A. J. and Jensen, O. M.,** International Agency for Research on Cancer, Annual Report, Lyon, 1976.
10. **Tuyns, A. J., Pequingnot, G., and Jensen, O. M.,** Le cancre de l'oesophage en Ille-et-Vilaine en fonction des niveaux de consomation d'alcool et de tabac, Des risques qui se multiplient, *Bull. Cancer,* 64, 45, 1977.
11. **Cook, P.,** Cancer of the oesophagus in Africa, *Br. J. Cancer,* 25, 853, 1971.
12. **Cook-Mozaffari, P. J., Azordegan, F., Day, N. E., Ressican, A., Sarah, C., and Aramesh, B.,** Oesophageal cancer studies in the Caspian littoral of Iran. Results of a case-control study. *Br. J. Cancer,* 39, 293, 1979.
13. **Hewer, T., Rose, E., Ghadirian, P., Castegnaro, M., Bartsch, H., Malaveille, C., and Day, N.,** Ingested mutagens from opium and tobacco pyrolysis products and cancer of the oesophagus, *Lancet,* ii, 494, 1978.

14. **Wynder, E. L., Hultberg, S., Jacobsson, F., and Bross, I. J.,** Environmental factors in cancer of the upper alimentary tract, *Cancer,* 10, 470, 1957.
15. **Hirayama, T.,** Diet and cancer, *Nutri. Cancer,*1(3), 67, 1979.
16. **Wahi, P. N., Bodkhe, R. R., Shashi, A., and Srivastava, M. C.,** Serum vitamin A studies in leukoplakia and carcinoma of the oral cavity, *Ind J. Pathol., Bactiol.,* 5, 10, 1962.
17. **Ibrahim, J., Jafarey, N. A., and Zuberi, S. J.,** Plasma vitamin A and carotene level in squamous cell carcinomas of oral cavity and oropharynx, *Clin. Oncol.,* 3, 38, 1977.
18. **Armstrong, B. and Doll, R.,** Environmental factors and cancer incidence and mortality in different countries, with special reference to dietary practices, *Int. J. Cancer,* 15, 617, 1975.
19. **Segi, M., Fukushima, I., Fujisaku, S., Kurihara, M., Saito, S., Anano, K., and Kamoi, M.,** An epidemiological study of cancer in Japan, *Gann,* Suppl. 48, 1957.
20. **Stocks, P.,** Cancer Incidence in North Wales and Liverpool Region in Relation to Habits and Environment, British Empire Cancer Campaign, 35th Annual Report, 1957.
21. **Wynder, E. L., Kmet, J., Dungal, N., and Segi, M.,** An epidemiological investigation of gastric cancer, *Cancer,* 16, 1461, 1963.
22. **Meinsma, L.,** Voeding en Kanker, *Voeding,* 25, 357, 1964.
23. **Acheson, E. D. and Doll, R.,** Dietary factors in carcinoma of the stomach: a study of 100 cases and 100 controls, *Gut.,* 5, 126, 1964.
24. **Higginson, J.,** Etiologic factors in gastrointestinal cancer in man, *J. Natl. Cancer Inst.,* 37, 527, 1966.
25. **Graham, S., Lilienfeld, A. M., and Tidings, J. E.,** Dietary and purgation factors in the epidemiology of gastric cancer, *Cancer,* 20, 2224, 1967.
26. **Hirayama, T.,** The epidemiology of cancer of stomach in Japan with special reference to the role of diet, in *Proc. 9th Intl. Cancer Congr.,* Harries, R. J. C., Ed., Sprigner-Verlag, Basel, 1967, 37.
27. **Paymaster, J. C., Sanghri, L. D., and Gangadharan, P.,** Cancer in the gastrointestinal tract in western India, *Cancer,* 21, 279, 1968.
28. **Hirayama, T.,** Epidemiology of stomach cancer, *Gass. Monogr.,* 11, 3, 1971.
29. **Haenszel, W., Kurihar, M., Segi, M., and Lee, R. K. C.,** Stomach cancer among Japanese in Hawaii, *J. Natl. Cancer Int.,* 49, 969, 1972.
30. **Graham, S., Schotz, W., and Martino, P.,** Alimentary factors in the epidemiology of gastric cancer, *Cancer,* 30, 927, 1972.
31. **Bjelke, E.,** *Epidemiologic studies of Cancer of the Stomach, Colon, and Rectum,* Vol. 1-4, Univ. Microfilms Intl., Ann Arbor, Michigan.
32. **Modan, B., Lubin, F., Barell, V., Greenberg, R. A., Modan, M., and Graham, S.,** The role of starches in the etiology of gastric cancer, *Cancer,* 34, 2087, 1974.
33. **Haenszel, W., Kurihara, M., Locke, F. B., Shimuzu, K., and Segi, M.,** Stomach cancer in Japan, *J. Natl. Cancer Inst.,* 56, 265, 1976.
34. **Bjelke, E.,** Dietary factors and the epidemiology of cancer of the stomach and large bowel, *Aktual. Probl. Klinischen Diatetik,* Suppl. 2, 1978.
35. **Cuello, C., Correa, P., Haenszel, W., Gordillo, G., Brown, C., Archer, M., and Tannenbaum, S.,** Gastric cancer in Colombia I. Cancer risk and suspect environmental agents, *J. Natl. Cancer Inst.,* 57, 1015, 1976.
36. **Hill, M. J., Hawksworth, G., and Tattersall, G.,** Bacteria, nitrosamines and cancer of the stomach, *Br. J. Cancer,* 28, 562, 1973.
37. **Davies, J. M.** Stomach cancer mortality in Worksop and Nottinghamshire mining towns, *Br. J. Cancer,* 41, 438.
38. **Kinlen, L. J., Scott, A., and Forbes, W.,** Cancer mortality in rural Scotland in relation to bracken coverage, in preparation.
39. **Smith, R. L.,** Recorded and expected mortality among Japanese of the United States and Hawaii, with specific reference to cancer, *J. Natl. Cancer Inst.,* 17, 459, 1956.
40. **Haenszel, W. and Kurihara, M.,** Studies of Japanese migrants. 1. Mortality from cancer and other diseases among Japanese in the United States, *J. Natl. Cancer Inst.,* 40, 43, 1968.
41. **Wynder, E. L., Kajitani, T., Ishikawa, S., Dodo, H., and Takono, A.,** Environmental factors of cancer of the colon and rectum. II. Japanese epidemiological data, *Cancer,* 23, 1210, 1969.
42. **Staszewski, J. and Haenszel, W.,** Cancer mortality among the Polish-born in the United States, *J. Natl. Cancer Inst.,* 35, 291, 1968.
43. **Haenszel, W.,** Cancer mortality among foreign born in the United States, *J. Natl. Cancer Inst.,* 26, 37, 1961.
44. **Staszewski, J., McCall, M. G., and Stenhouse, N. S.,** Cancer mortality in 1962-66 among Polish immigrants to Australia, *Br. J. Cancer,* 25, 599, 1971.
45. **Burkitt, D. P.,** Epidemiology of cancer of the colon and rectum, *Cancer,* 28, 3, 1971.
46. **Wynder, E. and Shigematsu, T.,** Environmental factors of cases of cancer of the colon and rectum, *Cancer,* 20, 1520, 1967.

47. **Phillips, R. L.,** Role of life style and dietary habits in risk of cancer among Seventh-Day Adventists, *Cancer Res.,* 35, 3513, 1975.
48. **Hill, M. J., Drasar, B. S., Ares, V. C., Crowther, J. S., Hawkesworth, G. M., and Williams, R. E. O.,** Bacteria and aetiology of cancer of the large bowel, *Lancet,* i, 95, 1971.
49. **Hill, M. J., Drasar, B. S., Williams, R. E. O., Meade, T. W., Cox, A. G., Simpson, J. E. P., and Mason, B. C.,** Faecal bile-acids and clostridia in patients with cancer of the large bowel, *Lancet,* i, 353, 1975.
50. **Mastromarino, A. J., Reddy, B. S., and Wynder, E. L.,** Fecal profiles of anaerobic microflora of large bowel cancer patients and patients with nonhereditary large bowel polyp, *Cancer Res.,* 38, 4458, 1978.
51. **Finegold, S. M., Flora, D. J., Atteberg, J. R., and Sutter, V. L.,** Fecal bacteriology of colonic polyp patients and control patients, *Cancer Res.,* 35, 3407, 1975.
52. **Watne, A. L., Lai, H.-Y., L., Mance, T., and Core, S.,** Fecal steroids and bacterial flora in patients with polyposis coli, *Am. J. Surg.,* 131, 42, 1976.
53. **Mudd, D. G., McKelvey, S. T. D., and Elmore, D. T.,** Fecal bile acid concentrations in patients at increased risk of large bowel cancer, *Br. J. Surg.,* 65, 357, 1978.
54. **Mudd, D. G., McKelvey, S.T. D., Norwood, W., and Elmore, D. T.,** Carcinoma of the large bowel and faecal bile acids, *Br. J. Surg.* 65, 355, 1979.
55. **Murrey, W. R., Blackwood, A., Trotter, J. M., Calman, K. C., and MacKay, C.,** Faecal bile acids and clostridia in the aetiology of colorectal cancer, *Br. J. Cancer,* 41, 923, 1980.
56. **I.A.R.C.,** Dietary fibre, transit-time, faecal bacteria, steroids and colon cancer in two Scandanavian populations, *Lancet,* ii, 207, 1977.
57. **Haeuszel, W., Berg, J. W., Segi, M., Kurihara, M., and Locke, F. H.,** Large bowel cancer in Hawaiian Japanese, *J. Natl. Cancer Inst.,* 51, 1765, 1973.
58. **Lyon, J. L. and Sorenson, A. W.,** Colon cancer in a low risk population, *Am. J. Clin. Nutr.* 31, 5227, 1978.
59. **Kinlen, L. J.,** Mortality in relation to abstinence from meat in certain orders of religious sisters in Britain, *Cancer Incidence in Defined Populations,* Report No. 4, Cold Spring Harbor Laboratory, Cold Spring Harbor, N.Y., 1980.
60. **Modan, B., Barell, V., Lubin, F., Modan, M., Greenberg, R. A., and Graham, S.,** Low-fibre intake as an etiologic factor in cancer of the colon, *J. Natl. Cancer Inst.,* 55, 15, 1975.
61. **Graham, S., Dayal, H., Swanson, M. Mittelman, A., and Wilkinson, G.,** Diet in the epidemiology of cancer of the colon and rectum, *J. Natl. Cancer Inst.,* 61, 709, 1978.
62. **Pomare, E. W. and Heaton, K. W.** Alteration of bile salt metabolism by dietary fibre (bran), *Br. Med. J.* 4, 262, 1973.
63. **Bingham, S., Williams, D. R. R., Cole, T. J., and James, W. P. T.,** Dietary fibre and regional large-bowel cancer mortality in Britain, *Br. J. Cancer,* 40, 456, 1979.
64. **Modan, B., Cuckle, H., and Lubin, F.,** Dietary retinol and carotene in the etiology of human gastrointestinal cancer, 1981.
65. **Breslow, N. E. and Enstrom, J. E.,** Geographic correlations between cancer mortality rates and alcohol-tobacco consumption in the United States, *J. Natl. Cancer Inst.,* 53, 631, 1974.
66. **Enstrom, J. E.,** Colorectal cancer and beer drinking, *Br. J. Cancer,* 35, 674, 1977.
67. **Dean, G., MacLennan, R., McLoughlin, H., and Shelley, E.,** Causes of death of blue-collar workers at a Dublin brewery, 1954-73, *Br. J. Cancer,* 40, 581, 1979.
68. **Jensen, O. M.,** Cancer morbidity and causes of death among Danish brewery workers, *Int. J. Cancer,* 23, 454, 1979.
69. **Asplin, F. D. and Callaghan, R. B. A.,** The toxicity of certain groundnut meals for poultry with special reference to their effect on ducklings and chickens, *Vet. Rec.* 73, 1215, 1961.
70. **Peers, F. G. and Linsell, C. A.,** Aflatoxin and liver cell cancer, *Trans. R. Soc. Trop. Med. Hyg.,* 71., 471, 1977.
71. **Keen, P. and Martin, P.,** Is aflatoxin carcinogenic in man? *Trop. Geogr. Med.,* 23, 44, 1971.
72. **Alpert, M. E., Hutt, M. S. R., Wogan, G. N., and Davidson, C. S.,** The association between aflatoxin content of food and hepatoma frequency in Uganda, *Cancer,* 28, 253, 1971.
73. **Van Rensberg, S. J., Vander Watt, J. J., Purchase, I. F. H., Coutinho, L. P., and Markham, R.,** Primary liver cancer rate and aflatoxin intake in a high cancer area, *S. Afr. Med. J.* 48, 2508a, 1974.
74. **Shank, R. C., Gordon, J. E., Wogan, G. N., Nondasuta, A., and Subhamani, B.,** Dietary aflatoxins and human liver cancer. III. Field Survey of rural Thai families for ingested aflatoxins, *Food Comset. Toxicol.* 40, 71, 1972.
75. **Lea, A. J.,** Dietary factors associated with death rates from certain neoplasmas in man, *Lancet,* ii, 332, 1966.
76. **Hirayama, T.,** Epidemiology of breast cancer with special reference to the role of diet, *Prev. Med.* 7, 173, 1978.
77. **Huell, P.,** Changing incidence of breast cancer in Japanese American women, *J. Natl. Cancer Inst.,* 51, 1479, 1973.

78. **Nomura, A., Henderson, B. E., and Lee, J.,** Breast cancer and diet among the Japanese in Hawaii, *Am. J. Clin. Nutr.* 31, 2020, 1978.
79. **Phillips, R. L.,** Conference on Cancer in Low Risk Populations, Utah, August 1978.
80. **Miller, A. B., Kelly, A., Choi, N. W., Matthews, V., Morgan, R. W., Munan, L., Burch, J. D., Feather, J., Howe, G. R., and Jain, M.,** A study of diet and breast cancer, *Am. J. Epidemiol,* 107, 499, 1978.
81. **Choi, N. W., Howe, G. R., Miller, A. B., Matthews, V., Morgan, R. W., Munan, L., Burch, J. D., Feather, J., Jain, M., and Kelly, A.,** An epidemiological study of breast cancer, *Am. J. Epidemiol.,* 107, 510, 1978.
82. **De Waard, F., and Baanders-van Halewiju, E. A.,** A prospective study in general practice on breast cancer in post menopausal women, *Int. J. Cancer,* 14, 163, 1974.
83. **MacMahon, B., Cole, P., and Brown J.,** Etiology of human breast cancer. A review, *J. Natl., Cancer Inst.,* 50, 21, 1973.
84. **Bjelke, E.,** Dietary vitamin A and human lung cancer. *Int. J. Cancer,* 15, 561, 1975.
85. **Maclennon, R., DaCosta, J., Day, N. E., Law, C. H., Ng, Y. K., and Shanmugaratnam, K.,** Risk factors for lung cancer in Singapore Chinese, a population with high female incidence, *Int. J. Cancer,* 20, 854, 1977.
86. **Mettlin, C., Graham, S., and Swanson, M.,** Vitamin A and lung cancer, *J. Natl. Cancer Inst.,* 62, 1453, 1979.
87. **Wald, N., Idle, M., Boreham, J., and Bailey, A.,** Low serum-vitamin-A and subsequent risk of cancer, *Lancet,* ii, 813, 1980.
88. **Kark, J. D., Smith, A. H., Switzer, B. R., and Hames, C. G.,** Serum vitamin A (retinol) and cancer incidence in Evans County, Georgia, *J. Natl. Cancer Inst.,* 66, 7, 1981.
89. **Wynder, E. L., Bross, I. J., and Day, E.,** A study of environmental factors in cancer of the larynx, *Cancer* 9, 86, 1956.
90. **Cole, P.,** Coffee-drinking and cancer of the lower urinary tract, *Lancet, i,* 1335.
91. **Fraumeni, J. F., Scotto, J., and Dunham, L. J.,** Coffee-drinking and bladder cancer, Lancet ii, 1204, 1971.
92. **Bross, I. D. and Tidings, J.,** Another look at coffee drinking and cancer of the urinary bladder, *Prev. Med.,* ii, 445, 1973.
93. **Mettlin, C. and Graham, S.,** Dietary risk factors in human bladder cancer, *Am. J. Epidemiol.,* 110, 255, 1979.
94. **Pamukeu, A. M.,** Epidemiologic studies on urinary bladder tumors in Turkish cattle, *Ann. N.Y. Acad. Sci.,* 108, 938, 1963.
95. **Hoover, R. N. and Strasser, P. H.,** Artificial sweeteners and human bladder cancer: preliminary results, *Lancet,* i, 387, 1980.
96. **Armstrong, B., Garrod, A., and Doll, R.,** A retrospective study of renal cancer with special reference to coffee and animal protein consumption, *Br. J. Cancer,* 33, 127, 1976.

Chapter 7

CARCINOGENIC MYCOTOXINS

R. Schoental

TABLE OF CONTENTS

I. INTRODUCTION

Since the discovery that certain secondary metabolites of various microorganisms have antibiotic activities (e.g., streptomycin, penicillin, etc.), much attention has been directed to the isolation of such substances. Many of such "antibiotics" have been found to be useful as drugs for the treatment of infectious diseases, of tumors, etc.[1] However, some other of the isolated products, which proved not effective, or too toxic in vivo, were usually not tested further for chronic or carcinogenic action, except in a few cases. Already in 1960 a compilation of substances and crude materials isolated from microorganisms exceeded 1000 items,[2] many more have been isolated in the intervening years, and their numbers are continuously increasing. There are more than 100,000 species of molds known, and though not all are toxigenic, they represent a rich source of interesting substances. The secondary metabolites of molds (microfungi) which cause toxic or otherwise deleterious effects in animals are known as mycotoxins. A number of books and reviews dealing with molds and mycotoxins have been published in recent years.[3-13]

Microorganisms (including molds) have been on earth probably longer than animals and man, and sporadically must have affected human and animal health, especially when the climatic and other environmental conditions were conducive to their growth and to the production of toxic secondary metabolites. However, only relatively recently have mycotoxins been recognized as possible causes of certain disorders and tumors, when they contaminate animal feeds or man's foods and drinks. Most of the relevant mycotoxins have been isolated and their chemical structures established within the last 20 years or so; only few have been tested for carcinogenic activity.

The mycotoxins which have already been found to be carcinogenic in experimental animals have a great variety of chemical structures (Table 1). Some of these compounds are representatives of groups of substances of related structures (but of modulated biological action), which may be produced by the same or by different strains or species of microorganisms. The formation and prevalence of any particular mycotoxin in foodstuffs and in any other substrate is a dynamic process changing with time and with environmental conditions, such as the availability of specific nutrients, the moisture content, the red-ox potential, the temperature, the presence of and interaction with the accompanying microorganisms, etc. Field contamination of foods is usually due to a number of organisms and to more than one mycotoxin, which may act additively or synergistically; the effects of exposure to multimycotoxins may differ from these induced experimentally by using single pure compounds.

Levels of mycotoxins, too low to have immediately recognizable effects, could have cumulative action and lead to tumors, to progressive changes in the biochemical processes, and contribute to a general decline and to premature senility. However, the effects of carcinogens including carcinogenic mycotoxins depend on the genetic predisposition, immunological competence, the nutritional and hormonal status, and the sex and the age of the individual at the time of exposure. The susceptibility to various carcinogenic agents at the perinatal age is particularly striking. Although mycotoxins are usually classified by the organ in which they cause the predominant acute effects (e.g., aflatoxins, sterigmatocystin, elaiomycin — as hepatotoxic, ochratoxins — as nephrotoxic, trichothecenes — as irritants and gastrotoxic, zearalenone — as estrogenic), each will affect also some of the other, interrelated organs, and can induce tumors at more than one organ or type of tissue.

Like other xenobiotics, mycotoxins undergo stepwise metabolic degradation in the course of which some of the formed intermediates may be effective initiators of the carcinogenic process, while others may be detoxification products or even inhibitory. Outbreaks of mycotoxicoses, whether in humans or livestock, which have been attributed

Table 1
EXAMPLES OF METABOLITES OF MICROORGANISMS
WHICH INDUCED TUMORS IN EXPERIMENTAL ANIMALS[8]

Compound	Parent microorganism	Animal spp.	Tumors in tissues
Actinomycins (A,L,S)	Streptomyces	Mouse	s.c. sarcoma
Aflatoxins (B_1,G_1,M_1)	*Aspergillus flavus*	Many spp. including monkeys	Liver, kidney, etc., s.c. sarcoma
Azaserine	Streptomycetes	Rat	Pancreas
Daunomycin	Streptomyces	Rat	Kidney, sex organs
Elaiomycin	*Streptomyces hepaticus*	Rat	Kidney, liver, etc.
Ethionine	Pseudomonas *E. coli*	Rat	Liver
Griseofulvin	*Penicillium griseofulvum*	Mouse	Liver
Luteoskyrin	*P. islandicum*	Mouse	Liver
Ochratoxin A	*P. ochraceum*	Mouse	Liver, kidney
Patulin	*P. patulum* Aspergillus spp.	Rat	s.c. sarcoma
Sterigmatocystin	*A. versicolor*	Rat, monkey	Liver, s.c. sarcoma
Streptozotocin	*Streptomyces achromogenes*	Rat	Liver, kidney, pancreatic islets
T-2 toxin	*Fusarium* spp.	Rat	Digestive tract, brain

to the toxic products of cultures of isolated microorganisms, may have been due to several additional factors. The case of the outbreak of liver disease in Japan, due to the consumption of "yellow rice" imported from Burma after World War II, might have been due not only to luteoskyrin and cyclochlorotine produced by *Penicillium islandicum* Sopp.[14,15] which contaminated the "yellow rice". A possibility cannot be excluded that aflatoxins (not known at the time) and other hepatotoxic mycotoxins might also have been present, and that their effects were aggravated by the poor nutritional status of a population exposed to war conditions. The hepatotoxic effects of luteoskyrin are generally influenced by a variety of chemical agents.[16]

II. AFLATOXINS

Aflatoxins (Figures 1 and 2) have been the most extensively studied mycotoxins since 1960, when they have been found in moldy peanut meal, which caused heavy losses among turkey poults given this meal in their diet. A toxigenic strain of *Aspergillus flavus* Link ex Fries, isolated from this meal, produced in laboratory cultures, intensely fluorescent metabolites which were able to reproduce liver lesions similar to those that killed the turkey poults. The aflatoxins comprise a number of related compounds, having a characteristic difuranoid moiety attached to a coumarin nucleus; aflatoxins B_1 (Figure 1), G_1 (Figure 2), and M_1 represent the carcinogenic members of this group of substances. The presence of the isolated double bond between carbon 2,3 is essential for the hepatotoxic action of the aflatoxins (Table 2).

Aflatoxin B_1 is one of the most effective hepatocarcinogens, not only among this group of compounds, but also in comparison with other known hepatocarcinogens; it can induce tumors of the liver (and of certain other organs) in many animal species. Many reviews,

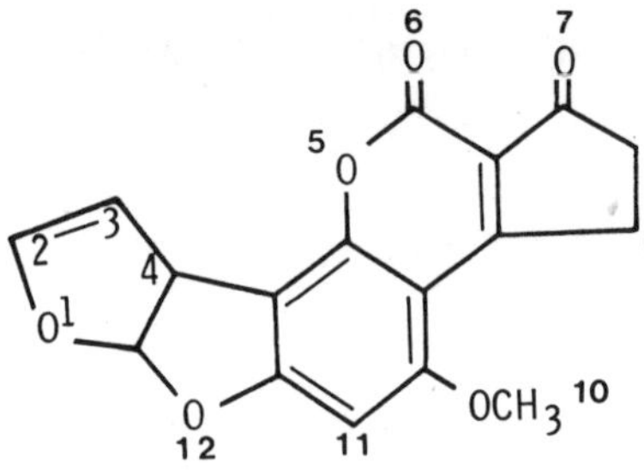

FIGURE 1.   The structure of aflatoxin B_1.

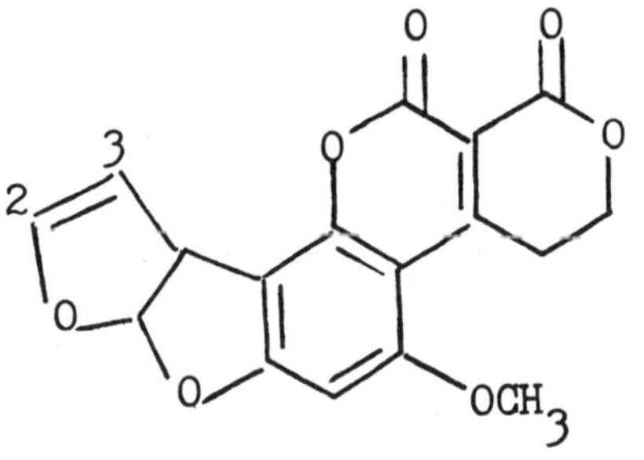

FIGURE 2.   The structure of aflatoxin G_1.

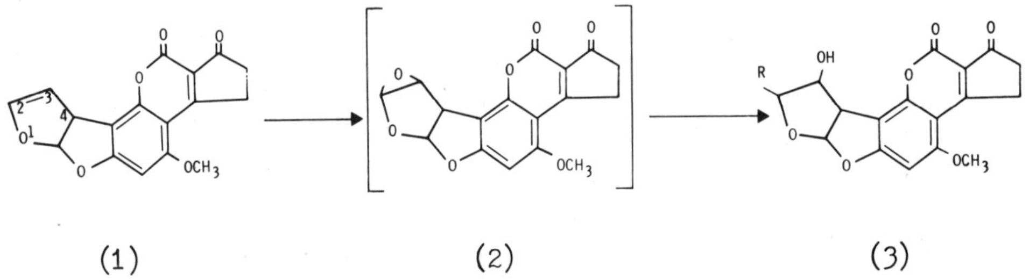

(1)   (2)   (3)

FIGURE 3.   Structures of aflatoxin B_1 and of certain of its metabolic products: (1) aflatoxin B_1; (2) aflatoxin B_1-2,3-epoxide; (3) metabolic products of aflatoxin B_1, (3a) 2,3-dihydroxy-2,3-dihydroaflatoxin B_1, R = OH, (3b) 2-glutathionyl-3-hydroxy-2,3-dihydroaflatoxin B_1, R = glutathionyl residue, (3c) 2,(N^7-guanyl)-3-hydroxy-2,3-dihydroaflatoxin B_1, R = guanyl residue.

symposia, and books have been published which deal with various aspects of aflatoxins, their natural occurrence, chemistry, biosynthesis, their biochemical and pathological effects in animals, and with some of the factors which can modify the response to their action.[17-22]

The conditions found to be optimal for the production of the carcinogenic aflatoxins by the common fungus *A. flavus* include aerobically growing them on appropriate substrates having 20 to 33% moisture content and pH about 5, at 28 to 32°C.[23] The climatic conditions which prevail in Africa, southeast Asia, and parts of America are therefore conducive to the production of aflatoxins in foodstuffs. The aflatoxin content of foods consumed by the people in Kenya, Swaziland, Mozambique, and Thailand has been

Table 2
STRUCTURE-TOXICITY RELATIONSHIPS OF VARIOUS AFLATOXINS

Compound	Structure	Toxicity
Aflatoxin B$_1$	Af B$_1$	+ + + +
Epoxide of Af B$_1$	2, 3-dihydro-2,3-epoxy-Af B$_1$	+ + + +
Aflatoxin B$_1$ 2,3-dihydrodiol	2,3-dihydro-2,3-dihydroxy aflatoxin B$_1$	−
Aflatoxin B$_1$ dichloride	2,3-dichloro-2,3-dihydro- aflatoxin B$_1$	+ + + +
Aflatoxin M$_1$	4-hydroxy-Af B$_1$	+ + + +
Aflatoxicol (AfRo)	7-hydroxy-Af B$_1$	+ +
Aflatoxin Q	9-hydroxy-Af B$_1$	+ +
Aflatoxicol H$_1$	7,9-dihydroxy-Af B$_1$	?
Aflatoxin P	10-0-demethyl-Af B$_1$	+ +
Aflatoxin B$_2$	2,3-dihydro-Af B$_1$	±
Aflatoxin M$_2$	2,3-dihydro-4-hyudroxy-Af B$_1$	±
Aflatoxin B$_{2a}$	2-hydroxy-2,3,dihydro-Af B$_1$	±
Aflatoxin G$_1$	Af G$_1$	+ + +
Epoxide of Af G$_1$	2,3-dihydro-2,3-epoxy-Af G$_1$	+ + +
Aflatoxin GM$_1$	4-hydroxy-Af G$_1$	+ + +
Aflatoxin G$_2$	2,3-dihydro-Af G$_1$	±
Aflatoxin G$_{2a}$	2-hydroxy-2,3-dihydro-Af G$_1$	±

investigated and appeared to show some correlation between the present intake of aflatoxins and the incidence of primary liver cancer in the respective areas.[24-26]

However, in these countries people may be exposed, besides aflatoxins, to other hepatocarcinogenic agents in their food or in their traditional herbal remedies, e.g., to sterigmatocystin, cycasin, the pyrrolizidine alkaloids, etc. Liver tumors affect a small proportion of the population of the respective countries and their etiology is likely to be multifactorial. Hepatocarcinogens of different chemical structures are known to act synergistically; they can reinforce each other's action. Nutritional factors can also influence the effects of liver damaging agents.[27]

Like other hepatocarcinogens, the aflatoxins become metabolically activated by liver enzymes (into the effective entities). As the presence of an isolated double bond in the structures of several types of carcinogens (including the pyrrolizidine alkaloids, the aflatoxins, and sterigmatocystins) is essential for their carcinogenic action, it has been suggested that their activation by hepatocytes involves the epoxidation of the isolated double bond in the dihydrofuranoid moiety.[28] Attempts to synthesize the 2,3-epoxides of aflatoxin B$_1$ for direct testing have as yet not been successful, but indirect evidence seems to support this possibility.[29-35] In vitro liver microsomal fractions activate aflatoxin B$_1$ to a mutagen.[29] The activated metabolite of aflatoxin B$_1$ reacts as a 2,3-epoxide.[30] Moreover, 2,3-dihydro-2,3-dichloro-aflatoxin B$_1$ considered as a model for the 2,3-epoxide of aflatoxin B$_1$, is an effective topocarcinogen.[31] Aflatoxin B$_1$ binds to DNA and to ribosomal RNA in vivo[32] and with glutathione forms a conjugate.[33] The major DNA adduct formed by aflatoxin B$_1$ in rat liver in vivo, or with calf thymus DNA in vitro (in the presence of phenobarbital-stimulated rat liver microsomes and NADPH generating system) has been shown to produce on hydrolysis the 2,3-dihydro-2-(N^7-guanyl)-3-hydroxy-aflatoxin B$_1$ (Figure 3).[34-36] The same guanyl-derivative was obtained from DNA-aflatoxin B$_1$ adducts formed in cultures of animal and human liver, bronchus and colon tissues.[37,38] The microsomes-mediated binding of aflatoxin B$_1$ to DNA can be inhibited by glutathione-S-transferase.[39]

The substitution of the N^7-position in the guanyl moiety of nucleic acids has been shown to occur in vitro and in vivo with various alkylating agents.[40-43] However, the significance for the carcinogenic process of N^7-guanyl alkylation of nucleic acids has been questioned when it was found that N-[^{14}C]-methyl-N-nitrosourethane methylated in vivo nucleic acids of the liver more effectively than those of the stomach, though N-methyl-N-nitrosourethane does not usually induce liver tumors in rats.[41] Subsequently using other carcinogens similar results have been reported by several groups of workers.[42,43] The mechanism of the initiation of tumors by aflatoxins, as in the case of other carcinogens, remains still unknown and open to further investigations.

Though aflatoxin B_1 is an extremely effective liver carcinogen for the rat, other species differ widely in their sensitivity to its action, while mice are refractory except when treated very early in life.[44] It is of interest that no liver damage could be detected in a woman, 14 years after her ingestion of several doses of aflatoxin (corresponding to 1.5 mg/kg) in attempts to commit suicide.[45]

Human liver disorders are likely to be caused by more than one agent. Hepatotoxic and hepatocarcinogenic substances occur naturally also in plants, and include cycasin (see Chapter 5) and pyrrolizidine alkaloids (see Chapter 4 and Appendix 2).

Human pyrrolizidine alkaloids poisoning has been recently reported to occur in the U.S.A. as a result of treatment of childhood disorders with commercial "herbal teas", which included plants containing toxic pyrrolizidine alkaloids.[46-48]

Commercial preparations imported from Mexico and sold in Arizona by herbalists under the name of *gordolobo yerba,* supposing to consist of *Gnapholium* spp., have been found to consist of *Senecio longilobus* (a plant which closely resembles the former) and to contain high concentrations (about 2%) of hepatotoxic pyrrolizidine alkaloids. The victims included a 2-month-old boy, given gordolobo as a home remedy for colds, who initially has been considered to suffer from the Reye's syndrome.[47,48] The Reye's syndrome has often been correlated with aflatoxin poisoning,[26] but like many other disorders can be caused by various, unrelated agents.[49]

Similarly, primary liver cancer in Africa and southeast Asia has been suggested to be due to aflatoxins contaminating foodstuffs. However, in these parts of the world herbal medicines are used,[50] some of which include plants of the *Crotalaria, Heliotropium, Senecio, Trichodesma* and certain other species which may contain hepatotoxic and hepatocarcinogenic pyrrolizidine alkaloids.[51] Aflatoxin B_1 has been shown to act synergistically with monocrotaline (a pyrrolizidine alkaloid) in inducing liver tumors in rats.[52] The hepatocytes of rats fed diets containing aflatoxin B_1 develop resistance to its cytotoxic, but not to its hepatocarcinogenic action, possibly due to an increased content of reduced gluthathione in the liver.[53]

III. AZASERINE

Azaserine (O-diazoacetyl-L-serine) (Figure 4) was isolated in 1954 from cultures of *Streptomyces fragilis* as an antibiotic and tumor inhibitor,[54] and synthesizes soon after,[55] to be used for the treatment of childhood leukemias. Its LD_{50} is about 150 mg/kg b.w.; it induces lesions in the liver and pancreas.[56] Repeated injections (5 mg/kg b.w., i.p.) induced in Wistar rats benign and malignant tumors in the pancreas and in the kidneys.[57] Intravenous injections induced kidney lesions in dogs.[58] Azaserine given to rats during the middle of pregnancy caused high mortality and abnormalities in the fetuses.[59]

The natural occurrence of azaserine in agricultural products has not yet been reported.

Azaserine, like other cytotoxic agents, has a striking effect on NAD coenzymes; in mouse liver, NAD becomes depleted within 1 to 2 hr after a single s.c. dose (200 mg/kg).[60] The decrease of NAD occurs mainly in the cytosol — the nuclei, microsomes, and mitochondria are less affected.[60] The effects of azaserine can be to some extent prevented

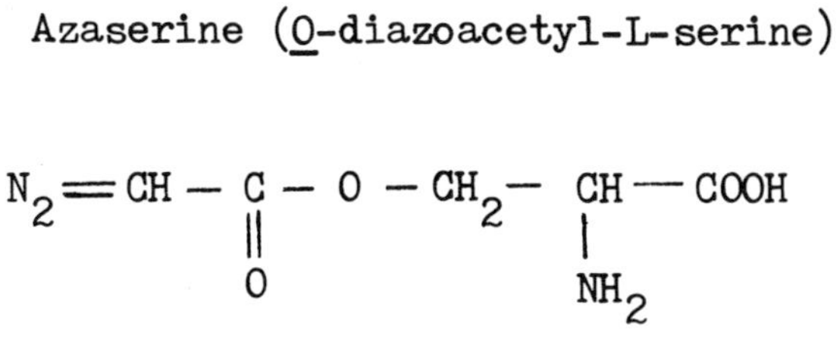

Azaserine (O-diazoacetyl-L-serine)

$$N_2 = CH - \underset{\underset{O}{\|}}{C} - O - CH_2 - \underset{\underset{NH_2}{|}}{CH} - COOH$$

FIGURE 4.   The structure of azaserine.

by pretreatment of the mice with nicotinamide; the nicotinamide moiety of the lost NAD is excreted in the form of the usual metabolites of nicotinamide, of which the proportion of N-methyl-nicotinamide is increased, but that of nicotinamide-N-oxide decreased.[61,62]

In isolated islets of Langerhans of the rat pancreas, azaserine causes depletion of NAD coenzymes and release of insulin; these effects can be prevented by nicotinamide.[63]

The role and fate of the adenosine-ribose moiety of the NAD coenzymes, lost by the action of azaserine, is not yet clear. As in the case of other carcinogenic agents which depress NAD, this moiety might be expected to undergo temporary polymerisation to poly (ADP-ribose), and then degradation into its constituent parts.[64]

Choline deficient diet made Wistar rats more susceptible to liver carcinogenesis by azaserine (repeated i.p. injections 30 mg/kg b.w.) and reduced its effect on the pancreas.[65]

A related compound 6-diazo-5-oxo-L-norleucine (DON), which was more effective as an antileukemic agent than azaserine[66] and also lowered NAD coenzymes in the mouse liver, would warrant testing for carcinogenic action.

IV. ELAIOMYCIN

Elaiomycin (4-methoxy-3-(1-octenyl-N-O-N-azoxy)-2-butanol) (Figure 5a) was isolated from cultures of *Streptomyces hepaticus* in the course of search for antibiotics in the laboratories of Park Davis & Co., and though it had tuberculostatic activity in vitro, it was not effective against experimental infections in mice or guinea pigs; moreover it caused liver damage.[67-70] Elaiomycin, like methylazoxymethanol (Figure 5c), the aglycon of cycasin[71] can induce in rodents, with one or a few doses, tumors benign and malignant of the liver, stomach, kidneys, brain, and thymus.[72-74] More recently another azoxy-compound was isolated in the Lederle Laboratories from cultures of *S. hinnulinus,* and is known as antibiotic LL-BH 872, 3R-1-hydroxy-3-(1'-cis-hexenyl-trans-azoxy)-2-butanone (Figure 5b).[75,76] Its long-term effects have not been reported, but the similarity of its structure to that of elaiomycin indicates the need to test it for carcinogenic activity. It is not yet known whether these azoxy-compounds occur in agricultural products. Screening of foodstuffs for their presence would be desirable.

V. OCHRATOXINS

Ochratoxins (Figure 6) are secondary metabolites of several *Aspergillus* and *Penicillium* species. They have been first isolated from cultures of a toxigenic *A. ochraceus* Wilh.,·in 1965 in South Africa,[77] where the structures of ochratoxin A, B, and C have been established[78] and confirmed by synthesis.[79]

Ochratoxin A is 7-carboxy-5-chloro-8-hydroxy-3, 4-dihydro-3-R-methyl isocoumarin amide of L-β-phenylalanine (Figure 6), ochratoxin B is its dechloro-derivative, while ochratoxin C is the ethyl-ester of ochratoxin A; all these isocoumarin compounds exhibit strong fluorescence, which is made use of in their detection and quantitation.

(a)

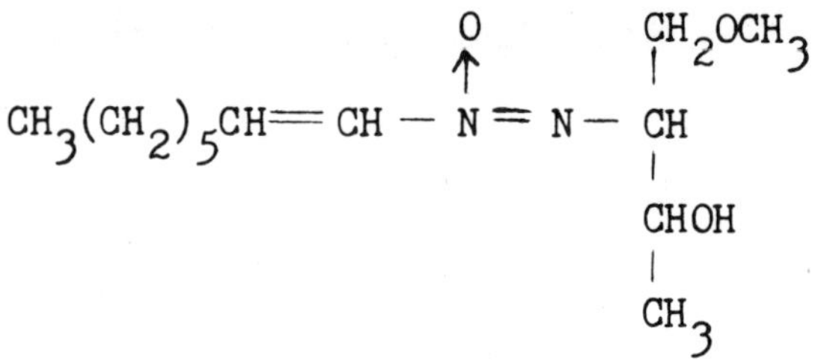

$$CH_3(CH_2)_5CH = CH - N \overset{\underset{\displaystyle \uparrow}{O}}{=} N - \underset{\underset{\displaystyle CH_3}{\overset{\displaystyle |}{CHOH}}}{\overset{\displaystyle CH_2OCH_3}{\overset{\displaystyle |}{CH}}}$$

(2$\underline{S}$,3$\underline{S}$)-4-methoxy-3-(1'-$\underline{cis}$-octenyl-$\underline{cis}$-azoxy)-2-butanol

Elaiomycin from <u>Streptomyces hepaticus</u>

(b)

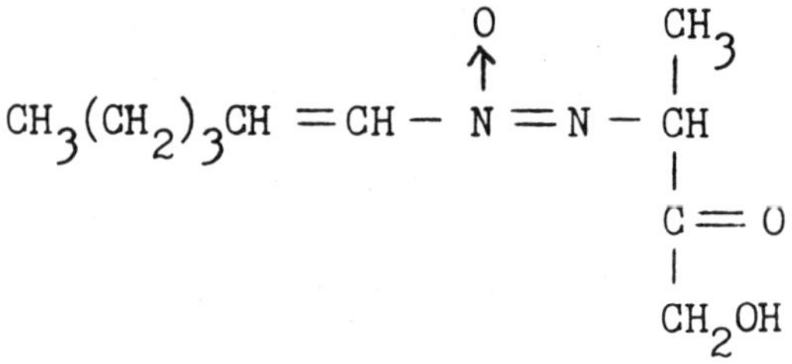

$$CH_3(CH_2)_3CH = CH - N \overset{\underset{\displaystyle \uparrow}{O}}{=} N - \underset{\underset{\displaystyle CH_2OH}{\overset{\displaystyle |}{C = O}}}{\overset{\displaystyle CH_3}{\overset{\displaystyle |}{CH}}}$$

(3$\underline{R}$)-1-hydroxy-3-(1'-$\underline{cis}$-hexenyl-$\underline{trans}$-azoxy)-2-butanone

Antibiotic LL-BH 872 from <u>Streptomyces hinnulinus</u>

(c)

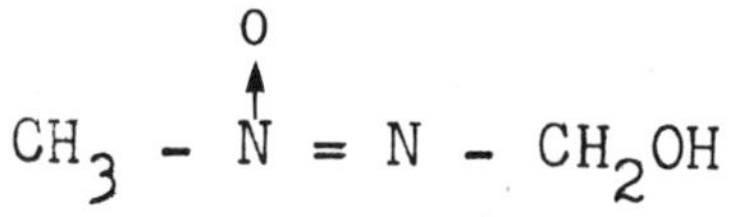

$$CH_3 - N \overset{\underset{\displaystyle \uparrow}{O}}{=} N - CH_2OH$$

Methylazoxymethanol

FIGURE 5.   The structures of elaiomycin, of antibiotic LL-BH 872, and of methylazoxymethanol.

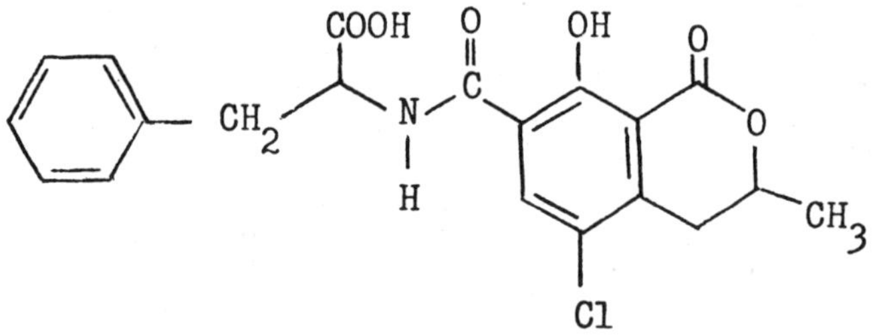

FIGURE 6.   The structure of ochratoxin A.

The chemistry, physical properties, occurrence, toxicology, teratogenicity, and the metabolism of ochratoxins have been reviewed;[80-84] the carcinogenic action of ochratoxin A in mice has only recently been reported[85] and warrants further studies.

Ochratoxin A, the most toxic of the naturally occurring compounds, is nephrotoxic and hepatotoxic for several animal species, including rodents,[86-90] fish (rainbow trout),[91,92] dogs,[93] poultry,[94-96] pigs,[97] and ruminants.[98] The LD_{50} of ochratoxin A depends on the species, age, sex, and the route of administration. Young animals and females are more susceptible than adult males. The sensitive species include pigs and poultry (LD_{50} below 6 mg/kg body weight), while rats and mice are more resistant, their LD_{50} are 2 to 3 times higher. For the rainbow trout the LD_{50} of ochratoxin A, by the intraperitoneal route, is about 5.3 mg/kg b.w., while that of its ethyl ester, ochratoxin C, is only 3 mg/ kg b.w.,[91] and that of ochratoxin B, the dechloroochratoxin, is more than 66.7 mg/kg b.w.[92] The acutely toxic effects include necrosis of the proximal tubules in the kidneys and necrosis of the periportal areas in the liver. On chronic exposure to nonfatal doses of the ochratoxins, the kidneys are the organs mainly affected, and develop structural and functional lesions, notably thickening of the tubular basement membrane, and interstitial fibrosis, causing polyuria, glucosuria, proteinuria, and increased excretion of a number of enzymes. The liver and the lymphoid tissues may also show lesions, but less specific.[84] When mice were given commercial diet to which crystalline ochratoxin A was added at a level of 40 ppm (40 mg/kg diet) for about 45 weeks, they developed hyperplastic lesions and tumors in the liver and kidneys.[85]

In certain areas of the Balkans (Bulgaria, Yugoslavia, and Rumania) the endemic incidence of nephropathies and of kidney tumors[99] is high. The possibility has been considered that these diseases may be related to the ingestion of food contaminated by ochratoxins[100] and other mycotoxins.[101] Estimation of ochratoxin A in cereals and meats showed higher levels in the areas affected by the endemic nephropathies than in control areas.[100]

Contamination with high levels of ochratoxin A has occasionally been detected in a proportion of examined samples of cereals, beans, stored peanuts, etc. in Canada,[102] and in oats and barley in Denmark (up to 27,500 ppb), especially when the grains caused disorders in livestock and were found moldy, contaminated by toxigenic species such as *A. ochraceus, P. viridicatum,* etc.[83]

Using ^{14}C labeled ochratoxin A, a large proportion of it has been found to be bound to serum albumin in blood, where it persists for several weeks. Ochratoxin A is partly excreted in the feces and urine unchanged, some undergoes metabolic hydroxylation at the carbon (4); some becomes hydrolyzed at the peptide bond to give L-β-phenylalanine and the isocourmarin moiety, known as ochratoxin α, which is not toxic.[103] The persistence of ochratoxin A in the blood of pigs at the time of slaughter has been used to evaluate the degree of contamination of their fodder with this mycotoxin in various parts of Sweden. A spectrophotometric procedure was used, based on the estimation of the decrease in the intensity of fluorescence at 380 nm, when ochratoxin A in the chloroform extract from pig's blood was hydrolyzed at 37°C for 2 hr by the enzymatic action of carboxypeptidase A in tris-(hydroxymethyl)-aminomethane-sulphuric acid buffer.[104]

Ochratoxin A from moldy fodder is carried over into various tissues of pigs. At slaughter of animals suffering from nephropathy the kidneys were found to contain the highest level of ochratoxin A, followed by the liver, the muscle, and the adipose tissue.[105] The Agricultural Board in Denmark issued instructions in 1978 to condemn the whole carcass, if at slaughter the pig's kidney contains more than 10 μg/kg of ochratoxin A. There appears to be a correlation between the content of ochratoxin A in the blood and the kidney (50 ng/mℓ in blood corresponds approximately to 10 ng/g in the kidneys).[104]

Pigs given ochratoxin A in the diet (1 mg/kg) for 2 years had pale and enlarged kidneys, but no tumors. Most of the kidneys showed focal damage of proximal tubules, hyalization of glomeruli, thickening of the basement membranes surrounding the atrophic tubules, and interstitial fibrosis. The tissues from the pigs which survived 2 years contained only small concentrations of ochratoxin A, which were similar to the concentrations found in the tissues of pigs killed after 3 months.[97] When large doses of ochratoxin A were given to cows, their milk contained some unchanged ochratoxin A and also ochratoxin α.[98]

However, the finding that ochratoxin A and B penetrated about 0.5 cm into a country cured ham from the surface-grown *A. ochraceus* points to the possibility of additional sources of contamination of food with these mycotoxins.[106] Ochratoxin A induced teratogenic effects when given during the middle of gestation to pregnant mice,[107] rats,[108,109] and hamsters.[110] Chick embryos, treated with ochratoxin A, also developed abnormalities.[111] A decrease of enzymatic activity in the kidneys was histochemically demonstrated to coincide with the sites of atrophy of the tubular epithelium.[112]

VI. PATULIN AND PENICILLIC ACID

A number of *Aspergillus, Byssochlamys,* and *Penicillium* species produce patulin (Figure 7) (synonyms: clavicin, clavatin, claviformin, expansin, penicidin, etc.), isolated (as an antibiotic) from cultures of *P. patulum*[113] and as claviformin from *A. giganteus* Wehm.[114] Patulin was intended to be used for the treatment of the common cold, but proved not effective and rather toxic.[115] Its LD_{50} depends on the route of entry, in rodents the LD_{50} by s.c. or i.p. administration being 10 mg/kg b.w. but higher when given orally.[116-118] The LD_{50} of patulin given intravenously to dogs was 10 mg/kg b.w.[119]

Patulin causes pulmonary edema, congestion, hemorrhages, and gastrointestinal and brain lesions. In long term tests, patulin induced sarcomas in rats at the site of repeated s.c. injections,[120] but no tumors have been induced in rats or mice when patulin was given orally[121] or intragastrically to rats in doses up to 1.5 mg/kg b.w., repeated three times weekly for 12 months.[122]

Patulin occurs naturally in many cereals, vegetables, meat, cheese, etc., also in fruits, especially apples contaminated by the "blue rot disease" caused by *P. expansum*.[123] Apple juice can contain up to 1000 ppm of patulin, but in the course of fermentation the levels of patulin decrease; cider has been reported to contain up to 45 ppm, depending on the method used for its preparation.[124]

Patulin was synthesised by Woodward; it contains an α,β-unsaturated lactone moiety.[125] The lactone group in patulin is readily opened by thiol-compounds to form various adducts, which are almost nontoxic. Long-term effects of the adducts are not known, but adducts with cysteine retained some teratogenic potential for the chick embryo.[126]

Penicillic acid (Figure 8) was isolated from cultures of *P. puberulum* Bainier and *P. cyclopium* Westling.[127] Penicillic acid occurs naturally in stored corn and other foodstuffs; levels up to 230 μg/kg have been reported.[128] Its acute toxicity to mice is not very high (LD_{50} 600 mg/kg b.w. orally and 250 mg/kg b.w. on i.v. injections).[129] On repeated s.c. injections, penicillic acid induced sarcomas in rats and in mice.[116,120] As an α,β-unsaturated lactone, penicillic acid behaves not unlike patulin, and reacts with thiol and amino-groups with loss of toxicity.[130] Penicillic acid increases the sensitivity of dogs to patulin on simultaneous injections, causing death from acute lung edema.[119]

A. Various Secondary Metabolites of Microorganisms

Among the many known secondary metabolites of microorganisms, only a few have been tested in pure form in long-term animal experiments. Evidence of potential carcin-

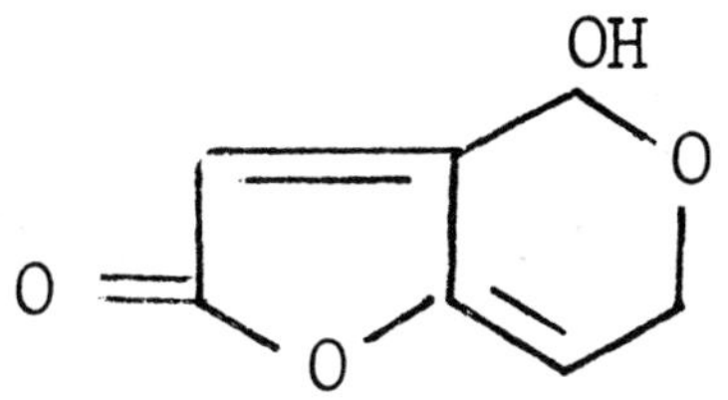

FIGURE 7. The structure of patulin.

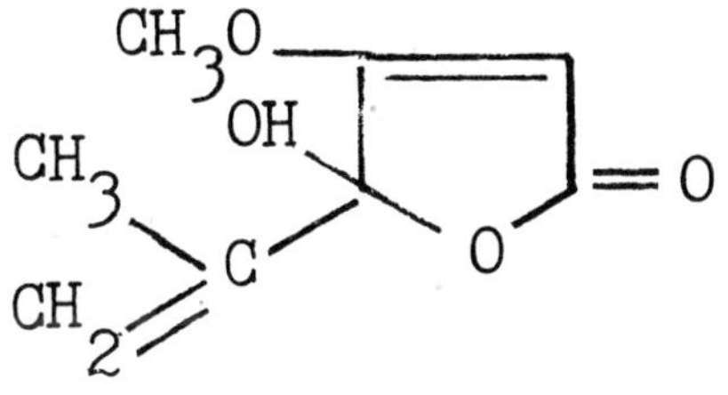

FIGURE 8. The structure of penicillic acid.

ogenicity have been reported for a number of compounds (Table 1). However, more data would be required in order to assess the potential hazards of several of these substances to human and animal health. It has been hoped that by testing the mutagenic activity of compounds, it would be possible to predict their carcinogenic potential. The methods so far used for this purpose have not yet proved sufficiently reliable to replace the expensive and time-consuming carcinogenicity tests in experimental animals, which remain essential for investigations of the induction and development of tumors.

VII. STERIGMATOCYSTIN

Sterigmatocystin (Figure 9) (3α, 12c-dihydro-8-hydroxy-6-methoxy-7H-furo[3',2':4,5] furo [2,3-c] xanthen-7-one), a secondary metabolite of *A. versicolor* (Vuillemin) Tiraboshi, of *Bipolaris* spp. and of certain other microfungi, was isolated from laboratory cultures and its structure established.[131-133] It has been found to occur naturally in wheat, peanuts, coffee beans, and on country cured hams, in levels of the order 1 ppm. However, cultures of *Bipolaris* on cornmeal have been found to give high yields (g/kg) of sterigmatocystin.[134,135] The strong fluorescence of sterigmatocystin and its derivatives allows its detection (from 0.01 μg) by thin layer chromatography and also by other methods.[136] Sterigmatocystin is about 20 to 200 times less toxic and less effective as carcinogen than aflatoxin B_1. It can induce liver tumors, benign and malignant, in rats on gastric intubation by feeding (1 to 10 ppm in the diet), by application to the skin, or by repeated s.c. injections[137-139] — and lung tumors in mice by feeding 5 ppm in diet.[140] In newborn mice, a single intraperitoneal injection induced tumors, mostly mesotheliomas.[141] Sterigmatocystin induced papillomas and epitheliomas when applied to the skin and sarcomas at the site of s.c. injections and mesotheliomas by i.p. injections in rats.[142]

Sterigmatocystin is eliminated by the rat mainly in the feces (about 70% of the dose within 12 hr),[143] but by vervet monkeys as a glucuronide in the urine.[144]

As in the case of aflatoxin B_1, the isolated double bond of the bifuranoid moiety of sterigmatocystin appears to undergo epoxidation and to form an adduct with DNA in vitro (in the presence of liver microsomal fraction from phenobarbital treated rats and NADPH-generating system). On hydrolysis the adduct gave a derivative identified as

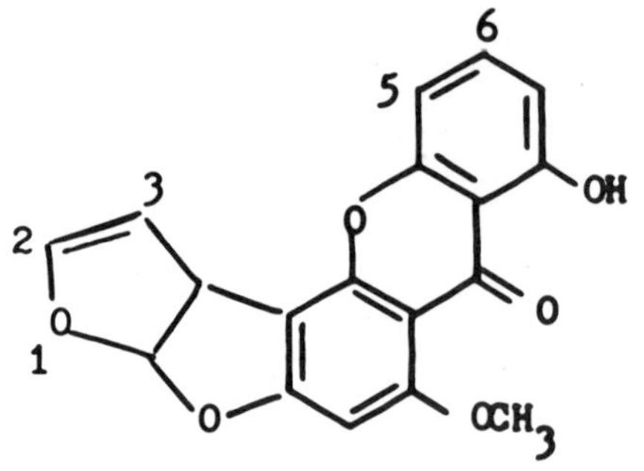

FIGURE 9.   The structure of sterigmatocystin.

1, 2-dihydro-2-(N^7-guanyl)1-hydroxysterigmatocystin.[145] The significance for the initiation of tumors of the substitution of guanine in DNA is not clear.

Sterigmatocystin has been shown to be a precursor of aflatoxin B_1 in cultures of *A. parasiticus*.[146]

The reported formation of sterigmatocystin on bread (but not on rye bread)[147] indicates the need for more studies of this mycotoxin, which may be of no less importance than aflatoxins in relation to human liver tumors.

VIII. STREPTOZOTOCIN

Steptozotocin (Figure 10), a 2-desoxy-D-glucose derivative of *N*-methyl-*N*-nitrosourea, a secondary metabolite of *Streptomyces achromogenes,* was isolated as antibiotic and antitumor agent in the laboratories of Upjohn Company,[148] where its structure was established.[149] Streptozotocin is diabetogenic and can induce tumors of the pancreas and the kidneys in rats[150-152] and liver tumors in the Chinese hamsters.[153] A single dose, 65 mg/kg b.w. (or less), is effective in inducing diabetes due to lesions in the pancreatic islet cells which become depleted of NAD coenzymes.[154,155] Pretreatment with nicotinamide (350 mg/kg b.w.) will prevent the diabetic lesions, allow better survival of the animals, and increase the incidence of pancreatic tumors.[156,157] Using [^{14}C-methyl]-streptozotocin, it has been shown by the elegant method of whole body autoradiography that its radioactivity concentrates and is retained in the mouse pancreatic islet-cells at a higher level than in other organs.[158] Using [^{14}C]-labeled nicotinamide, nicotinic acid, and tryptophan, it has been found by a similar autoradiograhic procedure that the mouse pancreatic islets take up only nicotinamide, which explains its ability to prevent diabetes by streptozotocin.[159] Investigations on the natural occurrence of streptozotocin in agricultural products would be desireable, as well as epidemiological studies on whether the increase of the incidence of human pancreatic tumors[160] may be related to the high protein and high B-vitamins diet in the U.S.A.

Streptozotocin has been used for the treatment of human insulinomas and certain other tumors. In the treated patients nephrotoxic effects related to streptozotocin have been observed, as have occasional neoplastic kidney lesions.[1606]

IX. T-2 TOXIN

T-2 toxin (Figure 11) (3α-hydroxy-4β,15-diacetoxy-8α-(3-methylbutyryloxy)-12, 13-epoxy-trichothec-9-en) belongs to a group of about four dozen tetracyclic sesquiterpenoid compounds, known as trichothecenes,[161] in recognition of the fact that the first member of this group was trichothecin, isolated from cultures of *Trichothecium roseum,*

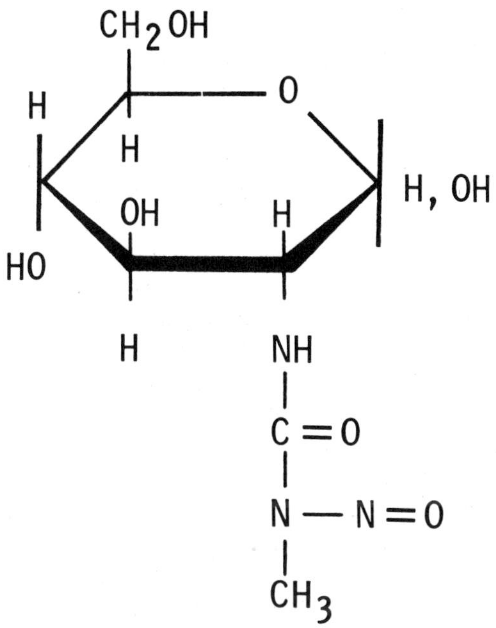

FIGURE 10. The structure of streptozotocin.

T - 2 Toxin: $R^1 = H$; $R^2 = R^3 = CH_3 CO$; $R^4 = (CH_3)_2 CHCH_2CO$

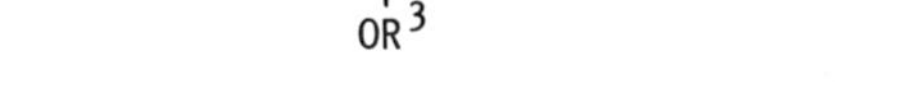

FIGURE 11. The structure of T-2 toxin.

in the course of a search for antibiotics.[162] The features of the trichothecenes responsible for their toxicity are the isolated double bond at C-9, 10, the epoxy-ring on C-12,13, and the presence of at least some esterified alcoholic hydroxyls. In T-2 toxin three of its four hydroxyls are esterified, two by acetic acid moieties at C-4,15, and one at C-8 by that of 3-methylbutyric acid.

T-2 toxin was first isolated from cultures of *Fusarium tricinctum,* a toxigenic contaminant of moldy corn, which caused cattle losses in Wisconsin from a hemorrhagic syndrome.[163] At a subsequent outbreak of similar hemorrhagic syndrome among cattle in Wisconsin, T-2 toxin was found to occur naturally in the moldy corn, at a level of approximately 2 ppm.[164] T-2 toxin has been detected in moldy fodder also in other outbreaks of similar mycotoxicoses in livestock in several countries including Canada,[165,166] Hungary,[167] Japan,[168] Scotland,[169] and the U.S.[170]

T-2 toxin has been identified as a constituent of "poaefusarin", obtained from cultures of *F. poae* in the U.S.S.R.[170] It has been isolated together with some of its hydrolysis products, HT-2 toxin and neosolaniol, from cultures of *F. sporotrichioides,*[171] which together with *F. poae* was identified as being involved in an outbreak of disorders among the human population of the Orenburg district in the U.S.S.R. during World War II, the people of which consumed bread made from moldy millet. These often fatal disorders came to be known as "alimentary toxic aleukia" (ATA) or "septic angina".[172-174]

Steroidal fractions obtained from cultures of these *Fusarium* species reproduced some features of ATA;[175] recently workers in the U.S.S.R., however, have confirmed that the toxicity of *F. sporotrichiella* cultures was due to their content of trichothecenes, consisting mainly of T-2 toxin, HT-2 toxin, and neosolaniol.[176]

Pure T-2 toxin reproduced in cats some of the features of ATA, including the characteristic leukopenia.[177,178] T-2 toxin is one of the most toxic among the trichothecenes.

The trichothecenes, their chemistry, their relative acute and chronic toxicities, and other aspects of their effects on animals in vivo, and on isolated cells in vitro, have been reviewed.[179-184] A recent bibliography already lists 2978 references.[185]

In long term experiments, T-2 toxin induced in the digestive tract of white Wistar rats lesions and tumors (benign and malignant), which included ulcers and adenocarcinomas of the stomach and duodenum, multiple pancreatic tumors (of the acinar and islet cells), and also brain tumors and cardiovascular lesions (Figures 12 to 23).

The neoplastic lesions were found in rats, which survived more than a year after the first of a few, relatively large, intragastric doses of T-2 toxin. In experiments in which rats were killed 8 months after the start of feeding them with diets containing 5 to 15 ppm of T-2 toxin, no neoplastic lesions have been seen.[187]

As it is now established that cultures of *F. sporotrichiella* Bilai var *poae* (Pk) Bilai contain T-2 toxin and some of its hydrolysis products, it is of interest that papillomas with hyperkeratoses in the squamous part of the rat's forestomach have been reported previously;[188] various lesions in the esophagus and in the squamous part of the rat stomach, the pancreas, and other organs have been induced in rats by crude alcoholic extracts from *F. poae* and *F. sporotrichioides.*[189]

T-2 toxin does not appear to require metabolic activation by specific liver enzymes and is not hepatotoxic. It exerts direct cytotoxic action on several types of cells, including the endothelial cells lining the arteries, as evidenced by the thickening of the arterial walls in some of the rats surviving large doses of T-2 toxin (Figures 21 to 23).[186] Synergistic effects on the acute toxicity was observed when the treatment with T-2 toxin was combined with that of aflatoxin B_1 in mice.[190]

It is not yet known whether the carcinogenic action is due to T-2 toxin per se, or whether some of its metabolic products play a role in this process. Low incidence of tumors was found in rats given in diet, fusarenon-X as well as in their controls.[190a]

Like most trichothecenes, T-2 toxin is not mutagenic in in vitro tests, without and with fraction S-9,[191,192] but is radiomimetic.[193] It can inhibit the synthesis of proteins and DNA and exerts its cytotoxic effects on actively proliferating cells. T-2 toxin and certain other trichothecenes cause similar acute and subacute effects in a number of animal species including: cats, mice, rats, guinea pigs, cattle, pigs, dogs, monkeys, chicken, turkeys, geese, trout, and man.

Direct evidence as regards the toxic effects of trichothecenes in humans has been obtained from Phase I and II treatment of cancer patients with diacetoxyscirpenol (Anguidine, NSC-141537) given intravenously (4.5 mg/M^2 to 6 mg/M^2) daily for 5 days and repeated after intervals.[194] The effects on the tumors were mainly disappointing; the toxic effects included "nausea, vomiting, phlebitis, erythema of skin, confusion, mental obtundation, hypotension, chills, fever, diarrhea, stomatitis, alopecia, blurred

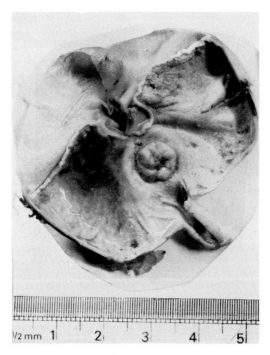

FIGURE 12. · Stomach showing a nodule on the glandular part. Male rat killed 24.5 months after the first and 8 months after the last of 5 doses of T-2 toxin. (Magnification × 1.28.) (From Schoental, R., Joffe, A. Z., and Yagen, B., *Cancer Res.,* 39, 2179, 1979. With permission.)

vision, ataxia, and weakness."[195] Myelosuppression, cardiovascular, gastrointestinal, and CNS symptoms were common.

Radiolabeled [3-^{3}H]-T-2 toxin has been synthesized, with specific activity 790 mCi/ mmol.[196] Using this tritium labeled preparation, a number of metabolites were detected in the excreta of broiler chicken, including T-2 toxin, HT-2 toxin, deacetyl HT-toxin (triol), neosolaniol, 4-deacetyl neosolaniol, and T-2 tetraol, each in amounts corresponding to less than, or about 1% of the administered dose. An additional eight metabolites as yet unidentified, have also been detected, and these represented the greater part of the administered dose, 80% of which was excreted within 48 hr after dosing.[197]

Though the epoxide ring in the trichothecenes is sterically hindered, it will react enzymically with thiol groups, e.g. of the reduced glutathione in the presence of glutathione-*S*-transferase.[198] Monodeacetyl nivalenol has been reported to bind to the active site of alcohol dehydrogenase, which contains four thiol groups in the active center and binds four molecules of this trichothecene.[199] Trichothecenes have been shown to inhibit protein and DNA synthesis in rabbit reticulocytes, Ehrlich ascites cells, protozoa, etc.[193] More recently T-2 toxin and HT-2 toxin have both been found to inhibit the incorporation of tritiated thymidine also into DNA of human fibroblasts in vitro.[200] The mechanism of the cytotoxic and carcinogenic action of trichothecenes requires further investigation.

X. ZEARALENONE

Zearalenone (Figure 24 [2]) (6-[10-hydroxy-6-oxo-trans-1-undecenyl]-β-resorcylic acid lactone), a metabolite of *F. graminearum, (Gibberella zeae),* a common contaminant

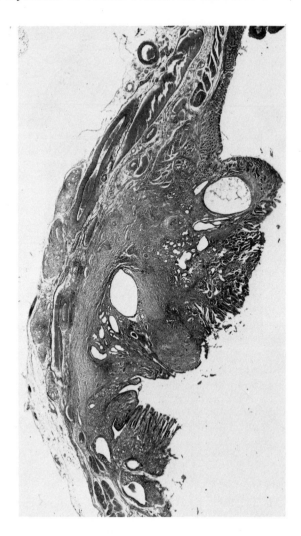

FIGURE 13.   Section through the nodule of the stomach in Figure 12, showing adenocarcinoma penetrating through the muscular layer. (H.&E.; magnification × 15.) (From Schoental, R., Joffe, A. Z., and Yagen, B., *Cancer Res.,* 39, 2179, 1979. With permission.)

of cereals (and of a number of other *Fusarium* species), was isolated as a result of a search for estrogenic agent(s) responsible for sporadic outbreaks of hyperestrogenism among pigs consuming moldy feed. Such pigs showed "vulvar hypertrophy and occasional vaginal eversion in females, preputial enlargment in castrated males, and prominent mammary glands in both sexes".[201] According to Stob et al., the active principle in the moldy feed was effective in improving growth rate and feed efficiency in sheep.[201] This presented a possibility for the use of zearalenone (or its derivatives) as anabolic agents in animal husbandry to replace diethylstilbestrol (DES). The structure of zearalenone as been established;[202] it has been synthesized by several groups of workers[203-207] as well as a number of its derivatives and analogs.

F. graminearum Schwabe, grown on maize (45% moisture) for about 10 weeks at 12°C, produces, besides zearalenone, four additional metabolites: 5-formylzearalenone, 7'-dehydrozearalenone, and the two epimeric 8'-hydroxyzearalenones.[208] Zearalenol, the

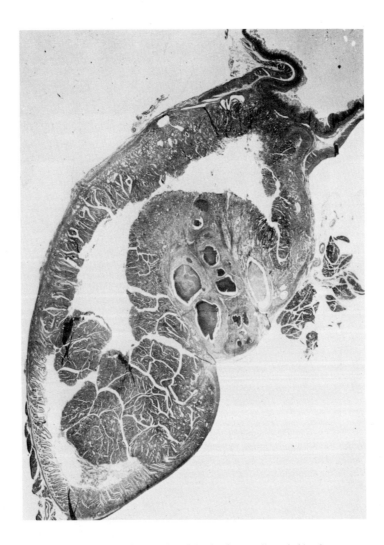

FIGURE 14. Longitudinal section of the duodenum, distended by the presence of an ulcerated papillary adenocarcinoma penetrating the serosa. Female rat killed 21 months after the first and 4 months after the last of five doses of T-2 toxin. (H. & E.; magnification × 6.) (From Schoental, R., Joffe, A. Z., and Yagen, B., *Cancer Res.*, 39, 2179, 1979. With permission.)

α isomer of the reduction products of zearalenone, has been reported in animal feeds.[209] Its levels 1.5, 4.0, and 0.15 mg/kg were only a fraction of those of zearalenone present in the two samples of oats, 25 mg/kg and 135 mg/kg, and in one of corn, 18 mg/kg, respectively. The estrogenic activity of α zearalenol is about three times higher than that of zearalenone; the contribution of zearalenol present in cereals to the biological effects may not be negligible.[209] Other minor metabolites of *F. roseum (graminearum)* include 6',8'-dihydroxyzearalenone,[210] two 3'-hydroxyzearalenones, and some other unidentified compounds.[211]

Another isolate, *F. roseum* "Gibbosum", produced optimally zearalenone when grown at temperatures 20 to 25°C on parboiled polished rice of 53 to 60% moisture for more than 9 days, and has been used for the preparation of [^{14}C]-labeled zearalenone with high specific activity, 1.63 to 46.5 μCi/mmol from [^{14}C]-acetate.[212]

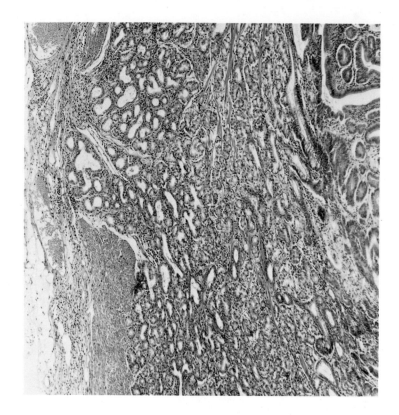

FIGURE 15.   Higher magnification of the adenocarcinoma from Figure 14, showing the site of its penetration through the muscle layer. (H. & E.; magnification
× 60.) (From Schoental, R., Joffe, A. Z., and Yagen, B., *Cancer Res.*, 39, 2179,
1979. With permission.)

A number of review articles have been published which deal with the chemistry of
zearalenone and some of its derivatives and analogs, with its biosynthesis, and with the
biological effects of zearalenone and certain related compounds.[213-219]

The detection and estimation of zearalenone among the various other mycotoxins,
which are usually present in moldy cereals and in other feeds and foodstuffs, is a difficult
problem. The various procedures used for the "clean-up" of crude extracts and for thinlayer chromatography (TLC) have been reviewed[220] and additional improvements described.[221,222] Attention has been drawn to the possibility of mistaking the methyl ether
of alternariol for zearalenone on TLC.[223]

Gas chromatography/mass spectrometry, as well as high pressure liquid chromatography, have also been in use,[224] and the sensitivity of detection of zearalenone apparently
increased to 2 μg/kg.[225] The biological method for the detection of uterotrophic activity,
though not specific for zearalenone and its estrogenic derivatives, is very valuable.[226]
However, the presence of T-2 toxin in the extracts could abolish the response to the
estrogenic agents present, and under such conditions the biological test can be mislead-
ing.[226-228]

The acute oral toxicity of zearalenone for the rat is very low, exceeding 16 g/kg body
weight. Subacute and chronic effects in rats and in their progeny have been reported,
mostly in abstracts. Inclusion of zearalenone in diet at levels of 0, 0.1, 1.0, and 10 mg/
kg body weight showed that the "only no effect level was 0.1 mg/kg." "Adverse effects
of zearalenone were reduced fertility and reproductive ability, increased numbers of
resorptions and stillborn fetuses and increased medullary trabeculae in bone".[229]

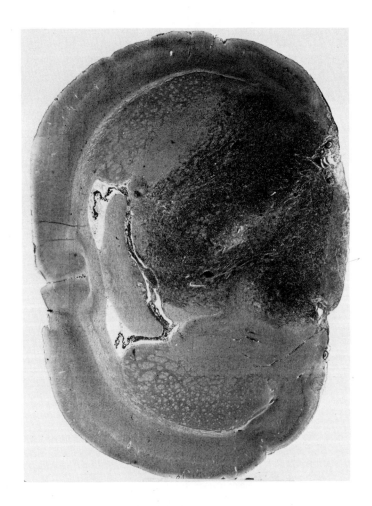

FIGURE 16.   Section of brain with a large tumor in a frontal lobe. Male rat killed 12.5 months after the first and 1 month after the last of eight doses of T-2 toxin given in conjunction with nicotinamide treatment. (H. & E.; magnification × 5.) (From Schoental, R., Joffe, A. Z., and Yagen, B., *Cancer Res.*, 39, 2179, 1979. With permission.)

Carcinogenic effects of the estrogenic zearalenone have not yet been published. In experiments still in progress, exposing rodents to large doses of zearalenone, chronic lesions and neoplasias in the target organs have been found.[228] Natural contamination of cereals with zearalenone can exceed 10 mg/kg and occasionally levels of more than 100 mg/kg have been reported.[230] The frequency of contamination of maize with zearalenone in southern Ontario, Canada, correlated with rainy weather conditions especially during August.[231]

When rats were given zearalenone by intragastric intubation 1, 0, 5.0, and 10.0 mg/kg/day on days 6 to 15 of gestation, skeletal abnormalities were found in some of the fetuses. The incidence of malformations increased with the dosage level from 12.8% at 1.0 mg/kg to 36.8% at 10 mg/kg.[232]

In mice significant transplacental effects on the survival of the fetuses were observed after doses of a synthetic derivative of zearalenol exceeding 1 mg/kg b.w., given by subcutaneous injections between the 10th and 16th day of gestation.[233]

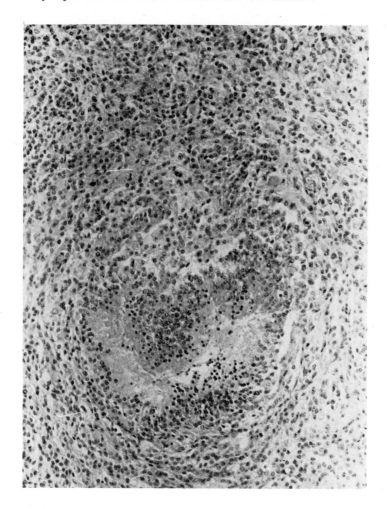

FIGURE 17.   Higher magnification of the neuroblastoma shown in Figure 16. (H. & E.; magnification × 120.) (From Schoental, R., Joffe, A. Z., and Yagen, B., *Cancer Res.*, 31, 2179, 1979. With permission.)

For the induction of tumors in rodents, it is known that relatively high doses of estrogenic substances, whether the physiological hormones or synthetic preparations, are needed.

Pigs are more sensitive to the estrogenic action of zearalenone. It has been estimated that a pig, which consumes daily 2 kg of feed, will develop abnormalities of sex organs within 8 days when 80% of the ration consists of moldy maize containing 0.6 ppm zearalenone.[231,234] This would indicate that zearalenone in doses of approximately 1 mg/pig/day might cause signs of hyperestrogenism.

The naturally occurring zearalenone is uterotrophic and estrogenic.[219] It becomes reduced to the more active zearalenol by the liver enzyme system, α-hydroxy-steroid dehydrogenase (which reduces steroids to estrogens) (Figure 24 [1]), and in part, conjugated to the respective glucuronide.[235-237] In the target tissues, the uterus, and the mammary glands, zearalenol becomes bound by the cytoplasmic estrogen receptors which transport it to the nucleus, where it binds to the same nuclear receptors as the physiological hormone.[238-240] This competitive binding to the receptors of the physiological estrogens is characteristic of many substances which have estrogenic activity regardless

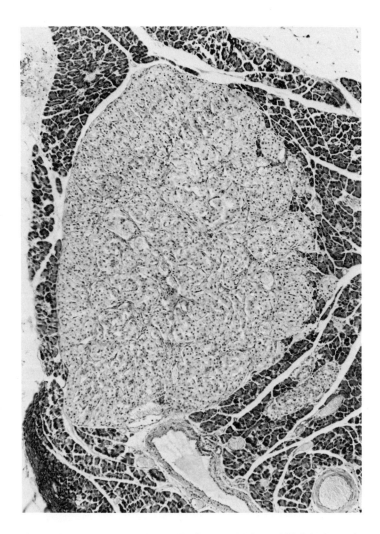

FIGURE 18.   Pancreatic islet cell adenoma. Male rat killed 23.5 months after the first and 13 months after the last of eight doses of T-2 toxin given in conjunction with nicotinamide treatment. (H. & E.; magnification × 70.) (From Schoental, R., Joffe, A. Z., and Yagen, B., *Cancer Res.*, 39, 2179, 1979. With permission.)

of their chemical structures (some are shown in Figure 24) and can be demonstrated not only in animals but also in human breast cancer cells, cultured in vitro.[241,242] The biological activity of the various estrogenic substances, whether natural or synthetic, depends on the presence, or on the biochemical formation in the course of their metabolism, of the two hydroxyls at the ends of their molecules, at a distance between 10 to 11 Å, and of the appropriate conformation.[217,218]

The estrogenic efficacy of the various compounds varies greatly[243] (Table 3). The oral doses of equivalent estrogenic potency vary by a factor of more than 100,000.

Zearalenone stimulates the biosynthesis of macromolecules, proteins, and nucleic acids in the uterus[244] and in other target organs, but excessive doses can lead to sterility and degeneration of genital organs in both males and females.

A teratogenic action and transplacental induction of tumors by estrogenic agents in humans has been known since the astute observations by Herbst and his colleagues,[245,246]

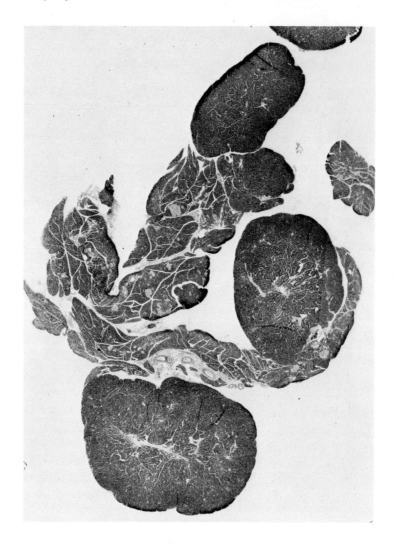

FIGURE 19.   Pancreas with multiple nodules of exocrine adenocarcinoma. Male rat killed 22 months after the first and 11 months after the last of seven doses of T-2 toxin. (H. & E.; magnification × 10.) (From Schoental, R., Joffe, A. Z., and Yagen, B., *Cancer Res.,* 39, 2179, 1979. With permission.)

who correlated the finding of vaginal tumors in girls and in young women with the medication of their mothers for threatened abortion with relatively large doses of synthetic estrogens. This treatment is now known to have induced abnormalities and tumors of sex organs not only among the female, but also among the male offspring resulting from such pregnancies.[247-249] Similar results would be expected to follow transplacental exposure to large equiestrogenic doses of other estrogenic agents including zearalenone and its analogs.

The synthetic zeranol (under the name of Frideron[250]) is now being used in oral contraceptives and as an anabolic in animal husbandry; equiestrogenic dosage should be compared when considering the respective roles of the various estrogenic agents in the induction of tumors in the target organs. Estrogens differ from other carcinogens in the mechanism by which they induce tumors, which is more akin to that of cocarcinogenic agents.[251] Regardless of the mode of action of estrogenic agents, it is worth pointing out

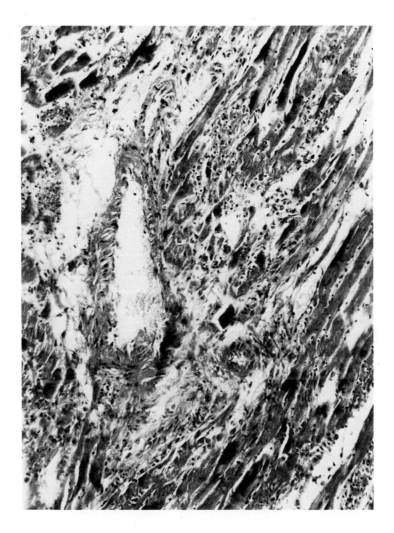

FIGURE 20.   Section of heart showing degeneration of the muscle fibers, cellular infiltration, and fibrosis. Male rat died 24 months after the first and 8 months after the last of five doses of T-2 toxin. (Phosphotungstic Mallory (PM); Magnification × 125.) (From Schoental, R., Joffe A. Z., and Yagen, B., *Cancer Res.*, 39, 2179, 1979. With permission.)

that the carcinogenic effects of oral contraceptives became epidemiologically discernible only about 20 years after their introduction and wide use; the high and geographically variable incidence of "idiopathic" tumors of sex organs makes it difficult to attribute small increases to particular causative agents. Zearalenone and its congeners have probably been responsible for many of the abnormalities and tumors of sex organs that have afflicted men and women (as well as animals) from time immemorial. It appears imperative to develop appropriate preventive measures in order to minimize the natural contamination of foodstuffs with *Fusaria* and their metabolites, for the sake of future generations.[252] Deliberate increase of the intake of estrogenic agents for inessential reasons is to be greatly deplored.

Oral contraceptives (especially their estrogenic components) have been shown to increase the retinol binding protein and the plasma concentration of vitamin A;[253,254] they depress the levels of pyridoxine, folic acid, and vitamin C.[255] In order to restore the levels

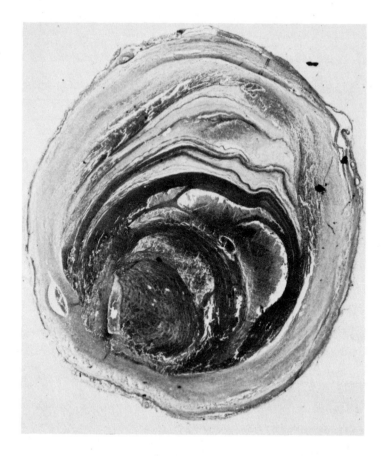

FIGURE 21.   Cross section of the coronary artery greatly distended and partly occluded by fibrinoid swelling of collagen. Male rat killed 21.5 months after the first and 10.5 months after the last of seven doses of T-2 toxin. (PM; magnification × 13.) (From Schoental, R., Joffe, A. Z., and Yagen, B., *Cancer Res.,* 39, 2179, 1979. With permission.)

of the water soluble vitamins to normal, about tenfold higher intake of these vitamins than usually recommended appears necessary.[255]

It would be of interest to investigate the effects of zearalenone and of its estrogenic derivatives (as well as other mycotoxins) on the various vitamin levels in relation to coenzymes, to the permeability of cellular membrane, etc. Mycotoxins may be contributing factors to the vitamin deficiencies observed among populations, especially in the developing countries.

XI. THE EFFECTS OF MYCOTOXINS ON IMMUNITY

Many carcinogens can affect the immune processes in the body.[256-258] Certain carcinogenic mycotoxins have been shown to impair immunity in experimental animals and livestock, cause involution of the thymus, affect the antibody formation, phagocytosis, production of interferon, etc.[259] This has been shown in the case of aflatoxins,[260,261] ochratoxin A,[262] diacetoxyscirpenol,[263] T-2 toxin,[264-266] and the trichothecenes responsible for stachybotryotoxicosis,[267-268] which include the macrocyclic satratoxin.[269] The possibility has been suggested that impairment of immune processes by aflatoxins and acti-

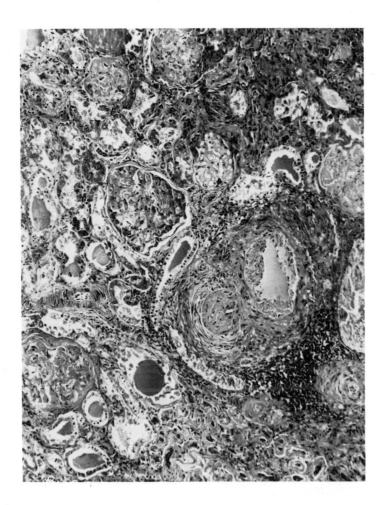

FIGURE 22.   Section of a kidney from the same rat as Figure 20 showing the
thick-walled, almost occluded arteries, degeneration of most of the renal elements, casts, fibrosis, and cellular infiltration. (H. & E.; magnification × 115.)
(From Schoental, R., Joffe, A. Z., and Yagen, B., *Cancer Res.,* 39, 2179, 1979.
With permission.)

vation of the endemic hepatitis-B virus, might explain the distribution of primary liver
cancer in humans in Africa, Southeast Asia, and elsewhere.[270]

Immunosuppression by mycotoxins can present serious problems in relation to bacterial
and viral diseases in livestock and man,[271] and requires further studies.

The immunosuppressive trichothecenes may play a role in relation to digestive tract
neoplasias in animals and man,[272] and may possibly be responsible for the activation of
some common viruses, e.g., the Epstein-Barr virus.[273]

The relations between the immunological functions, disease, and nutritional deficiencies are complex and show some inconsistencies.[274] Reduction of food intake (calories)
often appears to have favorable effects on the immunological responses, and on the
survival of mice.[274] The incidence of "spontaneous" adenocarcinomas in C3H/Umc mice
has been reported to decrease following caloric restrictions.[275] However, with reduction
of food intake, the amount of ingested carcinogenic contaminants, which may be present
in the animal diets (e.g., in the fat) will also decrease, and will affect the incidence of
tumors. This may explain the decrease in the incidence of "spontaneous" tumors reported

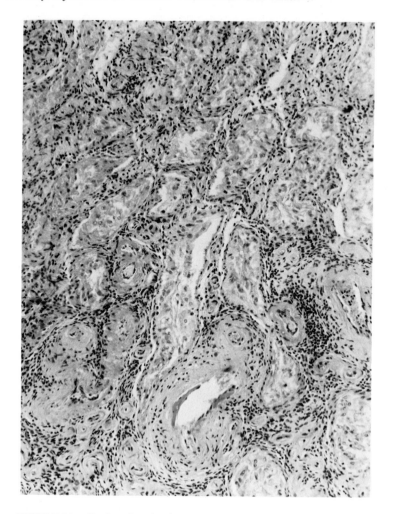

FIGURE 23.   Section of testis of the same rat as Figures 20 and 22, showing thick-walled partly occluded arteries, cellular infiltration, and degeneration. (H. & E.; magnification × 115.)(From Schoental, R., Joffe, A. Z., and Yagen, B., *Cancer Res.,* 39, 2179, 1979. With permission.)

in C3H-A^{vy} mice, when these were bred in Australia, and did not grow as large as when bred in the National Cancer Institute in the United States.[276]

XII. THE ROLE OF VITAMINS AND COENZYMES IN THE CYTOTOXIC AND CARCINOGENIC ACTION OF MYCOTOXINS

As yet no satisfactory explanation exists regarding the mechanism by which carcinogens can initiate tumors which may become apparent a long time after exposure to such agents.

Carcinogenic chemicals, like other xenobiotics, undergo stepwise metabolic degradation by more than one pathway in the animal body, with the formation of various intermediates which depend on the chemical structure of the particular agent, and on the enzymic endowment of the individual.

Carcinogens are usually divided into those which induce tumors at the site of application (usually known as proximate carcinogens, but should be referred to as *topocar-*

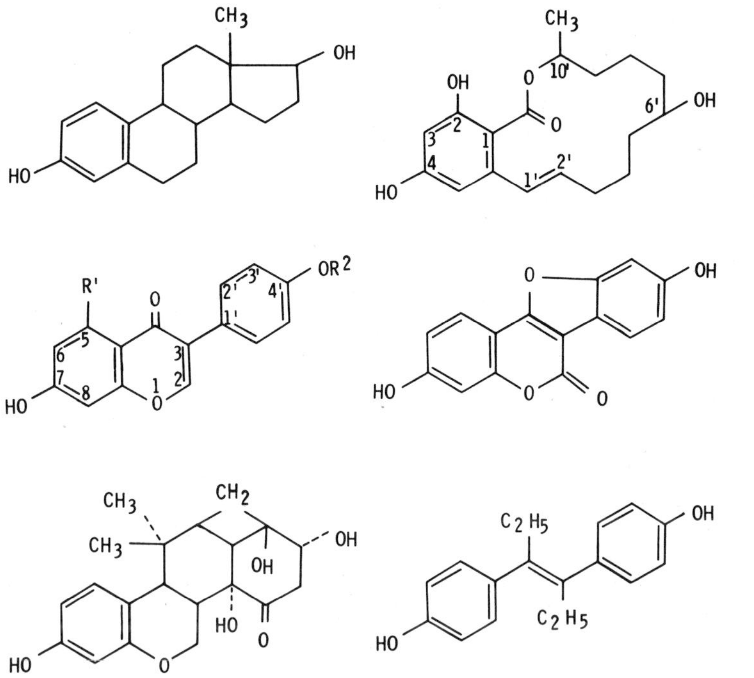

FIGURE 24. The structures of estrogenic agents. (1) estradiol-17-β ; (2) zearalenol; (3a) genistein, R_1 = OH; R_2 = H; (3b) biochanin A, R_1 = OH; R_2 = CH$_3$; (3c) daidzein, R_1 = H; R_2 = H; (3d) formononetin, R_1 = H; R_2 = CH$_3$; (4) coumestrol; (5) mirestrol; (6) diethylstilbestrol.

Table 3
RELATIVE ESTROGENIC ACTIVITY OF
ESTROGENIC COMPOUNDS (ON ORAL DOSING)

Zearalenone	100
Estrone	6,900
Zearalenol–α	200—300
Estradiol-17–β	10,000—20,000
Diethylstilbestrol	100,000
Coumestrol	35
Genistein	1
Daidzein	0.75
Biochanin A	0.46
Formononetin	0.26

cinogens) and those which induce mainly liver tumors and undergo activation in the liver cells. The induction of tumors at the site of application does not imply, however, that the parent compound is active per se, but indicates that the carcinogenic entity can be formed by biochemical processes operating in the affected cells.

The nature of the carcinogenic entities and the cellular constituents which are involved in the initiation of the carcinogenic process are still a matter of conjecture.

It had been assumed that alkylation (substitution of a hydrogen by a monofunctional alkylating entity) of nucleic acids, mainly DNA, may be related to the carcinogenic process. Many carcinogens form alkylating entities able to substitute reactive positions in certain amino acids of proteins and in purines, pyrimidines, and phosphate-ester moieties of nucleic acids in the tissues of the treated animals.[40,277,278]

However, the relevance of such "alkylations" (most extensively studied using various carcinogenic nitroso compounds) to the carcinogenic process is not clear.[279] Similarly alkylated species have been isolated from nucleic acids of tissues which develop tumors as a result of treatment with the respective agent, and also from tissues which remain free from neoplasias.[41-43] Moreover, the "alkylated" nucleic acids do not persist in the tissues, but mostly disappear within days or weeks; excision of the alkylated moieties and repair of the nucleic acids follows, and appears to be complete as far as it is possible to detect by the methods at present available.[278-280]

Another type, addition reactions, in which di- or more functional entities derived from the parent carcinogens bridge apposite reactive sites of cell's constituents, have been considered.[281,282] Such reactions, being more exclusive, may explain better than simple alkylations the rarity in molecular terms of the interactions which lead to an irreversible carcinogenic process. Like in the case of estrogenic agents, the particular reactive groups in the carcinogenic species probably have to be at an appropriate distance and of certain configuration to fit into a tridimensional space and to react with the appropriate apposite receptor groups.

The carcinogenic entities probably simulate some physiological metabolites and act as antimetabolites, and once attached to cell constituents, might not readily be dislocated or "digested" — hence would "stick" and remain *in situ*. When tissue homogenates are fractionated, such structures are likely to remain among the insoluble debris, hence are difficult to study.[283]

As for the carcinogenic mycotoxins, their structures suggest that they might be metabolized to polyfunctional intermediates. The aflatoxins and the sterigmatocystins have reactive carbonyl groups besides the epoxidisable bonds in the bifuranoid parts of their structures; the trichothecenes have, besides the 12,13-epoxide ring, an allylic methyl group, which on oxidation via hydroxymethyl, would yield an aldehydic function; the same would apply to the methyl group in streptozotocin, to the side chain in elaiomycin, etc., which are potential sites of reactive functional groups, in addition to the already present nitroso- or azoxy-functions. Methylazoxymethanol, the aglycone of cycasin, could be considered a model compound, which on dehydrogenation by the action of NADPH dependent alcohol dehydrogenase forms methylazoxymethanal.[281,284,285] The action of methylazoxymethanol has been shown to be modified by pyrazole, disulfiram,[284] or by butylated hydroxyanisole,[285] which interfere with its oxidation.

Metabolic activation of the hepatotoxic dialkylnitrosamines leads to alkyl-hydroxy-alkylnitrosamines; some of the more stable ones have been detected as urinary rat metabolites.[286,287] The less stable homologues have been synthesized in the form of their more stable acetyl esters,[288,289] which act as effective topocarcinogens and can induce tumors of the gastrointestinal tract and of other tissues.[290-292] The acetoxyalkyl-alkylnitroso compounds are mutagens for *Drosophilia*[293] and microorganisms.[294,295]

NAD coenzymes (comprising NAD, NADP, and their respective reduced forms) play essential roles in more than 50 vital intracellular processes; depletion of these coenzymes would lead to cell death and tissue necrosis. The cellular levels of NAD coenzymes differ depending on the type of tissue and on the age of the animal from which the tissue is derived. Fetal, regenerating tissues, and tumors have low levels of NAD coenzymes.[296-298]

Nicotinamide is the limiting constituent in the biosynthesis of NAD coenzymes. Except for small quantities derived from the metabolism of tryptophane, dietary vitamins (nicotinic acid and nicotinamide) usually supply the requirements, due to the wear and tear of the coenzymes and to the formation of N-methylnicotinamide and other N-methylated derivatives, which can serve no more for the biosynthesis of the NAD coenzymes and are excreted in the urine.

Many antitumor and carcinogenic agents lower the levels of NAD coenzymes in vivo and/or in vitro in those tissues in which they inhibit glycolysis and cause necrosis, including radiation,[299] antitumor agents,[300-302] carbon tetrachloride,[303,304] heliotrine,[305,306] streptozotocin,[156,307-309] dialkylnitrosamines,[310] azaserine,[62] N–methyl-N-nitroso-urea,[309,310] N–methyl-N-nitroso-N'-nitro-guanidine,[311,312] methylmethanesulphonate,[313] N-acetoxy-2-acetylaminofluorene,[312] 7-bromomethylbenz(a)anthracene,[312] and the diol-epoxides of benzo(a)pyrene.[312] The lowering of NAD coenzymes can be prevented by pretreatment with large concentrations of nicotinamide; this procedure has been found to change the localization of the tumors induced by a single dose of streptozotocin and by certain other carcinogens.[156,157,315,316]

The depression of NAD coenzymes by carcinogens occurs rapidly, within 1 to 2 hr in vivo and within 10 to 20 min in vitro, which indicates that this may be one of the primary intracellular effects of carcinogens. The concomitant formation of poly(ADP-ribose) suggests the removal of the nicotinamide moiety. Increased urinary excretion of alkylated derivatives of nicotinamide, including N-methylnicotinamide, have been reported after azaserine,[62] methylmethane sulfonate,[313] and a number of nitroso compounds.[314] However, though [14C-methyl-nicotinamide was detected in the urine of rats given [14C-methyl]-methyl-methane sulfonate, the quantities were very small and corresponded to about 3% of the excreted N-methylnicotinamide.[313] The possibility has to be considered that the released nicotinamide moiety might become polymerized (like the ADP-ribose moiety) or bound to cell constituents.

Other types of cofactors, though less investigated, appear to be also depleted by carcinogenic agents. The significance of this depletion, and the fate of the released moieties of the respective B vitamins warrant further studies.[317,318]

REFERENCES

1. **Garrod, L. P. and O'Grady, F., Eds.**, *Antibiotics and Chemotherapy,* 3rd ed., E. & S. Livingstone, Edinburgh, 1971.
2. **Miller, M. W.,** *The Pfizer Handbook of Microbioal Metabolites,* McGraw-Hill, New York, 1961.
3. **Christensen, C. M.,** *Molds, Mushrooms and Mycotoxins,* University of Minnesota Press, Minneapolis, 1975.
4. **Forgacs, J. and Carll, W. T.,** Mycotoxicoses, *Adv. Vet. Sci.,* 7, 273, 1962.
5. **Ciegler, A., Kadis, S., and Ajl, S. J., Eds.,** *Microbial Toxins, A Comprehensive Treatise,* Vol. 1 to 8, Academic Press, New York, 1971 and 1972.
6. **Purchase, I. F. H., Ed.,** *Mycotoxins,* Elsevier, Amsterdam, 1974.
7. **Rodricks, J. V., Ed.,** Mycotixins and other fungal-related food problems, *Advances in Chemistry,* Ser. No. 149, American Chemical Society, Washington, D.C., 1976.
8. **Schoental, R.,** Carcinogens in plants and microorganisms, in *Chemical Carcinogens,* Monogr. 173, Searle, C. E., Ed., American Chemical Society, Washington, D.C., 1976, 626.
9. Evaluation of the carcinogenic risk of chemicals to humans. Some naturally occurring substances, IARC Monographs, Vol. 10, Int. Agency Res. Cancer, Lyon, 1976.
10. **Rodricks, J. V., Hesseltine, C. W., and Mehlman, M. A., Eds.,** *Mycotoxins in Human and Animal Health,* Pathotox Publ., Park Forest South, Ill., 1977.
11. **Uraguchi, K. and Yamazaki, M., Eds.,** *Toxicology, Biochemistry and Pathology of Mycotoxins,* John Wiley & Sons, New York, 1978.
12. **Wyllie, T. D. and Morehouse, L. G., Eds.,** *Mycotoxic Fungi, Mycotoxins, Mycotoxicoses. An Encyclopedic Handbook,* Vol. 1-3, Marcel Dekker, New York, 1977.
13. **Moreau, C.,** *Moulds, Toxins and Food* (transl.), Moss, M. O., Ed., John Wiley & Sons, New York, 1979.
14. **Uraguchi, K., Tatsuno, T., Sakai, F., Tsukioka, M., Sakai, Y., Yonemitsu, O., Ito, H., Miyake, M., Saito, M., Enomoto, M., Shikata, T., and Ishiko, T.,** Isolation of two toxic agents, luteoskyrin and chlorine containing peptide from the metabolites of *Penicillium islandicum* Sopp, with some properties thereof, *Jpn. J. Exp. Med.,* 31, 19, 1961.

15. **Uraguchi, K., Saito, M., Noguchi, Y., Takahashi, K., Enomoto, M., and Tatsuno, T.,** Chronic toxicity and carcinogenicity in mice of the purified mycotoxins, luteoskyrin and cyclochlorotine, *Food Cosmet. Toxicol.,* 10, 193, 1972.
16. **Ueno, I., Horiuchi, T., and Enomoto, M.,** Effects of chemical agents on the hepatotoxicity and hepatic accumulation of luteoskyrin, *Toxicol. Appl. Pharmacol.,* 52, 278, 1980.
17. **Wogan, G. N.,** Chemical nature and biological effects of aflatoxin, *Bacteriol. Rev.,* 30, 460, 1966.
18. **Schoental, R.,** Aflatoxins, *Ann. Rev. Pharmacol.,* 7, 343, 1967.
19. **Goldblatt, L. A.,** *Aflatoxin, Scientific Background, Control and Implications,* Academic Press, New York, 1969.
20. **Detroy, R. W., Lillehoj, E. B., and Ciegler, A.,** Aflatoxin and related compounds, in *Microbiol Toxins,* 6, 4, 1971.
21. **Butler, W. H.,** Aflatoxin, in *Mycotoxins,* Purchase, I. F. H., Ed., Elsevier, Amsterdam, 1974, 1.
22. **Patterson, D. S. P.,** Aflatoxin and related compounds, in *Mycotoxic Fungi, Mycotoxins, Mycotoxicoses: An Encyclopedic Handbook,* Wyllie, T. D. and Morehouse, L. G., Eds., Marcel Dekker, New York, 1977, 131.
23. **Diener, U. L. and Davis, N. D.,** Aflatoxin formation by *Aspergillus flavus,* in *Aflatoxin,* Goldblatt, L. A., Ed., Academic Press, New York, 1969, 13.
24. **Linsell, C. A. and Peers, F. G.,** Field studies on liver cell cancer, in *Origins of Human Cancer,* Hiatt, H. H., Watson, J. D., and Winsten, J. A., Eds., Cold Spring Harbor Laboratory, Cold Spring Harbor, N.Y., 1977, 549.
25. **van Rensburg, S. J.,** Role of epidemiology in the elucidation of mycotoxin health risk, in *Mycotoxins in Human and Animal Health,* Rodricks, J. V., Hesseltine, C. W., and Mehlman, M. A., Eds., Pathotox Publ., Park Forest South, Ill., 1977, 699.
26. **Shank, R. C.,** Epidemiology of aflatoxin carcinogenesis, in Environmental cancer, Kraybill, H. F. and M. A. Mehlman, M. A., Eds., *Adv. Modern Toxicol.,* 3, 291, 1977.
27. **Newberne, P. M. and Gross, R. L.,** The role of nutrition in aflatoxin injury, in *Mycotoxins in Human and Animal Health,* Rodricks, J. V., Hesseltine, C. W., and Mehlman, M. A., Eds., Pathotox Publ., Park Forest South, Ill., 1977, 51.
28. **Schoental, R.,** Hepatotoxic activity of retrorsine, senkirkine and hydroxysenkirkine in newborn rats, and the role of epoxides in the carcinogenesis by pyrrolizidine alkaloids and aflatoxins, *Nature (London),* 227, 401, 1970.
29. **Garner, R. C., Miller, E. C., and Miller, J. A.,** Liver microsomal metabolism of aflatoxin B_1 to a reactive derivative toxic to *Salmonella typhimurium* TA 1530, *Cancer Res.,* 32, 2058, 1972.
30. **Swenson, D. H., Miller, E. C., and Miller, J. A.,** Aflatoxin B_1-2,3-epoxide: evidence for its formation in rat liver in vivo and by human liver microsomes in vitro, *Biochem. Biophys. Res. Commun.,* 60, 1036, 1974.
31. **Swenson, D. H., Miller, J. A., and Miller, E. C.,** The reactivity and carcinogenicity of aflatoxin B_1-2,3-dichloride, a model for the putative 2,3-oxide metabolite of aflatoxin B_1, *Cancer Res.,* 35, 3811, 1975.
32. **Swenson, D. H., Lin, J. K., Miller, E. C., and Miller, J. A.,** Aflatoxin B_1-2,3-epoxide as a probable intermediate in the covalent binding of aflatoxin B_1 and B_2 to rat liver DNA and ribosomal RNA in vivo, *Cancer Res.,* 37, 172, 1977.
33. **Degen, G. H. and Neumann, H-C.,** The major metabolite of aflatoxin B_1 in the rat is a glutathione conjugate, *Chem. Biol. Interactions,* 22, 239, 1978.
34. **Essigmann, J. M., Croy, R. G., Nadzan, A. M., Busby, W. F., Jr., Reinhold, V. N., Büchi, G., and Wogan, G. N.,** Structural identification of the major DNA adduct formed by aflatoxin B_1 in vitro, *Proc. Natl. Acad. Sci., U.S.A.,* 74, 1870, 1977.
35. **Lin, J., Miller, J. A., and Miller, E. C.,** 2,3-Dihydro-2-(guan-7-yl)-3-hydroxy-aflatoxin B_1, a major acid hydrolysis product of aflatoxin B_1-DNA or ribosomal RNA adducts formed in hepatic microsome-mediated reactions and in rat liver in vivo, *Cancer Res.,* 37, 4430, 1977.
36. **Croy, R. G., Essigmann, J. M., Reinhold, V. N., and Wogan, G. N.,** Identification of the principal aflatoxin B_1-DNA adduct formed in vivo in rat liver, *Proc. Natl. Acad. Sci. U.S.A.,* 75, 1745, 1978.
37. **Roebuck, B. D., Siegel, W. G., and Wogan, G. N.,** In vitro metabolism of aflatoxin B_1 by animal and human liver, *Cancer Res.,* 38, 999, 1978.
38. **Autrup, H., Essigmann, J. M., Croy, R. G., Trump, B. F., Wogan, G. N., and Harris, C. C.,** Metabolism of aflatoxin B_1 and identification of the major aflatoxin B_1-DNA adducts formed in cultured human bronchus and colon, *Cancer Res.,* 38, 694, 1979.
39. **Lotlikar, P. D., Insetta, S. M., Lyons, P. R., and Jhee, E.,** Inhibition of microsome-mediated binding of aflatoxin B_1 to DNA by glutathione-S-transferase. *Cancer Lett.,* 9, 143, 1980.
40. **Lawley, P. D.,** Carcinogenesis by alkylating agents, in *Chemical Carcinogens,* Searle, C. E., Ed., ACS Monogr., 173, Washington, D.C., 1976, 83.
41. **Schoental, R.,** Methylation of nucleic acids by N-[^{14}C]-methyl-N-nitrosourethan in vitro and in vivo, *Biochem. J.,* 102, 5C, 1967.

42. **Swann, P. F. and Magee, P. N.,** Nitrosamine-induced carcinogenesis. The alkylation of nucleic acids of the rat by N-methyl-N-nitrosourea, dimethylnitrosamine, dimethyl sulphate and methyl methanesulphonate, *Biochem. J.,* 110, 39, 1968.

43. **Lijinsky, W., Garcia, H., Keefer, L., Loo, J., and Ross, A. E.,** Carcinogenesis and alkylation of rat liver nucleic acids by nitrosomethylurea and nitrosoethylurea administered by intraportal injection, *Cancer Res.,* 32, 893, 1972.

44. **Vesselinovitch, S. D., Michailovich, N., Wogan, G. N., Lombard, L. S., and Rao, K. V. N.,** Aflatoxin B₁, a hepatocarcinogen in the infant mouse, *Cancer Res.,* 32, 2289, 1972.

45. **Willis, R. M., Mulvihill, J. J., and Hoofnagle, J. H.,** Attempted suicide with purified aflatoxin, *Lancet,* i, 1198, 1980.

46. **Stillman, A. E., Huxtable, R., Consroe, P., Kohnen, P., and Smith, S.,** Hepatic veno-occlusive disease due to pyrrolizidine (Senecio) poisoning in Arizona, *Gastroenterology,* 73, 349, 1977.

47. **Fox, D. W., Hart, M. C., Bergeson, P. S., Jarrett, P. B., Stillman, A. E., and Huxtable, R. J.,** Pyrrolizidine (Senecio) intoxication mimicking Reye syndrome, *J. Pediatr.,* 93, 980, 1978.

48. **Huxtable, R. J.,** New aspects of the toxicology and pharmacology of pyrrolizidine alkaloids, *Gen. Pharmacol.,* 10, 159, 1979.

49. **Reye, R. D. K., Morgan, G., and Baral, J.,** Encephalopathy and fatty degeneration of the viscera: a disease entity in childhood, *Lancet,* 2, 749, 1963.

50. **Watt, M. J. and Breyer-Brandwijk, M. G.,** *The Medicinal and Poisonous Plants of Southern and Eastern Africa,* Churchill Livingstone, Edinburgh, 1962.

51. **Schoental, R.,** Health hazards of pyrrolizidine alkaloids. A short review. *Toxicol. Lett.,* 1981, in press.

52. **Newberne, P. M. and Rogers, A. E.,** Nutrition, monocrotaline and aflatoxin B₁ in liver carcinogenesis, *Plant Foods Man,* 1, 23, 1973.

53. **Judah, D. J., Legg, R. F., and Neal, G. E.,** Development of resistance to cytotoxicity during aflatoxin carcinogenesis, *Nature (London),* 265, 343, 1977.

54. **Bartz, Q. R., Elder, C. C., Johnnessen, D. W., Haskell, T. H., Ryder, A., Frohardt, R. P., and Fusari, S. A.,** Azaserine, a new tumor-inhibitory substance. Isolation and characterization, *J. Am. Chem. Soc.,* 76, 2878, 1954.

55. **Wittle, E., Westland, R., Nicolaides, E., Dice, J., and More, J.,** Azaserine synthetic studies. I., *J. Am. Chem. Soc.,* 76, 2884, 1954.

56. **Hruban, Z., Swift, H., and Slesers, A.,** Effect of azaserine on the fine structure of the liver and pancreatic acinar-cells, *Cancer Res.,* 25, 708, 1965.

57. **Longnecker, D. S. and Curphey, T. J.,** Adenocarcinoma of the pancreas in azaserine-treated rats, *Cancer Res.,* 35, 2249, 1975.

58. **Fleischman, R. W., Baker, J. R., Schaeppi, U., Thompson, G. R., Rosenkrantz, H., Cooney, D. A., and Davis, R. D.,** Azaserine-induced pathology in dogs, *Toxicol. Appl. Pharmacol.,* 22, 595, 1972.

59. **Thiersch, J. B.,** Effects of O-diazo-acetyl-L-serine on rat litter, *Proc. Soc. Exp. Biol. (N.Y),* 94, 27, 1957.

60. **Narrod, S. A., Langan, T. A., Jr., Kaplan, N. O., and Goldin, A.,** Effect of azaserine (O-diazoacetyl-L-serine) on the pyridine nucleotide levels of mouse liver, *Nature (London),* 183, 1674, 1959.

61. **Narrod, S. A., Bonavita, V., Ehrenfeld, E. R., and Kaplan, N. O.,** Effect of azaserine on the biosynthesis of NAD in the mouse, *J. Biol. Chem.,* 236, 931, 1961.

62. **Bonavita, V., Narrod, S. A., and Kaplan, N. O.,** Metabolites of nicotinamide in mouse urine: effects of azaserine, *J. Biol. Chem.,* 236, 936, 1961.

63. **Deery, J. D. and Taylor, K. W.,** Effects of azaserine and nicotinamide on insulin release and NAD metabolism in isolated rat islets of Langerhans, *Biochem. J.,* 134, 557, 1973.

64. **Juarez-Salinas, H., Sims, J. L., and Jacobson, M. K.,** Poly(ADP-ribose) levels in carcinogen-treated cells, *Nature (London),* 282, 740, 1979.

65. **Shinozuka, H., Katyal, S. L., and Lombardi, B.,** Azaserine carcinogenesis: organ susceptibility change in rats fed a diet devoid of choline, *Int. J. Cancer,* 22, 36, 1978.

66. **Jacquez, J. A.,** Active transport of O-diazoacetyl-L-serine and 6-diazo-5-oxo-L-norleucine in Ehrlich ascites carcinoma, *Cancer Res.,* 17, 890, 1957.

67. **Haskell, T. H., Ryder, A., and Bartz, Q. R.,** Elaiomycin, a new tuberculostatic antibiotic, *Antibiot. Chemother.,* 4, 141, 1954.

68. **Ehrlich, J., Anderson, L. E., Coffey, G. L., Feldman, W. H., Fisher, M. W., Hillegas, A. B., Karlson, A. G., Knudsen, M. P., Weston, J. K., Youmans, A. S., and Youmans, G. P.,** Elaiomycin, a new tuberculostatic antibiotic, *Antibiot. Chemother.,* 4, 338, 1954.

69. **Stevens, C. L., Gillis, B. T., French, J. C., and Haskell, T. H.,** Elaiomycim. An aliphatic α, β-unsaturated azoxy compound, *J. Am. Chem. Soc.,* 80, 6088, 1967.

70. **Ohkuma, K., Nakamura G., and Yamashita, S.,** An antibiotic produced by Streptomyces strain No. 1252, identical with elaiomycin, *J. Antibiot. (Jpn.),* Ser. A, 10, 224, 1959.

71. **Laqueur, G. L. and Spatz, M.,** Toxicology of cycasin, *Cancer Res.,* 28, 2262, 1968.

72. **Schoental, R.,** Carcinogenic action of elaiomycin, *Nature (London),* 221, 765, 1969.

73. **Schoental, R.,** Gastric lesions including adenocarcinoma of the pylorus induced in rats by elaiomycin, a metabolite of *Streptomyces hepaticus, Gann Monogr.,* 8, 289, 1969.

74. **Schoental, R.,** Toxicity and carcinogenic action in rats of elaiomycin, a metabolite of *Streptomyces hepaticus,* in *Toxins of Animal and Plant Origin,* de Vries, A., and Kochva, E., Eds., Vol. 2, Gordon and Breach, London, 1972, 781.

75. **McGahren, W. J. and Kunstmann, M. P.,** A novel α, β-unsaturated azoxy-containing antibiotic, *J. Am. Chem. Soc.,* 91, 2808, 1969.

76. **McGahren, W. J. and Kunstmann, M. P.,** Circular dichroism. Studies of the azoxy chromophore of the antibiotic LL-BH872 and elaiomycin, *J. Am. Chem. Soc.,* 92, 1587, 1970.

77. **van der Merwe, K. J., Steyn, P. S., Fourie, L., Scott, de B., and Theron, J. J.,** Ochratoxin A, a toxic metabolite produced by *Aspergillus ochraceus* Wilh., *Nature (London),* 205, 1112, 1965.

78. **van der Merwe, K. J., Steyn, P. S., and Fourie, L.,** Mycotoxins. II. The constitution of ochratoxin A, B and C metabolites of *Aspergillus ochraceus* Wilh., *J. Chem. Soc.,* 7083, 1965.

79. **Steyn, P. S. and Holzapfel, C. W.,** The synthesis of ochratoxin A and B metabolites of *Aspergillus ochraceus* Wilh., *Tetrahedron,* 23, 4449, 1967.

80. **Steyn, P. S.,** Ochratoxin and other dihydroisocoumarins, in *Microbial Toxins,* Vol. 6, Ciegler, A., Kadis, S., and Ajl, S. J., Eds., Academic Press, New York, 1971, 179.

81. **Harwig, J.,** Ochratoxin A and related metabolites, in *Mycotoxins,* Purchase, I. F. H., Ed., Elsevier, Amsterdam, 1974, 345.

82. **Nesheim, S.,** The ochratoxins and other related compounds, in *Mycotoxins and Other Fungal Related Food Problems,* Rodrick, J. V., Ed., Am. Chem. Soc. Adv. Chem. Ser., Washington, D.C., No., 149, 276, 1976.

83. **Scott, P. M.,** *Penicillium* mycotoxins, in *Mycotoxic Fungi, Mycotoxins, Mycotoxicoses,* Vol. 2, Wyllie, T. D. and Morehouse, L. G., Eds., Marcel Dekker, New York, 1977, 283.

84. **Krogh, P.,** Causal associations of mycotoxic nephropathy, *Acta Pathol. Microbiol. Scand. Suppl.,* 269, 5, 1978.

85. **Kanisawa, M. and Suzuki, S.,** Induction of renal and hepatic tumors in mice by ochratoxin A, a mycotoxin, *Gann,* 69, 599, 1978.

86. **Purchase, I. F. H. and Theron, J. J.,** The acute toxicity of ochratoxin A to rats, *Food Cosmet. Toxicol.,* 6, 479, 1968.

87. **Purchase, I. F. H. and van der Watt, J. J.,** The long term toxicity of ochratoxin A to rats, *Food Cosmet. Toxicol.,* 9, 681, 1971.

88. **Munro, I. C., Moodie, C. A., Goodman, T. K., Scott, P. M., and Grice, H. C.,** Toxicological changes in rats fed graded dietary levels of ochratoxin A, *Toxicol. Appl. Pharmacol.,* 28, 180, 1974.

89. **Suzuki, S., Kozuka, Y., Satoh, T., and Yamazaki, M.,** Studies on the nephrotoxicity of ochratoxin A in rats, *Toxicol. Appl. Pharmacol.,* 34, 479, 1975.

90. **Sansing, G. A., Lillehøj, E. B., Detroy, R. W., and Miller, M. A.,** Synergistic toxic effect of citrinin, ochratoxin A and penicillic acid in mice, *Toxicon,* 14, 213, 1976.

91. **Doster, R. C., Sinnhuber, R. O., Wales, J. H., and Lee, D. J.,** Acute toxicity and carcinogenicity of ochratoxin in rainbow trout *(Salmo gairdneri), Fed. Proc. Fed. Am. Soc. Exp. Med.,* 30, 578, 1971.

92. **Doster, R. C., Sinnhuber, R. O., and Wales, J. H.,** Acute intraperitoneal toxicity of ochratoxin A and B in rainbow trout *(Salmo gairdneri), Food Cosmet. Toxicol.,* 10, 85, 1972.

93. **Szczech, G. M., Carlton, W. W., and Tuite, J.,** Ochratoxicosis in beagle dogs. II. Pathology, *Vet. Pathol.,* 10, 219, 1973.

94. **Choudhury, H. and Carlson, C. W.,** The lethal dose of ochratoxin for chick embryos, *Poultry Sci.,* 52, 1202, 1973.

95. **Huff, W. E., Wyatt, R. D., and Hamilton, P. B.,** Nephrotoxicity of dietary ochratoxin A in broiler chicken, *Appl. Microbiol.,* 30, 48, 1975.

96. **Galtier, P., Moré, J., and Alvinerie, M.,** Acute and short-term toxicity of ochratoxin A in 10-day-old chicks, *Food Cosmet. Toxicol.,* 14, 129, 1976.

97. **Krogh, P., Elling, F., Friis, C., Hald, B., Larsen, A. E., Lillehøj, E. B., Madsen, A., Mortensen, H. P., Rasmussen, F. and Ravnskov, U.,** Porcine nephropathy induced by long-term ingestion of ochratoxin A, *Vet. Pathol.,* 16, 466, 1979.

98. **Ribelin, W. E., Fukushima, K., and Still, P. E.,** The toxicity of ochratoxin to ruminants, *Can. J. Comp. Med.,* 42, 172, 1978.

99. **Chernozemsky, I. N., Stoyanov, I. S., Petkova–Bocharova, T. K., Nicolov, I. G., Draganov, I. V., Stoichev, I. I., Tanchev, Y., Naidenov, D., and Kalcheva, W. D.,** Geographic correlation between the occurrence of endemic nephropathy and urinary tract tumours in Vratza district Bulgaria, *Int. J. Cancer,* 19, 1, 1977.

100. **Krogh, P., Hald, B., Plestina, R., and Coevic, S.,** Balkan (endemic) nephropathy and foodborn ochratoxin A: preliminary results of a survey of foodstuffs, *Acta Pathol. Microbiol. Scand. Sect. B:* 85, 238, 1977.

101. **Barnes, J. M., Austwick, P. K. C., Carter, R. L., Flynn, F. V., Peristianis, G. C., and Aldridge, W. N.,** Balkan (endemic) nephropathy and a toxin-producing strain of *Penicillium verrucosum* var. *cyclopium:* an experimental model in rats, *Lancet,* i, 671, 1977.

102. **Scott, P. M., van Walbeek, W., Kennedy, B., and Anyeti, D.,** Mycotoxins (ochratoxin A, citrinin and sterigmatocystin) and toxigenic fungi in grains and other agricultural products, *Agric. Food Chem.,* 20, 1103, 1972.

103. **Chang, F. C. and Chu, F. S.,** The fate of ochratoxin A in rats, *Food Cosmet. Toxicol.,* 15, 199, 1977.

104. **Hult, K., Hökby, E., Gatenbeck, S., and Rutqvist, L.,** Ochratoxin A in blood from slaughter pigs in Sweden: use in evaluation of toxin content of consumed feed, *Appl. Environ. Microbiol.,* 39, 828, 1980.

105. **Krogh, P.,** Ochratoxin A residues in tissues of slaughter pigs with nephropathy, *Nord. Vet. Med.,* 29, 402, 1977.

106. **Escher, F. E., Koehler, P. E., and Ayres, J. C.,** Production of ochratoxin A and B on country cured ham, *Appl. Microbiol.,* 26, 27, 1973.

107. **Hayes, A. W., Hood, R. D., and Lee, H. L.,** Teratogenic effects of ochratoxin A in mice, *Teratology,* 9, 93, 1974.

108. **Brown, M. H., Szczech, G. M., and Purmalis, B. P.,** Teratogenic and toxic effects of ochratoxin A in rats, *Toxicol. Appl. Pharmacol.,* 37, 331, 1976.

109. **Moré, J. and Galtier, P.,** Toxicité de l'ochratoxine A. I. Effect embryotoxique et tératogenè chez le rat, *Ann. Rech. Vet.,* 5, 167, 1974.

110. **Hood, R. D., Naughton, M. J., and Hayes, A. W.,** Prenantal effects of ochratoxin A in hamsters, *Teratology,* 13, 11, 1976.

111. **Gilani, S. H., Bancroft, J., and Reily, M.,** Teratogenicity of ochratoxin A in chick embryos, *Toxicol. Appl. Pharmacol.,* 46, 543, 1978.

112. **Elling, F.,** Enzyme histochemical studies of ochratoxin A — induced mycotoxic porcine nephropathy, *Toxicon,* 17 (Suppl. 1), 42, 1979.

113. **Birkinshaw, J. H., Bracken, A., Michael, S. E., and Raistrick, H.,** Patulin in the common cold. II. Biochemistry and chemistry, *Lancet,* ii, 625, 1943.

114. **Florey, H. W., Jennings, M. A., and Philpot, F. J.,** Claviformin from *Aspergillus giganteus* Wehm, *Nature (London),* 153, 139, 1944.

115. **Stansfeld, J. M., Francis, A. E., and Stuart-Harris, C. H.,** Laboratory and clinical trials of patulin, *Lancet,* ii, 370, 1944.

116. **Ciegler, A.,** Patulin, in *Mycotoxins in Human and Animal Health,* Pathotox Publishers, Park Forest South, Ill., 1977, 609.

117. **Escoula, L., More, J., and Baradat, C.,** The toxins of *Byssochlamys nivea* Westling. I. Acute toxicity in rats and mice, *Ann. Rech. Vet.,* 8, 41, 1977.

118. **McKinley, E. R. and Carlton, W. W.,** Patulin mycotoxicosis in Swiss ICR mice, *Food Cosmet. Toxicol.,* 18, 181, 1980.

119. **Reddy, C. S., Chan, P. K., Hayes, A. W., and Williams, W. L.,** Acute toxicity of patulin and its interaction with penicillic acid in dogs, *Food Cosmet. Toxicol.,* 17, 605, 1979.

120. **Dickens, F. and Jones, H. E. H.,** Further studies on the carcinogenic action of certain lactones and related substances in the rat and mouse, *Br. J. Cancer,* 19, 392, 1965.

121. **Osswald, H., Frank, H. K., Komitowski, D., and Winter, H.,** Long-term testing of patulin administered orally to Sprague-Dawley rats and Swiss mice, *Food Cosmet. Toxicol.,* 16, 243, 1978.

122. **Becci, P. J., Knickerbocker, M., Cox, G. E., and Babich, J. G.,** Chronic toxicity study of patulin in the rat, *Toxicol. Appl. Pharmacol.,* 1980, in press.

123. **Frank, H. K.,** Occurrence of patulin in fruit and vegetables, *Ann. Nutr. Aliment.,* 31, 459, 1977.

124. **Stinson, E. E., Osman, S. F., Huhtanen, C. N., and Bills, D. D.,** Disappearance of patulin during alcoholic fermentation of apple juice, *Appl. Environ. Microbiol.,* 36, 620, 1978.

125. **Woodward, R. B. and Singh, G.,** The synthesis of patulin, *J. Am. Chem. Soc.,* 72, 1428, 1950.

126. **Ciegler, A., Beckwith, A. C., and Jackson, L. K.,** Teratogenicity of patulin and patulin adducts formed with cysteine, *Appl. Environ. Microbiol.,* 31, 664, 1976.

127. **Birkinshaw, J. H., Oxford, A. E., and Raistrick, H.,** Studies on the biochemistry of microogranisms. XLVIII. Penicillic acid, a metabolic product of *Penicillium puberulum* Bainier and *P. cyclopium* Westling, *Biochem. J.,* 30, 394, 1936.

128. **Thorpe, C. W. and Johnson, R. L.,** Analysis of penicillic acid by gas-liquid chromatography, *J. Assoc. Off. Anal. Chem.,* 57, 861, 1974.

129. **Murnaghan, M. F.,** The pharmacology of penicillic acid, *J. Pharmacol. Exp. Ther.,* 88, 119, 1946.

130. **Wilson, D. M.,** Patulin and pencillic acid, *in Mycotoxins and Other Fungal Related Problems,* Ser. 149, Rodricks, J. V., Ed., American Chemical Society, Washington, D.C., 1976, 90.

131. **Bullock, E., Roberts, J., and Underwood, J. G.,** Studies in mycological Chemistry. XI. The structure of isosterigmatocystin and an amended structure of sterigmatocystin, *J. Chem. Soc.,* p. 4179, 1962.

132. **Holzapfel, C. W., Purchase, I. F. H., Steyn, P. S., and Gouws, L.,** The toxicity and chemical assay of sterigmatocystin, a carcinogenic mycotoxin, and its isolation from two new fungal sources, *S. Afr. Med. J.,* 40, 1100, 1966.

133. **Cole, R. J.,** *Aspergillus* toxins other than aflatoxin, in *Mycotoxins and Other Fungal Related Food Problems,* Rodricks, J. V., Ed., Adv. Chem. Ser. 149, American Chemical Society, Washington, D.C., 1976, 68.

134. **Scott, P. M., vanWalbeek, W., Kennedy, B., and Anyeti, D.,** Mycotoxins (ochratoxin A, citrinin and sterigmatocystin) and toxigenic fungi in grains and other agricultural products, *J. Agric. Food Chem.,* 20, 1103, 1972.

135. **van der Watt, J. J.,** Sterigmatocystin, in *Mycotoxins,* Purchase, I. F. H., Ed., Elsevier, Amsterdam, 1974, 369.

136. **Vorster, L. J.,** A method for the analysis of cereals and groundnuts for three mycotoxins, *Analyst,* 94, 136, 1969.

137. **Purchase, I. F. H. and van der Watt, J. J.,** Carcinogenicity of sterigmatocystin, *Food Cosmet. Toxicol.,* 8, 289, 1970.

138. **Dickens, F., Jones, H. E. H. and Waynforth, H. B.,** Oral, subcutaneous and intratracheal administration of carcinogenic lactones and related substances: the intratracheal administration of cigarette tar in the rat, *Br. J. Cancer.,* 20, 134, 1966.

139. **Purchase, I. F. H. and van der Watt, J. J.,** Carcinogenicity of sterigmatocystin to rat skin, *Toxicol. Appl. Pharmacol.,* 26, 274, 1973.

140. **Zwicker, G. M., Carlton, W. W., and Tuite, J.,** Long term administration of sterigmatocystin and *Penicillium viridicatum* to mice, *Food Cosmet. Toxicol.,* 12, 491, 1974.

141. **Fujii, K., Kurata, H., Odashima, S., and Hatsuda, Y.,** Tumor induction by a single subcutaneous injection of sterigmatocystin in newborn mice, *Cancer Res.,* 36, 1615, 1976.

142. **Terao, K.,** Mesotheliomas induced by sterigmatocystin in Wistar rats, *Gann,* 69, 237, 1978.

143. **Nel, W., Kempff, P. G., and Pitout, M. J.,** The metabolism and some metabolic effects of sterigmatocystin, in *Mycotoxins in Human Health,* Purchase, I. F. H., Ed., MacMillan, London, 1971, 11.

144. **Thiel, P. G. and Steyn, M.,** Urinary excretion of the mycotoxin, sterigmatocystin by vervet monkeys, *Biochem. Pharmacol,* 22, 3267, 1973.

145. **Essigmann, J. M., Barker, L. J., Fowler, K. W., Francisco, M. A., Reinhold, V. N., and Wogan, G. N.,** Sterigmatocystin-DNA interactions: identification of a major adduct formed after metabolic activation in vitro, *Proc. Natl. Acad. Sci., U.S.A.,* 76, 179, 1979.

146. **Hsieh, D. P. H., Lin, M. T., and Yao, R. C.,** Conversion of sterigmatocystin to aflatoxin B_1 by *Aspergillus parasiticus, Biochem. Biophys. Res. Commun.,* 52, 992, 1973.

147. **Reiss, J.,** Mycotoxins in foodstuffs. VI. Formation of sterigmatocystin in bread by *Aspergillus vesicolor, Z. Lebensm. Unters. Forsch.,* 160, 313, 1976.

148. **Lewis, C. and Barbiers, A. R.,** Streptozotocin, a new antibiotic. In vitro and in vivo evaluation, *Antibiot. Ann.,* 247, 1959.

149. **Herr, R. R., Jahnke, H. K., and Argoudelis, A. D.,** The structure of streptozotocin, *J. Am. Chem. Soc.,* 89, 4808, 1967.

150. **Arison, R. N. and Feudale, E. L.,** Induction of renal tumor by streptozotocin in rats, *Nature (London),* 214, 1254, 1967.

151. **Mauer, S. M., Lee, C. S., Najarian, J. S., and Brown, D. M.,** Induction of malignant kidney tumors in rats with streptozotocin, *Cancer Res.,* 34, 158, 1974.

152. **Kazumi, T., Yoshino, G., Fujii, S., and Baba, S.,** Tumorigenic action of streptozotocin on the pancreas and kidney in male Wistar rats, *Cancer Res.,* 38, 2144, 1978.

153. **Berman, L. D., Hayes, J. A., and Sibay, T. M.,** Effect of streptozotocin in the Chinese hamster *(Cricetulus griseus), J. Natl. Cancer Inst.,* 51, 1287, 1973.

154. **Schein, P. S. and Loftus, S.,** Streptozotocin. Depression of mouse liver pyridine nucleotides, *Cancer Res.,* 28, 1501, 1968.

155. **Anderson, T., Schein, P. S., McMenamin, M. G., and Cooney, D. A.,** Streptozotocin diabetes. Correlation with extent of depression of pancreatic islet nicotinamide adenine dinucleotide, *J. Clin. Invest.,* 54, 672, 1974.

156. **Rakieten, N., Gordon, B. S., Beaty, A., Cooney, D. A., Davis, R. D., and Schein, P. S.,** Pancreatic islet cell tumors produced by the combined action of streptozotocin and nicotinamide, *Proc. Soc. Exp. Biol. Med.,* 137, 280, 1971.

157. **Rakieten, N., Gordon, B. S., Beaty, A., Cooney, D. A., and Schein, P. S.,** Modification of renal tumorigenic effect of streptozotocin by nicotinamide: spontaneous reversibility of streptozotocin diabetes, *Proc. Soc. Exp. Biol. Med.,* 151, 356, 1976.

158. **Tjälve, H., Wilander, E., and Johansson, E. B.,** Distribution of labelled streptozotocin in mice: uptake and retention in pancreatic islets, *J. Endocrinol.,* 69, 455, 1976.

159. **Tjälve, H. and Wilander, E.,** The uptake in the pancreatic islets of nicotinamide, nicotinic acid and tryptophan and their ability to prevent streptozotocin diabetes in mice, *Acta Endocrinol.,* 83, 357, 1976.
160. **Wynder, E. L.,** An epidemiological evaluation of the causes of cancer of the pancreas, *Cancer Res.,* 35, 2228, 1975.
160b. **Myerowitz, R. L., Sartiano, G. P., and Cavallo, T.,** Nephrotoxic and cytoproliferative effects of streptozotocin, *Cancer,* 38, 1550, 1976.
161. **Godtfredsen, W. O., Grove, J. F., and Tamm, C.,** On the nomenclature of a new class of sesquiterpenoids, *Helv. Chim. Acta,* 50, 1666, 1967.
162. **Freeman, G. G. and Morrison, R. I.,** Trichothecin: an antifungal metabolic product of *Trichothecium roseum* Link, *Nature (London),* 162, 30, 1948.
163. **Bamburg, J. R., Riggs, N. V., and Strong, F. M.,** The structure of toxins from two strains of *Fusarium tricinctum, Tetrahedron,* 24, 3329, 1968.
164. **Hsu, I. C., Smalley, E. B., Strong, F. M., and Ribelin, W. E.,** Identification of T-2 toxin in moldy corn associated with a lethal toxicosis in cattle, *Appl. Microbiol.,* 24, 684, 1972.
165. **Greenway, J. A. and Puls, R.,** Fusariotoxicosis from barley in British Columbia. I. Natural occurrence and diagnosis, *Can. J. Comp. Med.,* 40, 12, 1976.
166. **Puls, R. and Greenway, J. A.,** Fusariotoxicosis from barley in British Columbia. II. Analysis and toxicity of suspected barley, *Can. J. Comp. Med.,* 40, 16, 1976.
167. **Szathmary, C. I., Mirocha, C. J., Palyusik, M., and Pathre, S. V.,** Identification of mycotoxins produced by species of *Fusarium* and *Stachybotrys* obtained from Eastern Europe, *Appl. Environ. Microbiol.,* 32, 579, 1976.
168. **Yoshizawa, T. and Marooka, N.,** Trichothecenes from mold infected cereals in Japan, in *Mycotoxins in Human and Animal Health,* Rodricks, J. V., Hesseltine, C. W., and Mehlman, M. A., Eds., Pathotox Publ., Park Forest South, Ill., 1977, 309.
169. **Petrie, L., Robb, J., and Stewart, A. F.,** The identification of T-2 toxin and its association with haemorrhagic syndrome in cattle, *Vet. Rec.,* 101, 326, 1977.
170. **Mirocha, C. J., Pathre, S. V., Schauerhamer, B., and Christensen, C. M.,** Natural occurrence of *Fusarium* toxins in feedstuff, *Appl. Environ. Microbiol.,* 32, 553, 1976.
170a. **Mirocha, C. J. and Panthre, S.,** Identification of the toxic principle in a sample of poaefusarin, *Appl. Microbiol.,* 26, 719, 1973.
171. **Yagen, B., Joffe, A. Z., Horn, P., Mor, N., and Lutsky, I. I.,** Toxins from a strain involved in alimentary toxic aleukia, in *Mycotoxins in Human and Animal Health,* Rodricks, J. V., Hesseltine, G. W., and Mehlman, M. A., Eds., Pathotox Publ., Park Forest South, Ill., 1977, 329.
172. **Sarkisov, A. K.,** Etiology of "septic angina" in man, *J. Microbiol. Epidemiol. Immunobial.,* 1, 43, 1950.
173. **Mayer, C. F.,** Endemic panmyelotoxicosis in the Russian grain belt. I. The clinical aspects of alimentary toxic aleukia (ATA) — a comprehensive review, *Mil. Surg.,* 113, 173, 1953.
174. **Joffe, A. Z.,** *Fusarium poae* and *F. sporotrichioides* as principal causal agents of alimentary toxic aleukia, in *Mycotoxic Fungi, Mycotoxins, Mycotoxicoses. An Encyclopedic Handbook,* Vol. 3, Wyllie, T. D and Morehouse, L. G., Eds., Marcel Dekker, New York, 1978, 21.
175. **Olifson, L. E.,** The chemical nature of toxins isolated from overwintered cereals. Monitor Orenburg sect. of the U.S.S.R., *D. J. Mendeleyev Chem. Soc.,* 7, 37, 1957.
176. **Kotik, A. N., Chernoba, I. V. T., Komissarenko, N. F., and Trufanova, V. A.,** Isolation of *F. sporotrichiella* mycotoxin and a study of its physicochemical and toxic properties, *Mikrobiol. Zn.,* 41, 636, 1979.
177. **Sato, N., Ueno, Y., and Enomoto, M.,** Toxicological approaches to the toxic metabolites of Fusaria. Acute and subacute toxicities of T-2 toxin in cats, *Jpn. J. Pharmacol.,* 25, 263, 1975.
178. **Lutsky, I., Mor, N., Yagen, B., and Joffe, A. Z.,** The role of T-2 toxin in experimental alimentary toxic aleukia. A toxicity study in cats, *Toxicol. Appl. Pharmacol.,* 43, 111, 1978.
179. **Bamburg, J. R. and Strong, F. M.,** 12,13-Epoxytrichothecenes, in *Microbial Toxins, a Comprehensive Treatise, Algal and Fungal Toxins,* Vol. 7, Kadis, S., Ciegler, A., and Ajl, S. J., Eds., Academic Press, New York, 1971, 207.
180. **Smalley, E. B. and Strong, F. M.,** Toxic trichothecenes, in *Mycotoxins,* Purchase, I. H. F., Ed., Elsevier, Amsterdam, 1974, 199.
181. **Ohtsubo, K. and Saito, M.,** Chronic effects of trichothecene toxins, in *Mycotoxins in Human and Animal Health,* Rodricks, J. V., Hesseltine, C. W., and Mehlman, M. A., Eds., Pathotox Publ., Park Forest South, Ill., 1977, 255.
182. **Sato, N. and Ueno, Y.,** Comparative toxicities of trichothecenes, in *Mycotoxins in Human and Animal Health.* Rodricks, J. V., Hesseltine, C. W., and Mehlman, M. A., Eds., Pathotox Publ., Park Forest South, Ill., 1977, 295.
183. **Ueno, Y.,** Trichothecenes: overview address, in *Mycotoxins in Human and Animal Health,* Rodricks, J. V., Hesseltine, C. W., and Mehlman, M. A., Eds., Pathotox Publ., Park Forest South, Ill., 1977, 189.
184. **Palti, J.,** Toxigenic Fusaria, their distribution and significance as causes of disease in animals and man, *Acta Phytomedica,* Suppl. 6, 1, 1978.

185. **Meyer, H. and Frank, H. K.,** Bibliography of *Fusarium* toxins. A review with 2978 references, *Chem. Abstr.,* 92, 209649, 1980.

186. **Schoental, R., Joffe, A. Z., and Yagen, B.,** Cardiovascular lesions and various tumors found in rats given T-2 toxin, a trichothecene metabolite of *Fusarium, Cancer Res.,* 39, 2179, 1979.

187. **Marasas, W. F. O., Bamburg, J. R., Smalley, E. B., Strong, F. M., Ragland, W. L., and Degurse, P. E.,** Toxic effects on trout, rats and mice of T-2 toxin produced by the fungus *Fusarium tricinctum* (Cd) Snyd. Hans, *Toxicol. Appl. Pharmacol.,* 15, 471, 1969.

188. **Rubinshtein, I., Kukel, Yu P., and Kudinova, G. P.,** Papillomatosis with hyperkeratosis of the proventriculus in rats following their feeding on grain infested with the fungus *Fusarium sporotrichiella* Bilai var. *poae* (Pk) Bilai, *Vopr. Pitan.,* 26, 57, 1967.

189. **Schoental, R. and Joffe, A. Z.,** Lesions induced in rodents by extracts from cultures of *Fusarium poae* and *F. sporotrichioides, J. Pathol.,* 112, 37, 1974.

190. **Lindenfelsen, L. A., Lillehoj, E. B., and Burmeister, H. R.,** Aflatoxin and trichothecene toxins: skin tumor induction and synergistic acute toxicity in white mice, *J. Natl. Cancer Inst.,* 52, 113, 1974.

190a. **Saito, M., Horiuchi, T., Ohtsubo, K., Hatanaka, Y. and Ueno, Y.,** Low tumor incidence in rats with long-term feeding fusarenon-X, a cytotoxic trichothecene produced by *Fusarium nivale, Jpn. J. Exp. Med.,* 50, 293, 1980.

191. **Ueno, Y. and Kubota, K.,** DNA-attacking ability of carcinogenic mycotoxins in recombination-deficient mutant cells of *Bacillus subtilis, Cancer Res.,* 36, 445, 1976.

192. **Ueno, Y., Kubota, K., Ito, T., and Nakamura, Y.,** Mutagenicity of carcinogenic mycotoxins in *Salmonella typhimurium, Cancer Res.,* 38, 536, 1978.

193. **Ueno, Y.,** Mode of action of trichothecene mycotoxins, *Pure Appl. Chem.,* 49, 1737, 1977.

194. **Goodwin, W., Haas, C. D., Fabian, C., Heller-Bettinger, I., and Hoogstraten, B.,** Phase I evaluation of anguidine (diacetoxyscirpenol, NSC-141537), *Cancer,* 42, 23, 1978.

195. **Murphy, W. K., Burgess, M. A., Valdivieso, M., and Bodey, G. P.,** Anguidine: an early phase II study in colorectal adenocarcinoma, Abstr. C-419, *Proc. Am. Assoc. Cancer Res.,* 411, 1978.

196. **Wallace, E. M., Pathre, S. V., Mirocha, C. J., Robison, T. S., and Fenton, S. W.,** Synthesis of radiolabelled T-2 toxin, *J. Agric. Food Chem.,* 25, 836, 1977.

197. **Yoshizawa, T., Swanson, S. P., and Mirocha, C. J.,** T-2 metabolites in the excreta of broiler chickens administered ^{3}H-labeled T-2 toxin, *Appl. Environ. Microbiol.,* 39, 1172, 1980.

198. **Foster, P. M. D., Slater, T. F., and Patterson, D. S. P.,** A possible enzymic assay for trichothecene mycotoxins in animal feedstuffs, *Biochem. Soc. Trans.,* 3, 875, 1975.

199. **Ueno, Y. and Matsumoto, H.,** Inactivation of some thiol-enzymes by trichothecene mycotoxins from *Fusarium* species, *Chem. Pharmacol. Bull.,* 23, 2439, 1975.

200. **Agrelo, C. E. and Schoental, R.,** Synthesis of DNA in human fibroblasts treated with T-2 toxin and HT-2 toxin (the trichothecene metabolites of *Fusarium* species) and the effects of hydroxyurea, *Toxicol. Lett.,* 5, 155, 1980.

201. **Stob, M., Baldwin, R. S., Tuite, J., Andrews, F. N., and Gillette, K. G.,** Isolation of an anabolic, uterotropic compound from corn infected with *Gibberella zeae, Nature (London),* 196, 1318, 1962.

202. **Urry, W. H., Wehrmeister, H. L., Hodge, E. B., and Hidy, P. H.** The structure of zearalenone, *Tetrahedron Lett.,* 27, 3109, 1966.

203. **Taub, D., Girotra, N. N., Hoffsommer, R. D., Kuo, C. H., Slates, H. L., Weber, S., and Wendler, N. L.,** Total synthesis of the macrolide zearalenone, *Tetrahedron,* 24, 2443, 1968.

204. **Vlattas, I., Harrison, I. T., Tokes, L., Fried, J. H., and Cross, A. D.,** The synthesis of DL zearalenone, *J. Org. Chem.,* 33, 4176, 1968.

205. **Girotra, N. N. and Wendler, N. L.,** Knoevenagel condensation in the homophthalic acid series. A synthesis of zearalenone, *J. Org. Chem.,* 34, 3192, 1969.

206. **Hurd, R. N. and Shah, D. H.,** Total syntheses of the macrolide (R,S) zearalenone, *J. Med. Chem.,* 16, 543, 1973.

207. **Peters, C. A. and Hurd, R. N.,** A stereoselective synthetic route to (R) zearalenone, *J. Med. Chem.,* 18, 215, 1975.

208. **Bolliger, G. and Tamm, Ch.,** Vier neue Metabolite von *Gibberella zeae:* 5-Formyl-zearalenon,7'-Dehydrozearalenon, 8'-Hydroxy- und 8'-*epi*-Hydroxy-zearalenon, *Helv. Chim. Acta,* 55, 3030, 1972.

209. **Mirocha, C. J., Schauerhamer, B., Christensen, C. M., Niku-Paavola, M. L., and Nummi, M.,** Incidence of zearalenol (*Fusarium* mycotoxin) in animal feed, *Appl. Environ. Microbiol.,* 38, 749, 1979.

210. **Steele, J. A., Mirocha, C. J., and Pathre, S. V.,** Metabolism of zearalenone by *Fusarium roseum* "Graminearum", *J. Agric. Food Chem.,* 24, 89, 1976.

211. **Pathre, S. V., Fenton, S. W., and Mirocha, C. J.,** 3'-Hydroxyzearalenones, two new metabolites produced by *Fusarium roseum, J. Agric. Food Chem.,* 26, 421, 1980.

212. **Hagler, W. M. and Mirocha, C. J.,** Biosynthesis of [^{14}C]-zearalenone from [1-^{14}C]-acetate by *Fusarium roseum* "Gibbosum", *Appl. Environ. Microbiol.,* 39, 668, 1980.

213. **Mirocha, C. J., Christensen, C. M., and Nelson, G. H.,** F-2 (zearalenone) estrogenic mycotoxin from *Fusarium,* in *Microbial Toxins,* Vol. 7, Kadis, S., Ciegler, A., and Ajl, S. J., Eds., Academic Press, New York, 1971, 107.

214. **Mirocha, C. J. and Christensen, C. M.,** Oestrogenic mycotoxins synthesized by *Fusarium,* in *Mycotoxins,* Purchase, I.F.H., Ed., Elsevier, Amsterdam, 1974, 129.

215. **Shipchandler, M. T.,** Chemistry of zearalenone and some of its derivatives, *Heterocycles,* 3, 471, 1975.

216. **Pathre, S. V. and Mirocha, C. J.,** Zearalenone and related compounds, in *Mycotoxins and Other Fungi Related Food Problems,* Rodricks, J. V., Ed., Adv. Chem. Ser. 149, American Chemical Society, Washington, D.C., 1976, 178.

217. **Hidy, P. H., Baldwin, R. S., Gresham, R. L., Keith, C. L., and McMullen, J. R.,** Zearalenone and some derivatives: production and biological activities, in *Advances in Applied Microbiology,* Vol. 22, Perlman, D., Ed., Academic Press, New York, 1977, 59.

218. **Hurd, R. N.,** Structure relationships in zearalenones, in *Mycotoxins in Human and Animal Health,* Rodricks, J. V., Hesseltine, C. W., and Mehlman, M. A., Eds., Pathotox Publ., Park Forest South, Ill., 1977, 391.

219. **Mirocha, C. J., Pathre, S. V., and Christensen, C. M.,** Zearalenone, in *Mycotoxins in Human and Animal Health,* Rodricks, J. V., Hesseltine, C. W., and Mehlman, M. A., Eds., Pathotox Publ., Park Forest South, Ill., 1977, 345.

220. **Shotwell, O. L.,** Assay methods for zearalenone and its natural occurrence, in *Mycotoxins in Human and Animal Health,* Rodricks, J. V., Hesseltine, C. W., and Mehlman, M. A., Eds., Pathotox Publ., Park Forest South, Ill., 1977, 403.

221. **Gimeno, A.,** Improved method of thinlayer chromatographic analysis of mycotoxins, *J. Am. Off. Anal. Chem.,* 62, 182, 1979.

222. **Patterson, D. S. and Roberts, B. A.,** Mycotoxins in animal feedstuffs: sensitive TLC detection of aflatoxin, ochratoxin, sterigmatocystin, zearalenone and T-2 toxin, *J. Am. Off. Anal. Chem.,* 62, 1265, 1979.

223. **Seitz, L. M., Sauer, D. B., Mohr, H. E., Burroughs, R., and Paukstelis, J. V.,** Metabolites of *Alternaria* in grain sorghum. Compounds which could be mistaken for zearalenone and aflatoxin, *J. Agric. Food Chem.,* 23, 1, 1975.

224. **Engstrom, G. W., Richard, J. L., and Cysewski, S. J.,** High-pressure liquid chromatographic method for the detection and resolution of rubratoxin, aflatoxin and other mycotoxins, *J. Agric. Food Chem.,* 25, 833, 1977.

225. **Möller, T. E. and Josefsson, E.,** High pressure liquid chromatography of zearalenone in cereals, *J. Am. Off. Anal. Chem.,* 61, 789, 1978.

226. **Mirocha, C. J., Pathre, S. V., Behrens, J., and Schauerhamer, B.,** Uterotrophic activity of *cis* and *trans* isomers of zearalenone and zearalenol, *Appl. Environ. Microbiol.,* 35, 986, 1978.

227. **Palyusik, M., Harrach, B., Horvath, G., and Mirocha, C. J.,** Experimental Fusariotoxicosis of Swine Produced by Zearalenone and T-2 Toxin, Abstr. 705, 4th Int. IUPAC Symp. Mycotoxins and Phycotoxins, Lausanne, August 29 to 31, 1979.

228. **Schoental, R.,** unpublished results.

229. **Bailey, D. E., Cox, G. E., Morgareidge, K., and Taylor, J.,** Acute and subacute toxicity of zearalenone in the rat, *Toxicol. Appl. Pharmacol.,* Abstr. 126, 37, 144, 1976.

230. **Funnell, H. S.,** Mycotoxins in animal feedstuffs in Ontario, 1972-1977, *Can. J. Comp. Med.,* 43, 243, 1979.

231. **Sutton, J. C., Baliko, W., and Funnell, H. S.,** Relation of weather variables to incidence of zearalenone in corn in Southern Ontario, *Can. J. Plant Sci.,* 60, 149, 1980.

232. **Ruddick, J. A., Scott, P. M., and Harwig, J.,** Teratological evaluation of zearalenone administered orally to the rat, *Bull. Environ. Contam. Toxicol.,* 15, 678, 1976.

233. **Davis, G. J., McLachlan, J. A., and Lucier, G. W.,** Fetotoxicity and teratogenicity of zearanol in mice, *Toxicol. Appl. Pharmacol.,* Abstr. 19, 41, 138, 1977.

234. **Miller, J. K., Hacking, A., Harrison, J., and Gross, V. J.,** Stillbirth, neonatal mortality and small litters in pigs associated with ingestion of *Fusarium* toxin by pregnant sows, *Vet. Rec.,* 93, 555, 1973.

235. **Kiessling, K.-H., and Pettersson, H.,** Metabolism of zearalenone in rat liver, *Acta Pharmacol. Toxicol.,* 43, 285, 1978.

236. **Olsen, M., Pettersson, H., and Kiessling, K.-H.,** Hydroxysteroid dehydrogenase, a zearalenone reducing enzyme in rat liver, *Toxicon,* 17 (Suppl. 1), 134, 1979.

237. **Tashiro, F., Kawabata, Y., Ito, T., Shibata, S., and Ueno, Y.,** Biotransformation of zearalenone by hepatic enzyme in vitro, *Toxicon,* 17 (Suppl. 1), 187, 1979.

238. **Greenman, D. L., Boyd, P. A., Mehta, R. G., and Wittliff, J. L.,** Interaction of *Fusarium* mycotoxins with estradiol binding sites in target tissues, *J. Toxicol. Environ. Health,* 3, 348, 1977.

239. **Boyd, P. A. and Wittliff, J. L.,** Mechanism of *Fusarium* mycotoxin action in mammary gland, *J. Toxicol. Environ. Health,* 4, 1, 1978.

240. **Kiang, D. T., Kennedy, B. J., Pathre, S. V., and Mirocha, C. J.,** Binding characteristics of zearalenone analogs to estrogen receptors, *Cancer Res.,* 38, 3611, 1978.
241. **Katzenellenbogen, B. S., Katzenellenbogen, J. A., and Mordecai, D.,** Zearalenone Characterization of the estrogenic potencies and receptor interactions of a series of fungal β-resorcylic acid lactones, *Endocrinology,* 105, 33, 1979.
242. **Martin, P. M., Horwitz, K. B., Ryan, D. S., and McGuire, W. L.,** Phytoestrogen interaction with estrogen receptors in human breast cancer cells, *Endocrinology,* 103, 1860, 1978.
243. **Jukes, T. H.,** DES in beef production: science, politics and emotion, in *Origins of Human Cancer,* Hiatt, H. H., Watson, J. D., and Winsten, J. A., Eds., Cold Spring Harbor Laboratory, Cold Spring Harbor, N. Y., 1977, 1657.
244. **Ueno, Y. and Yagasaki, S.,** Toxicological approaches to the metabolites of Fusaria. X. Accelerating effect of zearalenone on RNA and protein syntheses in the uterus of ovariectomized mice, *Jpn. J. Exp. Med.,* 45, 199, 1975.
245. **Herbst, A. L., Ulfelder, H., and Poskanzer, D. C.,** Adenocarcinoma of the vagina: association of maternal stilbestrol therapy with tumor appearance in young females, *N. Engl. J. Med.,* 284, 878, 1971.
246. **Herbst, A. L., Scully, R. E., Robboy, S. J., and Welch, W. R.,** Abnormal development of the human genital tract following prenatal exposure to diethylstilbestrol, in *Origins of Human Cancer,* Hiatt, H. H., Watson, J. D., and Winsten, J. A., Eds., Cold Spring Harbor Laboratory, Cold Spring Harbor, N.Y., 1977, 399.
247. **Gill, W. B., Schumacher, G. F. B., and Bibbo, M.,** Structural and functional abnormalities in the sex organs of male offspring of mothers treated with diethylstilbestrol (DES), *J. Reprod. Med.,* 16, 147, 1976.
248. **Bibbo, M., Gill, W. B., Azizi, F., Blough, R., Fang, V. S., Rosenfield, R. L., Schumacher, G. F. B., Sleeper, K., Sonek, M. G., and Wied, G. L.,** Follow up study of male and female offspring of DES-exposed mothers, *Obstet. Gynecol.,* 49, 1, 1977.
249. **Henderson, B. E., Benton, B., Jing, J., Yu, M. C., and Pike, M. C.,** Risk factors for cancer of the testis in young men, *Int. J. Cancer,* 23, 598, 1979.
250. *The Extra Martindale Pharmacopoea,* 27th ed., Pharmaceutical Press, London, 1977, 1830.
251. **Lipsett, M. B.,** Interaction of drugs, hormones and nutrition in the causes of cancer, *Cancer,* 43, 1967, 1979.
252. **Schoental, R.,** Hazards of oral contraceptives to future generations, *Int. J. Environ. Stud.,* 9, 81, 1976.
253. **Gal, I., Parkinson, C., and Craft, I.,** Effects of oral contraceptives on human plasma vitamin A levels, *Br. Med. J.,* 2, 436, 1971.
254. **Anon.,** The effect of oral contraceptives on blood vitamin A levels and the role of sex hormones, *Nutr. Rev.,* 37, 246, 1979.
255. **Wynn, V.,** Vitamins and oral contraceptive use, *Lancet,* i, 561, 1975.
256. **Berenbaum, M. C.,** Effects of carcinogens on immune processes, *Br. Med. Bull.,* 20, 159, 1964.
257. **Stjernsward, J.,** Immunosuppression by carcinogens, *Antibiot. Chemother. (Basel),* 15, 213, 1969.
258. **Anon.,** Immunological deficiency and the risk of cancer, *Brit. Med. J.,* 3, 654, 1977.
259. **Richard, J. L., Thurston, J. R., and Pier, A. C.,** Effects of mycotoxins on immunity, in *Toxins.. Animal, Plant and Microbial,* Rosenberg, P., Ed., Pergamon Press, 1978; *Toxicon,* Suppl. 1, 801, 1978.
260. **Thaxton, J. P., Tung, H. T., and Hamilton, P. B.,** Immunosuppression in chicken by aflatoxin, *Poultry Sci.,* 53, 721, 1974.
261. **Giambrone, J. J., Ewert, D. L., Wyatt, R. D., and Eidson, C. S.,** Effect of aflatoxin on the humoral and cell mediated immune systems in the chicken, *Am. J. Vet. Res.,* 39, 305, 1978.
262. **Chang, C-F. and Hamilton, P. B.,** Impairment of phagocytosis by heterophils from chickens during ochratoxicosis, *Appl. Environ. Microb.,* 39, 575, 1980.
263. **Stähelin, H., Kalberer-Rusch, M. E., Signer, E., and Lazáry, S.,** Über einige biologische Wirkungen des Cytostaticum Diacetoxyscirpenol, *Arzneim. Forsch.,* 18, 989, 1968.
264. **Boonchuvit, B., Hamilton, P. B., and Burmeister, H. R.,** Interaction of T-2 toxin with *Salmonella* infections of chicken, *Poultry Sci.,* 54, 1693, 1975.
265. **Rosenstein, Y., Lafarge-Frayssinet, C., Lespinats, G., Loisillier, F., Lafont, P., and Frayssinet, C.,** Immunosuppressive activity of *Fusarium* toxins, *Immunology,* 36, 111, 1979.
266. **Lafarge-Frayssinet, C., Lespinats, G., Lafont, P., Loisillier, F., Mousset, S., Rosenstein, Y., and Frayssinet, C.,** Immunosuppressive effects of *Fusarium* extracts and trichothecenes: blastogenic response of murine splenic and thymic cells to mitogens, *Proc. Soc. Exp. Biol. Med.,* 160, 302, 1979.
267. **Bojan, F., Danko, Gy., and Krasznai, G.,** Immunological studies in experimental Stachybotryotoxicosis, *Acta Vet. Acad. Sci. Hung.,* 26, 223, 1976.
268. **Danko, Gy, and Krasznai, G.,** The effect of the toxin of *Stachybotrys alternans* on the immune response, *Magy. Allatorv. Lapja,* 31, 233, 1976.

269. **Eppley, R. M., Mazzola, E. P., Highet, R. J., and Bailey, W. J.,** Structure of satratoxin H, a metabolite of *Stachybotrys atra*. Application of proton and carbon-13 nuclear magnetic resonance, *J. Org. Chem.,* 42, 240, 1977.

270. **Lutwick, L. I.,** Relation between aflatoxin, hepatitis-B virus and hepatocellular carcinoma, *Lancet,* i, 575, 1979.

271. **Pier, A. C., Richard, J. L., and Cysewski, S. J.,** Implications of mycotoxins in animal disease, *J. Am. Vet. Med. Assoc.,* 176, 719, 1980.

272. **Yang, C. S.,** Research on Esophageal cancer in China: a review, *Cancer Res.,* 40, 2633, 1980.

273. **Epstein, M. A., Achong, B. G., and Barr, Y. M.,** Virus particles in cultured lymphoblasts from Burkitt's lymphoma, *Lancet,* i, 702, 1964.

274. **Good, R. A., Fernandes, G., Yunis, E. J., Cooper, W. C., Jose, D. C., Kramer, T. R., and Hansen, M. A.,** Nutritional deficiency, immunologic function, and disease, *Am. J. Pathol.,* 84, 599, 1976.

275. **Fernandes G., Yunis, E. J., and Good, R. A.,** Suppression of adenocarcinoma by the immunological consequences of calorie restriction, *Nature (London),* 263, 504, 1976.

276. **Schoental, R.,** Role of podophyllotoxin in the bedding and dietary zearalenone in the incidence of spontaneous tumors in laboratory animals, *Cancer Res.,* 34, 2419, 1974.

277. **Magee, P. N., Montesano, R., and Preussmann, R.,** *N*-nitroso compounds and related carcinogens, in *Chemical Carcinogens,* Searle, C. E., Ed., ACS Monogr. 173, American Chemical Society, Washington, D.C., 1978, 491.

278. **Pegg, A. E.,** Formation and metabolism of alkylated nucleosides: possible role in carcinogenesis by nitroso compounds and alkylating agents, *Adv. Cancer Res.,* 25, 195, 1977.

279. **Singer, B.,** *N*-nitroso alkylating agents: formation and persistence of alkyl derivatives in mammalian nucleic acids as contributing factors in carcinogenesis, *J. Natl. Cancer Inst.,* 62, 1329, 1979.

280. **Margison, G. P., Curtin, N. J., Snell, K., and Craig, A. W.,** Effect of chronic *N,N*-di-ethylnitrosamine on the excision of O^6-ethylguanine from rat liver DNA, *Br. J. Cancer,* 40, 809, 1979.

281. **Schoental, R.,** The mechanisms of action of the carcinogenic nitroso and related compounds, *Br. J. Cancer,* 28, 436, 1973.

282. **Schoental, R.,** Induction of tumours and bifunctional crosslinking metabolites of nitrosamines, *Br. J. Cancer,* 33, 668, 1976.

283. **Grunicke, H., Bock, K. W., Becher, H., Gäng, V., Schnierds, J., and Puschendorf, B.,** Effect of alkylating antitumor agents on the binding of DNA to protein, *Cancer Res.,* 33, 1048, 1973.

284. **Zedeck, M. S., Frank, N., and Wiessler, M.,** Metabolism of the colon carcinogen methylazoxymethanol acetate, *Frontiers Gastrointestinal Res.,* 4, 32, 1979.

285. **Wattenberg, L. W. and Sparnine, V. L.,** Inhibitory effects of butylated hydroxyanisole on methylazoxymethanol acetate-induced neoplasia of the large intestine and on nicotinamide adenine dinucleotide-dependent alcohol dehydrogenase activity in mice, *J. Natl. Cancer Inst.,* 63, 219, 1979.

286. **Okada, M. and Suzuki, E.,** Metabolism of butyl(4-hydroxybutyl)-nitrosamine in rats, *Gann,* 63, 391, 1972.

287. **Blattmann, L. and Preussmann, H.,** Structure of rat urinary metabolites of carcinogenic dialkylnitrosamines, *Z. Krebsforsch,* 79, 3, 1973.

288. **Wiessler, M.,** Chemie der Nitrosamine. II. Synthese α-Funktioneller Dimethylnitrosamine, *Tetrahedron Lett.,* 2575, 1975.

289. **Roller, P. P., Shimp, D. R., and Keefer, L. K.,** Synthesis and solvolysis of methyl (acetoxymethyl)nitrosamine. Solution chemistry of the presumed carcinogenic metabolite of dimethylnitrosamine, *Tetrahedron Lett.,* 2065, 1975.

290. **Wiessler, M. and Schmähl D.,** On the carcinogenic action of *N*-nitroso-compounds. 5th Communication. Acetoxymethyl-methylnitrosamine, *Z. Krebsforsch,* 85, 47, 1976.

291. **Joshi, S. R., Rice, J. M., Wenk, M. L., Roller, P. P., and Keefer, L. K.,** Selective induction of intestinal tumors in rats by methyl(acetoxymethyl) nitrosamine, an ester of the presumed reactive metabolite of dimethylnitrosamine, *J. Natl. Cancer Inst.,* 58, 1531, 1977.

292. **Wiessler, M., Habs, M., and Schmähl, D.,** 7th Communication: methyl-, trideuteromethyl-, ethyl-, *n*-propyl-, *n*-butyl-, acetoxymethyl–nitrosamine, and methyl-butyroxymethylnitrosamine, *Z. Krebsforsch,* 91, 317, 1978.

293. **Fahmy, O. G. and Fahmy, M. J.,** Genetic properties of *N*-α-acetoxy-*N*-methylnitrosamine. Relation to the metabolic activation of *N,N*-dimethylnitrosamine, *Cancer Res.,* 35, 3780, 1975.

294. **Okada, M., Suzuki, E., Anjo, T., and Mochizuki, M.,** Mutagenicity of α-acetoxy-dialkylnitrosamines: model compounds for the ultimate carcinogen, *Gann,* 66, 457, 1975.

295. **Moshizuki, M., Suzuki, E., Anjo, T., Wakabayashi, Y., and Okada, M.,** Mutagenic and DNA-damaging effects of *N*-alkyl-*N*-(α-acetoxyalkyl)nitrosamines, models for metabolically activated *N,N*-dialkylnitrosamines, *Gann,* 70, 663, 1979.

296. **Branster, M. V. and Morton, R. K.,** Comparative rates of synthesis of diphosphopyridine nucleotide by normal and tumour tissue from mouse mammary gland: studies with isolated nuclei, *Biochem. J.,* 63, 640, 1956.

297. **Morton, R. K.,** Enzymic synthesis of coenzyme 1 in relation to chemical control of cell growth, *Nature (London),* 181, 540, 1958.

298. **Kaplan, N. O.,** Regulation of enzyme and coenzyme levels, in *Current Aspects of Biochemical Energetics,* Kaplan, N. O. and Kennedy, E. P., Eds., Academic Press, New York, 1966, 447.

299. **Hilz, H., Gossler, M. V., Oldekop, M., and Scholz, M.,** Effects of X-ray irradiation in 4 ascites tumor cells: partial restoration of DPN content and DNA synthesis by nicotinamide, *Biochem. Biophys. Res. Commun.,* 6, 379, 1961.

300. **Roitt, I. M.,** The inhibition of carbohydrate metabolism in ascites-tumour cells by ethyleneimines, *Biochem. J.,* 63, 300, 1956.

301. **Borst, P., Grimberg, H., and Holzer, H.,** The DPN content of mitochondria isolated from ascites-tumour cells treated with a carcinostatic ethyleneimine, *Biochim. Biophys. Acta,* 74, 785, 1963.

302. **Grunicke, H., Richter, E., Hinz, M., Liersch, M., Puschendorf, B., and Holzer, H.,** Über den Einfluss von Trenimon (2,3,5-Trisäthylenimino-benzochinon-1,4) auf den NAD-Stoffwechsel von Ehrlich-Ascites-Tumorzellen, *Biochem. Z.,* 346, 60, 1966.

303. **Gibb, J. W. and Brody, T. M.,** The protective effect of nicotinamide on CCl$_4$ induced hepatotoxicity, *Biochem. Pharmacol.,* 16, 2047, 1967.

304. **Slater, T. F. and Sawyer, B. C.,** The effects of CCl$_4$ on the content of nicotinamide adenine dinucleotide phosphate in rat liver, *Chem. Biol. Interact.,* 16, 359, 1977.

305. **Christie, G. S. and Le Page, R. N.,** Liver damage in acute heliotrine poisoning. I. The intracellular distribution of pyridine nucleotides, *Biochem. J.,* 84, 25, 1962.

306. **Christie, G. S. and Le Page, R. N.,** Liver damage in acute heliotrine poisoning. II. The effect of nicotinamide on pyridine nucleotide concentrations, *Biochem. J.,* 84, 202, 1962.

307. **Schein, P. S. and Loftus, S.,** Streptozotocin: repression of mouse liver pyridine nucleotides, *Cancer Res.,* 28, 1501, 1968.

308. **Schein, P. S., Cooney, D. A., McMenamin, M. G., and Anderson, T.,** Streptozotocin diabetes — further studies on the mechanism of depression of nicotinamide adenine dinucleotide concentration in mouse pancreatic islets and liver, *Biochem. Pharmacol.,* 22, 2625, 1973.

309. **Gunnarsson, R., Berne, C., and Hellerstrom, C.,** Cytotoxic effects of streptozotocin and N-nitrosomethylurea on the pancreatic β cells with special regard to the role of nicotinamide-adenine dinucleotide, *Biochem. J.,* 140, 487, 1974.

310. **Schein, P. S.,** 1-Methyl-1-nitrosourea and dialkylnitrosamine depression of nicotinamide adenine dinucleotide, *Cancer Res.,* 29, 1226, 1969.

311. **Jacobson, M. K., Levi, V., Juarez-Salinas, H., Barton, R. A., and Jacobson, E. L.,** Effect of carcinogenic N-alkyl-N-nitroso compounds on nicotinamide adenine dinucleotide metabolism, *Cancer Res.,* 40, 1797, 1980.

312. **Rankin, P. W., Jacobson, M. K., Mitchell, V. R., and Busbee, D. L.,** Reduction of nicotinamide adenine dinucleotide levels by ultimate carcinogens in human lymphocytes, *Cancer Res.,* 40, 1803, 1980.

313. **Chu, B. C. F. and Lawley, P. D.,** Increased urinary excretion of pyrimidine and nicotinamide derivatives in rats treated with methyl methanesulphonate, *Chem. Biol. Interactions,* 8, 65, 1974.

314. **Chu, B. C. F. and Lawley, P. D.,** Increased urinary excretion of nucleic acid and nicotinamide derivatives by rats after treatment with alkylating agents, *Chem. Biol. Interactions,* 10, 333, 1975.

315. **Schoental, R.,** Pancreatic islet-cell and other tumors in rats given heliotrine, a monoester pyrrolizidine alkaloid, and nicotinamide, *Cancer Res.,* 35, 2020, 1975.

316. **Schoental, R.,** The role of nicotinamide and of certain other modifying factors in diethylnitrosamine carcinogenesis. Fusaria mycotoxins and spontaneous tumors in animals and man, *Cancer,* 40, 1833, 1977.

317. **Schoental, R.,** Alkylation of coenzymes and the acute effects of alkylating hepatotoxins, *FEBS Lett.,* 61, 111, 1976.

318. **Schoental, R.,** unpublished results.

Chapter 8

CARCINOGENIC CONTAMINANTS OF FOOD

R. Schoental

TABLE OF CONTENTS

I. INTRODUCTION

Cancer is the final manifestation of a cellular change brought about by exposure to carcinogenic agents. The exposure need not be continuous — a single or few exposures to significant levels of a carcinogenic agent may be sufficient to initiate the neoplastic process, which under appropriate conditions will result in clinically recognizable tumors long after the exposure took place. The type of change, and the biochemical processes involved are still unknown, and much remains to be learned about the factors which favor or inhibit the progressive stages in the development of tumors.

Epidemiological studies showed striking geographic variations in the incidence of certain types of cancer in man; thus the incidence of esophageal cancer varies more than 100-fold, of stomach cancer about 12-fold, of bowel about 40-fold, of breast about 8-fold, and of the prostate about 20-fold. These types of tumors have not yet been associated with specific causal factors, though environmental agents appear to be involved.[1,2]

The factors which have not received adequate consideration, but which may be able to explain some of these differences, are carcinogenic fungal metabolites of *Fusarium* and of certain other species. The presence of specific mycotoxins in the environment, especially in food and drink, depends critically on geographic and climatic conditions of a locality, and is as changeable as weather itself. Environmental temperatures and rainfall determine whether and which particular mycotoxins will be produced in agricultural products by the ubiquitous soil and storage fungi.

Among the 100,000 or so of the known fungal species, only a small proportion is toxigenic. The toxigenic organisms produce their toxic metabolites only under certain environmental conditions, which are critical for a particular fungal species. Many carcinogenic agents including certain mycotoxins, at high dosage levels, can cause recognizable acute and subacute effects.

High levels of mycotoxins occasionally contaminate livestock fodder and cause various types of mycotoxicoses which could give rise to mycotoxicoses "by proxy", or neoplasias, in people consuming products derived from the affected animals.

Most of the carcinogenic mycotoxins are lipophilic and therefore are likely to accumulate in the lipids of plants, seeds, and of other agricultural products, and after ingestion in the adipose tissues of animals.

The evidence for a sporadic contamination of food and drink with carcinogenic mycotoxin is at present fragmentary, especially as regards the toxic and estrogenic secondary metabolites of *Fusarium* species, as appropriate methods have not been available for their routine estimation. Yet, though the present evidence is scarce it clearly indicates that these mycotoxins may play an important role, especially in the Western world, in the etiology of certain disorders and tumors which have been considered idiopathic (Table 1). Mycotoxins, including those from *Fusaria,* are teratogenic.[29] It has already been recognized that disorders due to transplacental exposure of the fetus to carcinogenic agents are of particular significance in relation to the development of cancer in later life.

II. CONGENITAL DEFECTS

Most carcinogens are teratogenic in animals.[3] A relationship has also been demonstrated between cancer and congenital defects.[4] More evidence has since then been obtained which supports such a correlation in man.[5] Routine transplacental tests have become a part of toxicological and carcinogenic evaluation of chemical substances. However, regardless of their relationship to childhood and certain other tumors, congenital defects remain a most serious socioeconomic and humanitarian problem, and of great scientific interest.

Table 1
POSSIBLE INVOLVEMENT OF *FUSARIUM* MYCOTOXINS IN CERTAIN DISORDERS AND TUMORS OF UNKNOWN ETIOLOGY

Disorders and tumors	T-2 toxin	Zearalenone
Abortion	+	+
Fetal abnormalities	+	+
Sterility, hyperfertility	+ ,	+
Sex organ disorders (M and F) and tumors	+	+
Cardiovascular disorders	+	?
Blood disorders (ATA) leukemias, lymphomas	+	
Decreased immunity infections ("septic angina")	+	
Indigestion, ulcers, and tumors of the digestive tract	+	
Neurological disorders and brain tumors	+	
Diabetes (?); pancreatic tumors	+	

Due to better facilities and perinatal care, the infant mortality rate in the Western world has been declining, but not the incidence of congenital anomalies.[6] In the U.S.A. birth defects account for 7% of all live births, which means that 200,000 defective babies are born annually. The numbers of stillbirths and abortions are more than double this number.[7]

Only a very small proportion of congenital defects is hereditary. Environmental factors are responsible for most of such abnormalities, the incidence of which shows pronounced geographical and seasonal variations.[8] Higher incidence of congenital defects occurs in areas of high rainfall and among infants born during the winter months.[9-12] Babies born in winter have been conceived in spring, and their critical gestation time, the first trimester, falls at a time when the foodstuffs used have been in storage over the preceding autumn and winter. Stored cereals and other foods are likely to be more heavily contaminated with mycotoxins than when freshly harvested. Low temperatures prevailing during the winter months, high rainfall, and high humidity, which characterize the areas of high incidence of neonatal defects, are conditions favorable for the production of secondary metabolites by *Fusarium* and certain other fungal species. *Fusarium* mycotoxins are known to be teratogenic in experimental animals.[13,14] The teratogenic *Fusarium* mycotoxins have to be considered as risk factors also in relation to human fetal abnormalities — possibly even as the main risk factors.

Of the risk factors previously recognized,[15-17] transplacental exposure to viruses (rubella, in particular), diagnostic and medicinal X-ray irradiation, dietary vitamin deficiencies, and certain drugs (anticancer, anticoagulant, anticonvulsant, antivitamins, etc.) could account only for a small proportion (less than 5%) of the congenital defects. The environmental factors which are responsible for idiopathic, but not hereditary congenital defects have till now not been identified.[7] It has been suggested that a positive correlation exists between spina bifida and anencephaly and potato blight[18] and anencephaly and soft drinking water,[19] but these factors could not be consistently confirmed, and are open to other interpretation.[8,20]

In support of the *Fusarium* mycotoxins as some of the elusive causative agents, it is worth considering that "idiopathic" congenital anomalies, not unlike those seen in humans, also occur in livestock.[21-23] The occurrence of spay legs in newborn piglets has been correlated with ingestion of moldy feed contaminated by *Fusarium* species and could be reproduced with zearalenone,[24] the estrogenic metabolite of *Fusarium.*

In humans spina bifida and other congenital malformations have been correlated with excessive transplacental exposure to estrogenic and progestogenic agents during the first 4 to 6 weeks of pregnancy due to pregnancy tests[25] and to the use of oral contraceptives.[26-28]

Developmental abnormalities and cancer of the vagina in young women have been traced to the treatment of their mothers with diethylstilbestrol (DES) for threatened abortion.[29,30] The possibility has to be considered that the affected offspring, which constitute only a small proportion of the many derived from similarly treated mothers, might have been exposed in addition to fusarial mycotoxins, unknowingly present in the mother's diet; the latter might have been the decisive factor, and this explains the confusing epidemiological data.[31]

Pigs, which are particularly sensitive to the secondary metabolites of *Fusarium,* especially to zearalenone, would be a suitable test animal for the study of its long-term effects of resorcylic acid lactones, and would be of great value for the interpretation of their role in the etiology of animal and human disorders.

III. CONTAMINANTS OF ALCOHOLIC DRINKS

Epidemiological studies have correlated a number of disorders (excessive abortions, congenital defects, "fetal alcohol syndrome", brain damage, cardiovascular disease, liver cirrhosis[32-36]) and tumors (of the liver and of the alimentary tract) with alcoholic drinks.[37-41] Yet, when tested in experimental animals, the effects do not support the epidemiological evidence, especially as regards the induction of tumors.

Alcoholic beverages drunk by people do not consist of pure ethanol, but contain, besides this common ingredient, a variety of substances which vary with their type. Two main types of alcoholic drinks have to be distinguished: those which are direct products of alcoholic fermentation of carbohydrate-containing materials (such as beer, cider, wine, etc.) and have relatively low alcohol content, and spirits (such as arak, gin, liqueurs, vodka, whiskey, etc.) which are distillates from variously fermented brews, and usually contain higher concentrations of alcohol together with flavoring compounds, plant extractives, etc.

Sake, sherry, whiskey, and pure ethanol have been tested for carcinogenic activity and gave negative results.[42] In experiments in which rats were given brandy, gin, whiskey, or red wine for 12 to 15 weeks in conjunction with inadequate diet, no significant liver lesions were seen.[43]

The possibility has to be considered that the starting materials (grapes, maize, rice, barley, potatoes, etc.) which determine the type of the alcoholic drinks, may occasionally be contaminated by field or storage microfungi, and contain mycotoxins such as aflatoxins, patulin, ochratoxins, trichothecenes, zearalenone, etc.[44] Many of the mycotoxins are not volatile and would remain in the distillation residues. But when used in beer brewing, such lipophilic substances would be extracted into the alcoholic drinks and could be the cause of some of the disorders (acute or chronic) observed in heavy beer drinkers. Significant contaminations of cereals and other agricultural products with mycotoxins are likely to be sporadic, which could explain inconsistencies encountered in various studies intended to trace the correlation of the particular disorder with the consumption of alcohol.[38-43,45]

IV. BEER AND MYCOTOXINS

Barley harvested during wet weather will be contaminated by *Fusarium* and other microorganisms.[46] The microflora present on barley has been the subject of much research in relation to the properties and qualities of malt and of beer, especially of its "gushing".[47-55]

Excessive "gushing" of beer attracted attention during 1928.[48] The preceding year, 1927, is known for its unseasonal weather conditions, exceptional to such an extent that they warranted inclusion among the "historical weather events" in England[56] and in the U.S.A.[57] Outbreaks of disorders caused by moldy fodder were common among livestock, and vulvovaginitis, a condition of hyperestrogenism known to be due to the estrogenic metabolite of *Fusarium,* zearalenone, occurred in pigs.[58] Cereals and other agricultural products used for alcoholic fermentations are probably usually sound and only at times of inclement weather during storage, and following wet harvest would be heavily contaminated by mycotoxins of *Fusarium* and other species. This explains why it is so difficult, when testing alcoholic drinks,[59] to obtain experimental evidence for the ill effects reported in people who may not even be heavy drinkers[60-61] (as previously discussed[62]).

V. COBALT-BEER DRINKERS CARDIOMYOPATHY AND *FUSARIUM* MYCOTOXINS

Several outbreaks of fatalities have been reported among heavy beer drinkers, which have been attributed to the presence of traces of cobalt and which came to be known as "cobalt-beer drinkers cardiomyopathy". These occurred in the fall and winter of 1965 to 1966, in Quebec,[63,64] Omaha,[65,66] Minnesota,[67] and Belgium.[68] Though these outbreaks have been claimed to be caused by cobalt salts added to a particular brand of beer in order to stabilize its foaming qualities affected by the use of detergents, the small quantities of the cobalt salts (estimated to correspond to 8 mg of cobalt sulfate per 24 pt of beer, the amount a heavy beer drinker may consume per day!) could not have caused such fatalities,[63,67,69] neither could malnutrition or other factors.[70,71]

At necropsies of the fatal cases in Quebec, besides the eponymous heart lesions, acute necrotizing esophagitis and gastrointestinal abnormalities were also present.[72] Such lesions would be compatible with contamination, by trichothecene, the toxic metabolites of *Fusarium.*

Variations in the types of lesions observed in fatal cases of heavy beer drinkers could be interpreted as the result of variations in the microflora contaminating the cereals used for brewing, and in the relative proportions of the various mycotoxins possibly present in the beer, which may include aflatoxins, zearalenone, various trichothecenes, moniliformin, ochratoxin, etc. Of these, the intensely fluorescent aflatoxins are readily detectable, but the detection and estimation of other mycotoxins, especially the various trichothecenes, require the development of appropriate sensitive methods for routine use.

It may be significant that during the winter of 1965 to 1966 the weather in the U.S.A. was unusually severe[57] and conducive to the production of mycotoxins. An outbreak occurred of fatal hemorrhagic diathesis among cattle in Wisconsin in 1965, and this was traced to moldy fodder contaminated by *F. tricinctum,* which produces T-2 toxin.[73]

VI. TERATOGENIC EFFECTS OF ALCOHOL AND MYCOTOXINS

The "fetal alcohol syndrome" was described in offspring of alcoholic mothers,[35,36] but could not consistently be reproduced in experimental animals.[34,59,74] Only after prolonged administration of liquid diet containing very high concentrations of alcohol (correspond-ing to about 30% of the calories intake) have embryotoxic and teratogenic effects been observed.[75,76] These effects are likely to be nonspecific but related to the accumulation of acetaldehyde, an intermediate metabolite of ethanol, which usually is further oxidized to acetic acid.

The incidence of the "fetal alcohol syndrome", which comprises developmental retar-dation and facial anomalies, as well as of the more pronounced neonatal abnormalities like anencephaly and spina bifida, is higher among the poorer socioeconomic groups, whose living conditions may expose them more to dampness and to mycotoxins. More-over, beer, the cheaper alcoholic drinks, and other foodstuffs are more likely to be contaminated with mycotoxins than high quality ones.

A significant, up to threefold increase in the incidence of anencephaly and spina bifida occurred in Boston, Massachusetts during the prohibition, with a peak at about 1929 to 1932, and was attributed to parental consumption of "impure" alcoholic drinks.[77] Among the affected children, some must have been conceived about 1928; the preceding year, 1927, is known for its unusually severe weather conditons.[57] Alcoholic brews might have been made from grain, harvested during 1927, and kept in storage; impurities in alcoholic drinks made from such moldy grain would have included some mycotoxins.

Aflatoxin B_1, ochratoxin A, T-2 toxin, and zearalenone are relatively stable com-pounds. They are not completely inactivated or destroyed during brewing. In part they would remain in beer and in part in the spent grain.[53,78-80]

Several of the mycotoxins which were appropriately tested including aflatoxins, ochra-toxin, T-2 toxin, and zearalenone, have been found to be fetotoxic and teratogenic in experimental animals.[81] One or a few doses of the mycotoxins given at midpregnancy were effective in producing in experimental rodents a variety of skeletal and certain other fetal abnormalities. The type of lesions depends on the dose and on the stage of fetal organogenesis at the time of transplacental exposure.[81] Treatment of rats with T-2 toxin at the end of pregnancy led to high mortality among the offspring; brain congestion and hemorrhage was the main lesion.[257] Alcohol-induced brain damage has been reported in young males and arises early in the alcoholic career.[82]

VII. MYCOTOXINS IN FOOD

Epidemiological evidence has been reported which incriminated maize from which local beer is made in the incidence of esophageal cancer in Kenya.[83] More recently direct evidence has been obtained that maize, as well as kafir beer and other fermented foods made from maize, is sometimes contaminated with *Fusarium* species and with the es-trogenic metabolite, zearalenone, in Zambia, Swaziland, and Lesotho[84,85] (but trichoth-ecenes have not been looked for). Martin and Keen[85] found more zearalenone-containing samples (containing up to 53 mg/kg zearalenone) among those collected from the High-veld areas than from the Lowveld in Swaziland. In Transkei, in the areas in which esophageal cancer predominates, the incidence of *Fusarium* species which produce both zearalenone and a trichothecene, deoxynivalenol, appears to be rather high.[86]

The areas of high incidence of esophageal cancer in countries with warm climate are usually at higher altitude than the surrounding countryside. This applies to the south-western district of Transkei, to the highlands of Kenya, and to the eastern regions of the Caspian Littoral in Iran. At higher altitudes, the temperatures are lower and the rainfall higher than at sea level, and cereals are more likely to be contaminated by *Fusarium* molds and their metabolites.

Marasas[86] stresses that "moldy corn consumption is not only a matter of expediency depending on the success of the crop, but that moldy ears are actually preferred by many

Transkeians for beer making, because of the allegedly improved flavor." They found not only zearalenone (up to 10 mg/kg) but also a trichothecene metabolite deoxynivalenol, (in levels up to 4 mg/kg). The levels appeared to correlate with the incidence of esophageal cancer.[86]

In the north of Sweden, there used to be a high incidence of Plummer-Vinson syndrome (known also as Peterson-Kelly syndrome) among women, and appeared correlated with nutritional deficiencies, especially a deficiency of iron and vitamins. This syndrome includes atrophy of the epithelium of the upper alimentary tract and esophageal strictures, and is correlated with a tendency to develop tumors of the upper alimentary tract. Since the introduction of supplementation of flour with vitamins and iron in Sweden, the frequency of the syndrome decreased, but the incidence of tumors of the upper alimentary tract in these areas has been increasing.[87] *Fusarium* mycotoxins, zearalenone, and deoxynivalenol have been found in some samples of Swedish grain,[88] and also in other countries. *Fusarium* mycotoxins were likely to have been involved in the causation of pellagra,[89] and this would explain why pellagra-like conditions occur occasionally among alcoholics.

Epidemiological and other investigations have recently been reported in relation to the high incidence (exceeding 100 per 100,000) of esophageal cancer in China, among the population of the provinces Henan, Hepei, and Shansi; the highest incidence has been recorded in the southern part of the Taihon mountains, in the districts Linxian, Yangchen, and Dszxian.[90] The Chinese researchers obtained evidence that this type of tumor (which occurs locally also among chicken and other livestock) may be related to the contamination of foodstuffs with microfungi and their mycotoxins. *Aspergillus, Fusarium, Geotrichum, Penicillium,* and other species have been isolated. Rats were given maize inoculated with the various locally occurring microfungi; significant numbers of esophageal and forestomach neoplasias developed in the series in which *F. poae* Peck Wr. was the contaminating organism.[90]

Moreover, in the maize meal inoculated with the microfungi (with the addition of sodium nitrite), they detected nitrosamines by gas chromatography-mass spectrometry. Dimethyl- and diethyl-nitrosamine, methylbenzylnitrosamine, and the volatile new *N*-3-methylbutyl-*N*-1-methylacetonyl-nitrosamine were found, in levels 0.2 to 0.3 ppm. According to the Chinese researchers in the etiology of the esophageal tumors, nitroso compounds may be involved, as well as nutritional deficiencies, especially deficiency of vitamin C and of trace elements, such as molybdenum. They found that the frequency of esophageal cancer shows geographically declining gradients and that in the province Kiangsu, the incidence of esophageal cancer is inversely proportional to that of liver neoplasias.[90]

Lesions of the upper digestive tract have previously been reported in rats fed grain contaminated with *F. sporotrichiella* Bilae var. *poae*[91] and in rats given intragastrically extracts from cultures of *F. poae* and *F. sporotrichioides.*[92] Pure T-2 toxin isolated from such cultures induced in rats benign and malignant tumors of the digestive tract, brain, and certain other lesions.[93]

In Iran, much effort has been spent searching for the etiological agents responsible for the high incidence of esophageal cancer among a population which does not drink alcohol. A recent epidemiological case-control study in the northeastern Caspian Littoral did not confirm the previously found association with consumption of sheep milk and yogurt or of wild vegetables. An association remained positive with the consumption of bread, tea, and a low intake of vegetables and fruits. There appears also to be an association with storage of wheat in underground pits.[94] This potential source of fungal contamination has, however, still to be followed up.

Besides the secondary metabolites of *Fusarium,* aflatoxins, ochratoxin A, and patulin may be relevant in relation to cancers of various organs. There is need for continuous surveillance of foods and drinks (not only alcoholic) for the presence of the mycotoxins, though these may only sporadically be present in significant concentrations.

Mycotoxins present in food could cause acute and chronic "illness" regardless of alcoholic beverages.[95] The outbreak in the U.S.S.R. of "alimentary toxic aleukia" (ATA) after eating bread made from moldy cereals is a striking example.[96] The relatively more frequent occurrences of various disorders which may be caused by mycotoxins among heavy beer drinkers is a reflection of the fact that a person may drink up to 24 pt of beer per day, but he could hardly consume the equivalent amount (more than 10 kg) of food daily.

However, food as well as beer and other alcoholic beverages may contain a number of other contaminants in addition to mycotoxins. Such contaminants may include residues from pesticides, organic and inorganic impurities, nitroso compounds, etc.

An outbreak of poisoning involving about 500 people (and 13 deaths) occurred in 1900 in the Manchester area, mainly among poor workhouse inmates, and was attributed to the presence of arsenic in their beer (2 to 4 ppm), allegedly derived from sulfuric acid used to invert starch and cane sugars.[97] The toxic effects of arsenic have some similarities with those caused by T-2 toxin, especially as regards the symptoms seen in the digestive tract and the skin and some of the neurological disturbances. It is of interest that *Herpes zoster* was seen among the people involved in this Manchester outbreak of beer poisoning and was attributed to arsenic.[97] T-2 toxin is immunosuppressive and may cause spread and exacerbation of some dormant viruses.

Of the nitroso compounds, volatile alkylnitrosamines have occasionally been detected in beer and whiskey[98-100] in trace quantities, which though too small to be effective per se, could act synergistically and increase the carcinogenic action of mycotoxins.

VIII. NITROSO COMPOUNDS

Experimental animal studies on dimethylnitrosamine were originally initiated because acute and subacute toxicity was observed in workers exposed to this compound in industry (good evidence that man is susceptible to its hepatotoxic action).[101] More than 100 nitroso compounds have already been synthesized; most of these are able to induce various types of tumors in all of the species of animals so far tested.[102-104]

This class of carcinogens deserves attention, in view of their possible formation in the gastrointestinal tract of animals and man from nitrite (or nitrate) and nitrosatable amines.[105-109] Nitrates are present in many plants and can become reduced to nitrites by various microorganisms, including intestinal *Escherichia coli* and *Clostridia*. Nitrite is usually present in human saliva as a result of reduction of nitrate by the oral microflora.[110] The concentration of the reactants and the type of the amino compound will influence the amount of the nitroso compound formed. Under experimental conditions tumors resulted from the treatment of animals with nitrite and various nitrogen-containing compounds,[111] including certain drugs (notably aminopyrine).[112,113] The possibility has to be considered that under certain conditions alkylnitroso compounds may present carcinogenic health hazards to man.

Nitrates and nitrites have been traditionally used for the preservation of fish and meat.[114] Nitrite is also used in conjunction with sugar, spices, polyphosphates, and sodium ascorbate for the curing of meat products, as it is essential for producing the desired flavor in the cured products. Besides protecting them from spoilage by bacteria and from *Clostridium botulinum* (which can cause botulism), nitrite imparts the red color to the end product. It reacts with myoglobin to form nitrosylmyoglobin; when during cooking the protein becomes denatured, the color is retained because of the formation of nitrosylmyochrome.

In the U.K. the use of nitrate and nitrite is allowed, the mixture not exceeding 500 mg/kg (the upper limits for nitrite is 200 mg/kg). In the U.S. only 120 mg/kg of nitrite can be used in conjunction with sodium ascorbate (500 mg/kg). It has been proposed that the concentration of nitrite should be still more lowered (to 40 mg/kg) and that the upper limit of detectable nitrosamines in foodstuffs should not exceed 10 μg/kg.[114]

Traces of volatile nitrosamines (in ppb) have been occasionally detected in various products including fish and meat, most consistently in fried bacon, in which dimethyl-nitrosamine, N-nitrosopyrrolidine, 3-hydroxy-N-nitrosopyrrolidine, and sometimes other nitrosamines have been found.[115-118] In bacon the N-nitrosopyrrolidine is formed in the course of frying by decarboxylation of the noncarcinogenic nitrosoproline; the levels of nitrosamines do not appear to increase on frying other cured meats.[118]

Transnitrosation can also occur in the human stomach at its physiological acidity (pH 1 to 3), when catalyzed by thiocyanate, derived from saliva; some inactive aliphatic nitroso compounds could then form carcinogenic nitrosamines.[119] Human saliva is known to contain thiocyanate (about 110 mg/ℓ in nonsmokers, its concentration significantly higher in smokers (320 mg/ℓ). The formation of nitrosamines from secondary amines in human saliva may possibly be related to the presence of microorganisms.[110]

Traces of volatile nitroso compounds have been found in human blood. These increased sharply following an experimental meal consisting of bread, bacon, tomatoes, spinach, and beer.[116] In these same laboratories, volatile nitroso compounds have been detected in beer.[99]

From the point of view of human cancers, carcinogens which may be formed in the stomach or which may be present in food from "natural" sources from plants or microorganisms, or formed in the course of frying, smoking, or broiling (like polycyclic aromatic hydrocarbons),[120] deserve particular attention, as these might have been responsible for the incidence of tumors before large scale industrialization could affect human life. They contribute to the high tumor baseline, and add to the difficulties in the evaluation of the changes taking place in modern times.

IX. CARCINOGENS IN MILK

Mammalian life depends on milk, the food essential for the very young. Yet, milk could be harmful if the lactating female ingests, or is otherwise exposed to toxic, carcinogenic and unwholesome substances.[121] It has long been known that cows' milk may become tainted or unpalatable when cows graze on odorous or toxic plants.[122] A variety of drugs given to women during lactation have been detected in their milk,[123,124] as well as various pollutants,[125] insecticides,[126] hormones, oral contraceptives, etc.[127,128]

Carcinogenic substances are of particular importance in this connection because their action is often cumulative, and because the suckling and the very young are more susceptible than adults to their action, even if only minute amounts are present in the milk.[129,130] The lactating female is to some extent protected from the effects of noxious agents by excreting these into the milk.[131]

Many carcinogens, "natural" or synthetic (some of which are shown in Table 2) have been detected in the milk when given experimentally to lactating females or have induced lesions or tumors in the offspring.[131-163]

The pyrrolizidine alkaloids, retrorsine and lasiocarpine, given to lactating rats caused acute and delayed liver damage in the offspring.[131] Regrettably the surviving young were killed before tumors could develop. Transfer of such hepatocarcinogenic agents into cows' milk[132-133] may occasionally present a public health problem, as fatal poisoning of livestock due to plants containing pyrrolizidine alkaloids still occurs in the U.S. and in other parts of the world.[132] Grazing animals, when they have a choice, usually avoid

Table 2
**EXAMPLES OF CARCINOGENS, NATURAL AND SYNTHETIC, WHICH,
WHEN GIVEN TO LACTATING ANIMALS, HAVE BEEN DETECTED IN THEIR
MILK AND/OR CAUSED LESIONS OR TUMORS IN THE OFFSPRING**

Natural carcinogens	Synthetic carcinogens
Retrorsine and other pyrrolizidine alkaloids	Methylcholanthrene Urethane
Sanguinarine	N-methyl-N-nitroso urethane
Aflatoxins	Nitroquinoline-N-oxide
Cycasin	N-butyl-N-nitrosourea
Estradiol-17 β	Diethylnitrosamine
Bracken toxin	Dimethylnitrosamine
Ochratoxin A	Dipropylnitrosamine
T-2 toxion	Polychlorinated biphenyls
Zearalenone	Polychlorodibenzo-p-dioxin

eating the bitter toxic plants, but they may do it when the alkaloids are in the form of their less unpalatable N-oxides, or when no other forage plants are available.

The possible transfer of the hepatotoxic and hepatocarcinogenic pyrrolizidine alkaloids into human milk may affect the baby, especially in those parts of the world where nursing mothers use plants containing these alkaloids as herbal remedies. It has been estimated that a baby consumes about 600 mℓ of milk per day, thus it will consume within 12 days the amount of milk corresponding approximately to its body weight (approximately 6.8 kg).[132] The action of the hepatotoxic pyrrolizidine alkaloids present in the milk would be aggravated by malnutrition and lead to marasmus, kwashiorkor, and childhood liver diseases. These disorders remain often fatal in many parts of Africa, Asia, and South America. With improved nutritional conditions these disorders, which represent the more acute stages of liver damage, are less likely to be fatal, but may lead to an increased incidence of primary liver cancer, especially where food may be contaminated by hepatotoxic mycotoxins such as aflatoxins, sterigmatocystins, elaiomycin, etc.[130]

Of the carcinogenic mycotoxins, the transfer of aflatoxins into milk of cows and of other mammals has been extensively studied, and the excretion of about 0.3% of the ingested amount of aflatoxin B_1 in unchanged form, besides its metabolite, aflatoxin M_1, are well documented.[135-140] Less attention has so far been paid to the possible presence in milk of other carcinogenic mycotoxins, especially those produced by the *Penicillium* and *Fusarium* species. These appear to be of special importance in countries having temperate climates. Under experimental conditions, some of these mycotoxins have been detected in the milk of pigs and/or cows, including ochratoxin A,[146] T-2 toxin,[147,147a] and zearalenone,[148,149] as well as other carcinogens.[134,141,144,145,150-163]

In view of the presence of nitrates in plant materials, it might be expected that the digestive tract of ruminants with its copious microflora would present favorable conditions for the formation of alkylnitroso compounds in vivo. Several groups of workers have investigated nitrosamines in the cows' pooled milk and in dairy products, but the results were variable and inconclusive.[118,159] Such variability may be related to the ascorbic and tannic acids, phenolics and thiol compounds present in cows' fodder. These substances are known to interact with nitrous acid and to prevent nitrosylation reactions. However, when lactating animals were given nitrosamines experimentally, the milk contained some of the unchanged compounds.

After a single intraperitoneal dose of C^{14}-labeled diethylnitrosamine, 35 mg/kg, the milk removed by a special pump from the mammary glands of golden hamsters has been shown to contain the unchanged compounds and also some, as yet not identified metabolites.[158]

The milk removed from the stomachs of suckling rats at various intervals, after giving their mothers 40 mg diethylnitrosamine per rat (about 100 mg/kg b.w.) by stomach tube, contained up to 36 ppm of the unchanged compound.[159] It has been estimated that from such a dose, each suckling received about 20 μg diethylnitrosamine. In parallel experiments in which lactating female rats were given 3 to 4 similar doses of diethylnitrosamine (100 to 120 mg/kg b.w. each) by stomach tube and the young were allowed to survive, a high incidence of various tumors developed in the offspring, which survived longer than 7 months. The tumors were often multiple and included among others, hepatocellular carcinomas of the liver, papillary carcinomas of the kidneys, and esthesioneuroepitheliomas of the nasal turbinals, which spread into the brain.[160,251] Various multiple tumors developed also in the offspring of Syrian golden hamsters treated with diethylnitrosamine during lactation.[161,162]

After a single oral dose, 30 mg/kg body weight of each of dimethyl-, diethyl-, and dipropylnitrosamine given to lactating goats, these nitrosamines were secreted into the goat's milk. The amounts found after 30 min were 9.7, 4.9, and 5.8 ppm respectively. The nitrosamines were still detectable about 24 hr later. [163]

X. ORGANOHALOGEN AND OTHER MISCELLANEOUS COMPOUNDS

Among various xenobiotics which are potentially carcinogenic, certain organophosphorus and organohalogen compounds, introduced since World War II, cause much concern. In view of the presence and persistence of such compounds in the environment, including water,[164,164a] whether as a result of their use in agriculture as herbicides and pesticides or following industrial accidents, human errors, etc., the possibility exists of their entry into the food chain and to present health hazards to animals and man. Moreover, food such as meat (particularly animal fats), poultry, eggs, and milk and its various products may retain some of the chemical agents used to control field pests and storage fungi, when ingested by the animals with their feeds and water. Other chemicals which are used as drugs, prophylactically, or for the treatment of animal diseases, as anabolics for growth promotion, etc., may also be carried over into animal products.[165]

When large scale outbreaks of health disorders occur following some industrial accidents, these usually focus attention on the public health hazard of specific agents. Such were the cases of the industrial accidents involving polychlorinated biphenyls, dioxins, etc., which led to extensive investigations of these compounds in regard to their toxic and carcinogenic potentials.[166-171]

A recent experimental study of the distribution of technical pentachlorophenol contaminated with dioxins in lactating cows showed that these compounds could be detected in the cows' milk. On cessation of exposure, the levels of the compounds with polar groups declined rapidly, but the lipophilic dioxins and hexachlorobenzenes accumulated and persisted in the milk fat and in the adipose tissues longer than in other tissues.[172]

Of particular importance appears to be the dioxin, which is present as a minor contaminant of the herbicide, 2,4,5-trichlorophenol.

2,3,7,8-Tetrachlorodibenzo-p-dioxin (TCDD) is an effective poison and carcinogen for some species, more potent even than aflatoxin B_1.[167,171] In female rats daily doses corresponding to 0.1 μg/kg b.w. induced hepatocellular carcinomas in the liver and squamous carcinomas of the hard palate, of the nasal turbinals, and of the lung.[171] This dioxin is the most potent inducer of microsomal aromatic hydrocarbons hydroxylase, being about 30,000 times more potent than methylcholanthrene,[173] and also induces cytochrome P_1-450. TCDD appears to act in a hormone-like manner and to stimulate certain target tissues. TCDD is porphyrogenic.[167] The relation of the porphyrogenic action to the induction of tumors has not been systematically studied, but urinary excretion of porphyrins has been observed in rats given several types of carcinogens including lead acetate,[174] diethylnitrosamine, monocrotaline, T-2 toxin, and ethylmethanesulphonate.[175]

2,3,7,8-Tetrachlorodibenzo-*p*-dioxin does not appear to bind significantly to DNA; its mutagenic activity is doubtful,[176] but it induces reproductive disturbances in several species of animals including nonhuman primates.[177,178]

The toxicology of TCDD has been reviewed.[179] Various animal species show striking variations in sensitivity to its toxic action; the LD_{50} can vary 1000-fold or so. The hamsters appear the most resistant among the mammals, the LD_{50} (at 50 days) being more than 3000 μg/kg by i.p. and 1157 μg/kg by oral administration. The effects on the intestinal mucosa are probably responsible for the (unusual) higher susceptibility to the oral rather than to the intraperitoneal route of entry. TCDD is teratogenic[181,182] and can increase the tumor incidence in rats.[167,171,183] In humans exposed industrially or accidentally to TCDD, "chloracne" is a consistent lesion. This skin condition is characterized by erythema, edema, followed by pustules, hyperkeratoses, hyperpigmentation, etc., especially on the exposed parts of the body. Cardiovascular, pancreatic, and neurological disorders are sometimes present.[179]

Though carcinogenic, TCDD has been reported to inhibit skin tumorigenesis in mice treated with polycyclic aromatic hydrocarbons, but has to be applied 3 to 5 days before the hydrocarbons.[184] This effect is probably related to the striking ability of TCDD to induce the enzymes, arylhydrocarbon hydroxylase and uridine diphosphoglucuronyl transferase, not only in the liver, but also in extrahepatic tissues including the skin. The increased hydroxylation and conjugation with glucuronide would facilitate the removal of the parent hydrocarbon and lessen its activation to the carcinogenic entities. However, TCDD has been reported to enhance the formation of fibrosarcomas induced by s.c. injection of 3-methylcholanthrene in mice.[185]

Certain inorganic agents, including arsenic, lead, chromium, and other compounds used in agriculture or deposited on agricultural products from chimneys, car exhaust fumes, etc.,[186,187] as well as polycyclic aromatic hydrocarbons,[188,189] could contribute to the carcinogenic hazards possibly by their synergistic action with other carcinogenic agents. Idiopathic tumors that occur in man, livestock, or in any other domestic or wild animals are seldom caused by a single factor. Most carcinogenic agents act often synergistically. However, exclusion from the environment, even of a single carcinogenic agent, might be important for the prevention of cancer and would delay the onset of clinically detectable tumors. As for genetic, immunological and viral factors, these are not possible to evaluate and most difficult to counteract.

At a recent Royal Society Meeting for the discussion on long-term hazards to man from man-made chemicals in the environment, it has been reported that the trends in cancer mortality at 45 to 64 years of age in England and Wales during 1931 to 1975 showed a change of less than 1%/year since 1951 for most of the tumors.[190] Tumors of the sex organs and of the digestive tract accounted for about two thirds of all cancer cases in the western countries, already before the advent of synthetics and the impact of industrialization that followed World War II.[191] It is not unlikely that among the main unrecognized causes of these tumors might have been *Fusarium* mycotoxins, the estrogenic resorcylic acid lactones, and the carcinogenic trichothecenes.

The present state of knowledge and technological development in the western world indicates that a promising approach to cancer prevention would be to attempt to control the postharvest production of mycotoxins by appropriate drying to less than 15% moisture content or by freezing to $-15°C$ or so.[192]

XI. FATS AND FIBER

Most epidemiologists agree that high fat diets are positively correlated with the incidence of cardiovascular diseases and of certain tumors, such as of the breast, ovary, and endometrium in women, of the prostate in men, and possibly also of colo-rectal tumors and those of the pancreas. It remains a matter of controversy, however, whether fats of animal origin, with their more saturated fatty acids and high cholesterol content, are more deleterious than vegetable oils, containing polyunsaturated fatty acids and phytosterols.[193-207]

Much attention has been devoted to the study of the respective merits and demerits of various fats and of their constituents, but as yet little consideration has been given to their contaminants, which occasionally may be present in all types of fats, and which can contribute significantly to the variable effects observed.[208]

The chemical nature of the lipophilic contaminants will vary, as well as their respective concentrations, not only depending on the type of fat, but may vary also in different batches of the same type of fat. Inconsistent results in animal experiments have been reported sometimes even from one laboratory. These might have been related to variations in the contaminants present in the respective batches of the fats used.

A. Animal Fats

Animal fats are mixtures of various neutral triglycerides, containing saturated and unsaturated fatty acids, fat soluble vitamins, and variable levels of steroids, which besides cholesterol include small amounts of steroidal hormones, etc. Animal fats could contain also variable amounts of lipophilic mycotoxins and plant constituents, carried over from rations consumed by the animals before slaughter. In recent times pesticides used in agriculture and anabolics used in animal husbandry are possible sources of additional fat contaminants.

B. Vegetable Oils

Vegetable oils are mixtures of neutral triglycerides containing a variety of saturated mono- and polyunsaturated fatty acids, phytosterols, nonsteroidal phytoestrogens, tocopherols, etc. Contaminants in such oils will vary, not only depending on the oil seeds from which they were obtained (coconuts, cornseed, cottonseed, groundnuts, etc.), some of which might have been moldy or contaminated with pesticides, etc., but also depending on the methods used for the extraction of the oil and its subsequent treatment. Two types of methods are in use: hydraulic pressing of ground seedmeals, or solvent extraction, followed by solvent removal.[209] Each of these methods can give rise to the formation of undesirable products, such as residual impurities present in the solvents, products of oxidation, or of epoxidation of unsaturated compounds, phenolics, etc.

Vegetable oils used for human consumption are usually refined.[209] Peanut butter, used without refining, has been found occasionally to contain aflatoxins at relatively high levels (500 ppb or more), which gave rise to detectable aflatoxin M_1 in the urine after its consumption by children in the Philippines.[210]

The refining of vegetable oils includes washes with dilute sodium hydroxide and is usually followed by bleaching with adsorbing earth.[209] The alkaline washes remove not only free fatty acids but also phenolic compounds and xenobiotics (including mycotoxins) which contain readily hydrolyzable ester or lactone groups. The effects of the various refining stages on the content of such xenobiotics in the oils has been demonstrated in the case of aflatoxin B_1.[211] Hydraulic extraction of moldy peanut meal containing 5500 ppb of aflatoxin B_1 yielded a crude oil, which contained 812 ppb aflatoxin B_1 (a large part of the original mycotoxin remained in the spent meal, which contained about 7000 ppb aflatoxin B_1). After washing with sodium hydroxide, the oil retained 14 ppb, and after further bleaching with earth, the residual level of aflatoxin B_1 in the refined oil was less than 1 ppb. Aflatoxin B_1, present in corngerm meal at a level of 425 ppb, yielded on solvent extraction crude oils containing 8 ppb when hexane was used, or 135 ppb when chloroform was used; but after alkaline washes and bleaching less than 1 ppb remained in the refined oils.[211] The materials recovered from the alkaline refining of vegetable oils can represent about 40% of the crude oil. The soap stocks, like the extracted oilseed meals, will occasionally contain significant levels of (hydrolyzed?) mycotoxins. When used for animal feeds, some of the mycotoxins may be carried over into the animal tissues and into the milk of dairy cows.

As an example, a recent incident occurred in California: cows which consumed cottonseed meal containing 8840 ppb of aflatoxin B_1 for about 1 month (4 kg/cow/day) secreted in the milk aflatoxin M_1 at levels up to 8.8 μg/kg (as estimated by high pressure liquid chromatography).[212] Very high levels of aflatoxins in milk (up to 500 μg/kg) have been reported from small scale village producers in Iran, though cows' milk from large scale producers in Isfahan contained very low concentrations.[213] Bulking of milk will dilute toxic contaminants, which may occasionally be present in the milk from small farms in any country, where animal fodder may become moldy due to wet weather and inappropriate storage facilities.

So far most data on the presence of mycotoxins in feeds and in edible tissues of food producing animals have been obtained mainly in relation to the very widely studied aflatoxins,[214] and though some extrapolation to other contaminants, including other mycotoxins having similar lipophilic properties, may be justified, actual determinations in the case of each toxic compound would be desirable and necessary.

Thus, aflatoxin M_1 added experimentally to milk was shown to remain mainly in buttermilk, cheese, and whey. Only about 10% of the added amount might have been retained by the butter, as estimated by difference.[215] Contaminants more lipophilic than aflatoxin M_1 (including aflatoxin B_1) would be expected to concentrate to a larger extent in cream and butter. Actual data would be desirable to obtain. Similarly, all fats used for human consumption should be screened for the presence of lipophilic contaminants (pesticides, mycotoxins, etc.). These might be retained by the adipose tissues of livestock and not removed on rendering the fat. (Lipophilic contaminants which are not readily hydrolyzable. would remain also in vegetable oils, despite alkaline washes.)

Cottonseeds (especially those damaged by boll weevils) have been found to be contaminated by a number of microfungi, which included, besides *Aspergillus flavus, Alternaria, Cladosporium, Penicillium,* and *Fusarium* species.[216] Such spoilage fungi could produce a variety of toxic metabolites, besides aflatoxins, which have been estimated. It has recently been reported that glandless cottonseeds and cottonseed oil induced liver tumors in rainbow trout *(Salmo gairdnerii),* though no aflatoxins or nitrosamines could be detected.[217] Other hepatocarcinogens (mycotoxins or pesticides) might have been present in the cottonseeds and need to be identified.

Mycotoxins which are lipophilic are mainly present in high-fat fractions of cereals, oilseeds, and other contaminated biological materials. This has been found to be the case by estimating aflatoxins in various milling fractions of corn. Following wet or dry milling of aflatoxin-containing corn, the germ and the fiber fraction, which are used for oil extraction, contained the highest concentration of aflatoxins, while the starch retained less than 10% of the aflatoxin originally present in the grain.[218,219]

Similarly, when zearalenone was present in the corn kernels, it was concentrated in their outer fractions (which are used for the extraction of corn oil and the extracted meals for cattle feeds). The starch retained only about 12% of the zearalenone content of corn kernels.[220] Other lipophilic mycotoxins would be distributed in a similar way, and similarly on extraction of the outer coating of grains remain in the crude oils and the extracted meals. Refining of the crude oils by alkaline washings and bleaching processes will remove most of the mycotoxins which contain hydrolyzable lactone or ester groups in their structures (including *Fusarium* toxins).

It is of interest that people, who due to unfortunate circumstances had to consume bread or porridge made from moldy corn or other cereals, often developed pellagra.[221] Pellagra may be considered a mycotoxicosis due mainly to *Fusarium* mycotoxins.[89,222] Pellagra was not prominent among the Mexicans and certain other people of South America who consume corn in the form of tortillas. For making tortillas, the corn is treated with slaked lime, heated, and after cooling strained, washed with water, and mashed to a soft glutinous paste in a stone mortar. Small balls of this paste, known as "masa", are then pressed by a metallic press and the flat tortillas baked on a hot pan. Tortillas prepared by this process have been shown to retain less than 10% of aflatoxin B_1 present in the corn kernels.[223] Steeping of corn in slaked lime would similarly hydrolyze and remove other mycotoxins, such as trichothecenes, and explain the absence of pellagra among the people who eat tortillas. In general grits and white flour are less likely to be contaminated by significant levels of lipophilic mycotoxins as these remain mainly in the germ, fiber, and bran fractions.

The present tendency to encourage the eating of bran in order to supply roughage to the highly refined western diets may not be without hazards, unless such preparations are definitely free from mycotoxins.[222] Yet, no particular attention has been paid to this possibility. Sporadic contamination of such fiber preparations with mycotoxins may explain the variable effects of high fiber diets reported in epidemiological and experimental investigations.[224-228]

Sporadic contamination of animal fats with mycotoxins could also explain some of the inconsistent results obtained in experiments in which cholesterol[229] or other steroids have been tested, as these substances are notoriously difficult to purify.

As an example to serve the case of the alleged toxicity of certain steroidal fractions prepared from poaefusarin and sporofusarin, the steroidal glycosides were obtained from cultures of *F. poae* and *F. sporotrichioides*.[230] These steroidal substances were considered to be responsible for the toxicity of crude alcoholic extracts of the cultures, which were able to reproduce in experimental animals some of the characteristics of a disorder known as alimentary toxic aleukia (ATA) in the U.S.S.R. However, when a crude sample of poaefusarin prepared in the U.S.S.R.[96] was reinvestigated in the U.S.A., it was found to contain T-2 toxin and some zearalenone.[231] More recently, alcoholic extracts from cultures of *F. sporotrichioides* grown on autoclaved wheat have also been reinvestigated. These contained T-2 toxin and small amounts of related trichothecenes, HT-toxin, and neosolaniol, which accounted for all the toxicity of the extracts.[232] T-2 toxin reproduced in cats the hematological (and certain other lesions) characteristic of human ATA.[233]

A detailed study of the steroidal constituents of alcoholic extracts from cultures of *F. sporotrichioides* led to the isolation of six nontoxic steroids, four of which proved to be the known phytosteroids: β-sitosterol, camphesterol, stigmasterol, and ergosterol. The structure of a new, unknown steroid has been identified as 12β-acetoxy-4, 4-dimethyl-24-methylene-5α-cholesta-8,14-diene-3β, 11α-diol.[234]

The adventitious presence of carcinogenic mycotoxins in cereals and in other constituents of diet may be responsible for some of the tumors considered as "spontaneous" in man and animals, and may have confounded many of the epidemiological investigations in man, as well as some of the results of experimental studies in animals.[235-237]

High fat diets have been reported to enhance the incidence of spontaneous mammary tumors in mice,[238] of skin tumors induced in mice by the application of polycyclic aromatic hydrocarbons, of mammary tumors after treatment with 7,12-dimethyl-benz(a)anthracene[239,240] or with N-methylnitrosourea,[241] of colon tumors after treatment with dimethylhydrazine,[242] and others.[243]

These experiments have mostly been performed before the carcinogenic potentialities of *Fusarium* mycotoxins became known, and no attention had been paid to the possible presence of the latter in the fats or in other ingredients of the diets used. The effects attributed to, e.g., fats per se, might have been due to their contaminants, which could vary qualitatively and quantitatively from one batch of fat to another.

Recently, using labeled T-2 toxin, evidence was obtained as regards the extent of contamination of various animal tissues, including the adipose tissue[147a] by this mycotoxin.

When pigs were given tritium-labeled T-2 toxin (0.1 mg/kg b.w.), the kidneys, liver, fat, and muscle contained radioactivity corresponding at 18 hr after the treatment to 15.9, 13.8, 0.49, and 3.1 ppb T-2 toxin, respectively. When the dose was increased to 0.4 mg/kg b.w. the respective levels increased 3- to 4-fold.[244]

Chicken given 5 mg/kg b.w. of T-2 toxin excreted most of the dose in the feces, mainly as unchanged T-2 toxin and also some of its deacylated derivatives. The concentrations in the excreta of T-2 toxin, neosolaniol, HT-2 toxin, and T-2 toxin tetraol corresponded to 108, 40, 26, and 32 ppm, respectively.[245] These data indicate that T-2 toxin (and its derivatives) can concentrate in the chicken excreta. At present there is a tendency to recycle excreta by adding them to animal rations (at a level of 10%). This may introduce increasing hazard to animal health and may contribute to hemorrhagic disorders in livestock, the etiology of which is sometimes difficult to trace. T-2 toxin disappears rapidly from chicken liver and muscle, within less than 5 hr after dosing.[245] When tritium-labeled T-2 toxin was injected into hens, a small proportion of radioactivity was carried over into the eggs.[246]

When hens were exposed to high levels of T-2 toxin (about 20 mg/kg), they showed neural disturbances[247] and diminished egg production; the egg shells were thin and fragile,[248] and the feathering became altered.[249] Leukopenia, thrombocytopenia, and decreased immunity can follow.[250]

When [14C] zearalenone was given to laying hens (10 mg/kg; 1.54 μCi/Kg), the radioactivity was eliminated in the excreta; 94% of the administered dose within 72 hr, one third of the eliminated radioactivity represented unchanged zearalenone, third, a polar metabolite. Edible muscle tissue retained some activity, and lipophilic metabolite(s) persisted in the fat and in the egg yolk beyond 72 hr after dosing.[250a]

It is of interest that hen eggs, especially the egg yolk and its lipids, have been reported to be carcinogenic in some strains of mice and to induce lymphosarcomas, and tumors of the lung, of the mammary glands,[251] of the brain,[252] the stomach, etc.[253] The carcinogenic substances have not been identified, but it has been concluded that more than one carcinogen may be involved.[254] The distribution and the effects of the carcinogenic agents of these hen eggs would be not incompatible with the characteristics of the mycotoxins from *Fusarium.*

Attention has been drawn in this section to the possibility that extraneous contaminants of fats may be responsible for some of their deleterious effects. However, the intrinsic constituents of fats can undergo undesirable chemical changes such as hydrolysis, hy-droperoxidation, epoxidation, hydroxylation, etc., which may have some effects on the permeability of cellular membranes and on various biochemical processes. Whether and to what extent such changes might be involved in the carcinogenic process needs further investigation.

It has been found that reduction of food intake, especially at early age, will reduce the incidence of "spontaneous" tumors in laboratory animals.[255] This evidence may have to be reinterpreted in view of the possibility that the "spontaneous" tumors may be due to carcinogenic contaminants of diet.[256] The reduction of food intake would reduce also the amount of the ingested carcinogens.

REFERENCES

1. **Berg, J. W.,** World variations in cancer incidence as clues to cancer origin, in *Origins of Human Cancer,* Hiatt, H. H., Watson, J. D., and Winsten, J. A., Eds., Cold Spring Harbor Laboratory, Cold Spring Harbor, N.Y., 1977, 15.
2. **Miller, R. W.,** Ethnic differences in cancer occurrence: genetic and environmental influence with particular reference to neuroblastoma, in *Genetics in Human Cancer,* Mulvihill, J. J., Miller, R. W., and Fraumeni, J. F., Jr., Eds., Raven Press, New York, 1977, 1.
2a.**Schoental, R.,** Mycotoxins and fetal abnormalities, *Int. J. Environ. Stud.,* 17, 25, 1981.
3. **Di Paolo, J. A. and Kotin, P.,** Teratogenesis-oncogenesis. A study of possible relationships, *Arch. Pathol.,* 81, 3, 1966.
4. **Miller, R. W.,** Relation between cancer and congenital defects in man, *N. Engl. J. Med.,* 275, 87, 1966.
5. **Bolande, R. P.,** Childhood tumors and their relationship to birth defects, in *Genetics of Human Cancer,* Mulvihill, J., Miller, R. W., and Fraumeni, J. R., Jr., Eds., Raven Press, New York, 1977, 43.
6. **Scrimgeour, J. B. and Cockburn, F.,** Congenital abnormalities, *Lancet,* ii, 1349, 1979.
7. **Harbison, R. D.,** Teratogens, in *Toxicology, The Basic Science of Poisons,* 2nd ed., Casarett, J. and Doull, J., Eds., Macmillan, New York, 1980, 158.
8. **Smithells, R. W.,** Environmental teratogens of man, *Br. Med. Bull.,* 32, 27, 1976.
9. **MacMahon, B., Pugh, T. F., and Ingalls, T. H.,** Anencephaly, spina bifida and hydrocephalus incidence related to sex, race and seasonal birth and incidence in siblings, *Br. J. Prev. Soc. Med.,* 7, 211, 1953.
10. **Knox, E. G.,** Anencephaly and dietary intakes, *Br. J. Prev. Soc. Med.,* 26, 219, 1972.
11. **Laurence, K. M., Carter, C. O., and David, P. A.,** Major central nervous system malformations in South Wales. I. Incidence, local variations and geographical factors, *Br. J. Prev. Soc. Med.,* 22, 146, 1968.
12. **Laurence, K. M., Carter, C. O., and David, P. A.,** Major central nervous system malformations in South Wales. II. Pregnancy factors, seasonal variation and social class effects, *Br. J. Prev. Soc. Med.,* 22, 212, 1968.
13. **Stanford, G. K., Hood, R. D., and Hayes, A. W.,** Effect of prenatal administration of T-2 toxin to mice, *Res. Commun. Pathol. Pharmacol.,* 10, 743, 1975.
14. **Ruddick, J. A., Scott, P. M., and Harwig, J.,** Teratological evaluation of zearalenone administered orally to the rat, *Bull. Environ. Contam. Toxicol.,* 15, 678, 1976.
15. **Warkany, J. and Kalter, H.,** Congenital malformations, *N. Engl. J. Med.,* 265, 993, 1961.
16. **Wilson, J. G. and Fraser, F. C.,** Eds., *Handbook of Teratology,* Vol. 1, Plenum Press, New York, 1977.
17. **Persaud, T. V. N.,** *Problems of Birth Defects. From Hippocrates to Thalidomide and After,* MTP Press, Lancaster, England, 1977, 59.
18. **Renwick, J. H.,** Anencephaly and spina bifida are usually preventable by evidence of a specific, but unidentified substance present in certain potato tubers, *Br. J. Prev. Soc. Med.,* 26, 67, 1972.
19. **Fedrick, J.,** Anencephalus and maternal tea drinking. Evidence for a possible association, *Proc. R. Soc. Med.,* 67, 356, 1974.
20. **Crawford, M. D., Gardner, M. J., and Sedgwick, P. A.,** Infant mortality and hardness of local water supplies, *Lancet,* i, 988, 1972.
21. **Priester, W. A., Glass, A. G., and Waggoner, N. S.,** Congenital defects in domesticated animals: general considerations, *Am. J. Vet. Res.,* 31, 1871, 1970.
22. **Cho, D. Y. and Leipold, H. W.,** Congenital defects of the bovine central system, *Vet. Bull.,* 47, 489, 1977
23. **Cotchin, E.,** Comparative oncology: the veterinary contribution, Proc. R. Soc. Med., 69, 17, 1976.
24. **Miller, J. K., Hacking, A., Harrison, J., and Gross, V. J.,** Stillbirth, neonatal mortality and small litters in pigs associated with the ingestion of *Fusarium* toxin by pregnant sows, *Vet. Rec.,* 93, 555, 1973.
25. **Gal, I., Kirman, B., and Stern, J.,** Hormonal pregnancy tests and congenital malformations, *Nature, (London),* 216, 83, 1967.
26. **Nora, A. H. and Nora, J. J.,** A syndrome of multiple congenital anomalies associated with teratogenic exposure, *Arch. Environ. Health,* 30, 17, 1975.
27. **Janerich, D. T., Dugan, J. M., and Standfast, S. J.,** Congenital heart disease and prenatal exposure to exogenous sex hormones, *Br. Med. J.,* i, 1058, 1977.

28. **Rothman, K. J. and Louik, C.,** Oral contraceptives and birth defects, *N. Engl. J. Med.,* 299, 522, 1978.
29. **Herbst, A. L., Ulfelder, H., and Poskanzer, D. C.,** Adenocarcinoma of the vagina: association of maternal stilbestrol therapy with tumor appearance in young females, *N. Engl. J. Med.,* 284, 878, 1971.
30. **Herbst, A. L., Scully, R. E., Robboy, S. J., Welch, W. R., and Cole, P.,** Abnormal development of human genital tract following prenatal exposure to diethylstilbestrol, in *Origins of Human Cancer,* Hatt, H. H., Watson, J. D., and Winsten, J. A., Eds., Cold Spring Harbor Laboratorty, Cold Spring Harbor, N.Y., 1977, 339.
31. **Schoental, R.,** The importance of *Fusarium* toxins and oestrogenic metabolites in the aetiology of health disorders of animals and men, *Proc. 4th Mtg. Mycotoxins in Animal Disease,* Ministry Agr. Food. and Fisheries, Weybridge 1981, in press.
32. **Harlap, S. and Shion, P. H.,** Alcohol, smoking and incidence of spontaneous abortions in the first and second trimester, *Lancet,* ii, 173, 1980.
33. **Kline, J., Shrout, P., Stein, Z., Susser, M., and Warburton, D.,** Drinking during pregnancy and spontaneous abortion, *Lancet,* ii, 176, 1980.
34. **Streissguth, A. P., Landesman-Dwyer, S., Martin, J. C., and Smith, D. W.,** Teratogenic effects of alcohol in humans and laboratory animals, *Science,* 209, 353, 1980.
35. **Lemoine, P. H., Harousseau, H., Borteyru, J. P., and Menuet, J. C.,** Les enfants de parents alcoholiques: anomalies observees a propos de 127 cas, *Arch. Fr. Pediatr.,* 25, 830, 1967.
36. **Jones, K. L. and Smith, D. W.,** The fetal alcohol syndrome: an epidemiologic perspective, *Teratology,* 12, 1, 1975.
37. **McMichael, A. J.,** Increases in laryngeal cancer in Britain and Australia in relation to alcohol and tobacco consumption trends, *Lancet,* ii, 1244, 1978.
38. **Lieber, C. S., Seitz, H. K., Garro, A. J., and Worner, T. M.,** Alcohol-related diseases and carcinogenesis, *Cancer Res.,* 39, 2863, 1979.
39. **Tuyns, A. J.,** Epidemiology of alcohol and cancer, *Cancer Res.,* 39, 2840, 1979.
40. **Schottenfeld, D.,** Alcohol as a co-factor in the etiology of cancer, *Cancer,* 43, 1962, 1979.
41. **Kono, S. and Ikeda, M.,** Correlation between cancer mortality and alcoholic beverage in Japan, *Br. J. Cancer,* 40, 449, 1979.
42. **Kuratsune, M., Kohchi, S., Horu, A., and Nishizumi, M.,** Test of alcoholic beverages and ethanol solution for carcinogenicity and tumor-promoting activity, *Gann,* 62, 395, 1971.
43. **Jordö, L. and Olsson, R.,** The effect on the rat liver of long-term administration of different alcoholic beverages together with inadequate diet, *Acta Pathol. Microbiol. Scand. Sect. A.,* 83, 717, 1975.
44. **Lillehoj, E. B. and Hesseltine, C. W.,** *Mycotoxins in Human and Animal Health,* Rodricks, J. V., Hesseltine, C. W., and Mehlman, M. A., Eds., Pathotox Publishers, Park Forest South, Ill., 1977, 107.
45. **Dyer, A. R., Stamler, J., Paul, O., Lepper, M., Shekelle, R. B., McKean, H., and Garside, D.,** Alcohol consumption and 17-year mortality in the Chicago Western Electric Company study, *Prev. Med.,* 9, 78, 1980.
46. **Hacking, A., Rosser, W. R., and Dervish, M. T.,** Zearalenone-producing species of *Fusarium* on barley seed, *Ann. Appl. Biol.,* 82, 7, 1976.
47. **Sloey, W. and Prentice, N.,** Effects of *Fusarium* isolates applied during malting on properties of malt, *Am. Soc. Brew. Chem. Proc.,* 24, 1962.
48. **Gjertsen, P., Trolle, B., and Andersen, K.,** Studies on gushing. I. Weathered barley as a contributory cause of gushing in beer, in *Eur. Brew. Convention Proc. Congr.,* Elsevier, Amsterdam, 1963, 320.
49. **Gjertsen, P., Trolle, B., and Andersen, K.,** Studies on gushing. II. Gushing caused by microorganisms specially *Fusarium* species, in *Eur. Brew. Convention Proc. Congr.,* Elsevier, Amsterdam, 1965, 428.
50. **Trolle, B.,** Danish grain quality research, Eur. Brew. Convention Proc. 12th Congr., 1969, 99.
51. **Kieninger, H.,** Gushing of bottled beer—present state of research, *Brauwelt,* 116, 1600, 1976.
52. **Etchevers, G. C., Banasik, O. J., and Watson, C. A.,** Microflora of barley and its effects on malt and beer properties: a review, *Brew. Dig,* 52, 46, 1977.
53. **Mannio, M. and Enari, T.-M.,** Uber die Wirkung von Fusarium-Schimmelpilzen der Gerste bei der Bierherstellung, *Brauwissenschaft,* 26, 134, 1973.
54. **Nummi, M., Niku-Paevola, M.-L., and Enari, T.-M.,** Der Einfluss eines Fusarium-Toxins auf die Gersten-Vermälzung, *Brauwissenschaft,* 28, 130, 1975.
55. **Pollock, J. R. A.,** Ed., *Brewing Science,* Vol. 1, Academic Press, London, 1979.
56. **Lamb, H. H.,** *The English Climate,* Appendix 2, English University Press, London, 1964.
57. **Ludlum, D. M.,** *Weather Record Book: The Outstanding Events 1871-1970,* Weatherwise, Princeton, N. J., 1971.
58. **McNutt, S. H., Purwin, P., and Murray, C.,** Vulvovaginitis in swine: preliminary report, *J. Am. Vet. Med. Assoc.,* 73, 484, 1928.
59. **Øisund, J. F., Fjorden, A. F., and Morland, J.,** Is modern ethanol consumption teratogenic in the rat?, *Acta Pharmacol. Toxicol.,* 43, 145, 1978.

167

60. **Pawan, G. L. S.,** Metabolism of alcohol (ethanol) in man, *Proc. Nutr. Soc.,* 31, 83, 1972.
61. **Hinds, M. W., Kolonel, L. N., Lee, J., and Hirohata, T.,** Association between cancer incidence and alcohol/cigarette consumption among five ethnic groups in Hawaii, *Br. J. Cancer,* 41, 929, 1980.
62. **Schoental, R.,** Relationships of *Fusarium* mycotoxins to disorders and tumors associated with alcoholic drinks, *Nutr. Cancer,* 2(2), 88, 1980.
63. **Morin, Y. L. and Daniel, P.,** Quebec beer-drinkers cardiomyopathy etiological considerations, *Can. Med. Assoc. J.,* 97, 926, 1967.
64. **Morin, Y., Tetu, A., and Mercier, G.,** Quebec beer-drinkers' cardiomyopathy. Clinical and hemodynamic aspects, *Ann. N.Y. Acad. Sci.,* 156, 566, 1969.
65. **Sullivan, J. F., Egan, J. D., and George, R. P.,** A distinctive myocardiopathy occurring in Omaha, Nebraska: clinical aspects, *Ann. N.Y. Acad. Sci.,* 156, 526, 1969.
66. **Grinvalsky, H. T. and Fitch, D. M.,** A distinctive myocardiopathy occurring in Omaha, Nebraska: pathological aspects, *Ann. N.Y. Acad. Sci.,* 156, 544, 1969.
67. **Alexander, C. S.,** Cobalt-beer cardiomyopathy. A clinical pathological study in twenty-eight cases, *Am. J. Med.,* 53, 395, 1972.
68. **Kasteloot, A., Terryn, R., Bosmans, P., and Joossens, J. V.,** Alcoholic perimyocardiopathy, *Acta Cardiol.,* 21, 341, 1966.
69. **Grice, H. C., Goodman, T., Munro, I. C., Wiberg, G. S., and Morrison, A. B.,** Myocardial toxicity of cobalt in the rat, *Ann. N.Y. Acad. Sci.,* 156, 189, 1969.
70. **Anon.,** Alcoholic cardiomyopathy, *Br. Med. J.,* 2, 247, 1972.
71. **Rossi, M. A.,** Alcohol and malnutrition in the pathogenesis of experimental alcoholic cardiomyopathy, *J. Pathol.,* 130, 105, 1980.
72. **Bonenfant, J. L., Miller, F., and Roy, P. E.,** Quebec beer-drinkers cardiomyopathy. Pathological studies, *Can. Med. Assoc. J.,* 97, 910, 1967.
73. **Hsu, I. C., Smalley, E. B., Strong, F. M., and Ribelin, W. E.,** Identification of T-2 toxin in moldy corn associated with a lethal toxicosis in cattle, *Appl. Microbiol.,* 24, 684, 1972.
74. **Schwetz, B. A., Smith, F. A., and Staples, R. E.,** Teratogenic potential of ethanol in mice, rats and rabbits, *Teratology,* 18, 385, 1978.
75. **Chernoff, G. F.,** The fetal alcohol syndrome in mice: an animal model, *Teratology,* 15, 223, 1977.
76. **Randall, C. L. and Taylor, W. J.,** Prenatal alcohol exposure in mice: teratogenic effects, *Teratology,* 19, 305, 1978.
77. **MacMahon, B. and Yen, S.,** Unrecognized epidemic of anencephaly and spina bifida, *Lancet,* i, 31, 1971.
78. **Chu, F. S., Chang, C. C., Ashoor, S. H., and Prentice, N.,** Stability of aflatoxin B₁ and ochratoxin A in brewing, *Appl. Microbiol.,* 29, 313, 1975.
79. **Krogh, P., Hald, B., Gjertsen, P., and Myken, F.,** Fate of ochratoxin A and citrinin during malting and brewing experiments, *Appl. Microbiol.,* 28, 31, 1974.
80. **Nip, W. K., Chang, C. C., Chu, F. S., and Prentice, N.,** Fate of ochratoxin A in brewing, *Appl. Microbiol.,* 30, 1048, 1975.
81. **Hayes, A. W.,** Mycotoxin teratogenicity, *Toxicon,* 17 (Suppl. 1), 739, 1978.
82. **Lee, K., Moller, L., Hardt, F., Haubek, A., and Jensen, E.,** Alcohol-induced brain damage and liver damage in young males, *Lancet,* ii, 759, 1979.
83. **Cook, P.,** Cancer of the oesophagus in Kenya. A summary and evaluation of the evidence for the frequency of occurrence and a preliminary indication of the possible association with the consumption of alcoholic drinks made from maize, *Br. J. Cancer,* 25, 853, 1972.
84. **Lovelace, C. E. A. and Nyathi, C. B.,** Estimation of the fungal toxins zearalenone and aflatoxin, contaminating opaque beer in Zambia, *J. Sci. Food Agric.,* 28, 288, 1977.
85. **Martin, P. M. D. and Keen, P.,** The occurrence of zearalenone in raw and fermented products from Swaziland and Lesotho, *Sabouraudia,* 16, 15, 1978.
86. **Marasas, W. F. C., van Rensburg, S. J., and Mirocha, C. J.,** Incidence of *Fusarium* species and the mycotoxins, deoxynivalenol and zearalenone, in corn produced in esophageal cancer areas in Transkei, *J. Agric. Food Chem.,* 27, 1108, 1979.
87. **Larsson, L., Sandstrom, A., and Westling, P.,** Relationship of Plummer-Vinson disease to cancer of the upper alimentary tract in Sweden, *Cancer Res.,* 35, 3308, 1975.
88. **Pettersson, H. and Kiessling, K. H.,** Mycotoxins in Swedish grains and mixed feeds, *Chem. Rundschau,* 32 (35), 1979.
89. **Schoental, R.,** Mouldy grain and the aetiology of pellagra: the role of toxic metabolites of *Fusarium,* *Biochem. Soc. Trans.,* 8, 147, 1980.
90. **Lin, P. and Tang, W.,** The epidemiology and etiology of esophageal cancer in China, *J. Cancer Res. Clin. Oncol.,* 96, 121, 1980.
91. **Rubinstein, Y. I., Kukel Y. P., and Kudinova, G. P.,** Papillomatosis with hyperkeratosis of the proventriculus in rats following their feeding on grain infested with fungus *Fusarium sporotrichiella* Bilai var. *poae* (Pk) Bilai, *Voprosy Pitaniya,* 26, 57, 1967.

92. **Schoental, R. and Joffe, A. Z.,** Lesions induced in rodents by extracts from cultures of *Fusarium poae* and *F. sporotrichioides, J. Pathol.,* 112, 37, 1974.

93. **Schoental, R., Joffe, A. Z., and Yagen, B.,** Cardiovascular lesions and various tumours found in rats given T-2 toxin, a trichothecene metabolite of *Fusarium* species, *Cancer Res.,* 39, 2179, 1979.

94. **Cook-Mozaffari, P. J., Azordegan, F., Day, N. E., Ressicaud, A., Sabai, C., and Aramesh, B.,** Oesophageal cancer studies in the Caspian Littoral of Iran: results of a case-control study, *Br. J. Cancer,* 39, 293, 1979.

95. **Schoental, R.,** Possible public health significance of *Fusarium* toxins, Proc. 3rd Meet., *Mycotoxins in Animal Disease,* Ministry of Agriculture, Fisheries, and Food, Weybridge, 1979, 67.

96. **Joffe, A. Z.,** *Fusarium poae* and *F. sporotrichioides* as principal causal agents of alimentary toxic aleukia, in *Mycotoxic Fungi, Mycotoxins, Mycotoxicoses: An Encyclopedic Handbook,* Vol. 3, Wyllie, T. D. and Morehouse, L. G., Eds., Marcel Dekker, New York, 1978, 21.

97. **Reynolds, E. S.,** An account of the epidemic outbreak of arsenical poisoning occurring in beer drinkers in the north of England and the Midland Counties in 1900, *Lancet,* i, 166, 1901.

98. **Spiegelhalder, B., Eisenbrand, G., and Preussman, R.,** Contamination of beer with trace quantities of *N*-nitrosodimethylamine, *Food Cosmet. Toxicol.,* 17, 29, 1979.

99. **Goff, E. U. and Fine, D. H.,** Analysis of volatile *N*-nitrosamines in alcoholic beverages, *Food Cosmet. Toxicol.,* 17, 569, 1979.

100. **Scalan, R. A., Barbour, J. F., Hotchkiss, J. H., and Libbey, L. M.,** *N*-nitrosodimethylamine in beer, *Food Cosmet. Toxicol.,* 18, 27, 1980.

101. **Barnes, J. M. and Magee, P. N.,** Some toxic properties of dimethyl nitrosamine, *Br. J. Ind. Med.,* 11, 167, 1954.

102. **Magee, P. N. and Barnes, J. M.,** Carcinogenic nitroso compounds, *Adv. Cancer Res.,* 10, 163, 1967.

103. **Druckrey, H., Preussmann, R., Ivankovic, S., and Schmähl, D.,** Organotrope carcinogene Wirkungen bei 65 verschiedenen *N*-Nitroso-Verbindungen an BD-Ratten, *Z. Krebsforsch,* 69, 103, 1967.

104. **Magee, P. N., Montesano, R., and Preussmann, R.,** *N*-nitroso compounds and related carcinogens, *Am. Chem. Soc. Monogr.,* 173, 491, 1976.

105. **Sander, J., Schweinsberg, F., and Menz, H. P.,** Untersuchungen über die Entstehung cancerogener Nitrosamine im Magen, *Hoppe-Seyler's Z. Physiol. Chem.,* 349, 1691, 1968.

106. **Mirvish, S. S.,** *N*-nitroso compounds their chemistry and in vivo formation and possible importance as environmental carcinogens, *J. Toxicol. Environ. Health,* 2, 1267, 1977.

107. **Mirvish, S. S. and Chu, C.,** Chemical determination of methylnitrosourea and ethylnitrosourea in stomach contents of rats after intubation of the alkylureas plus sodium nitrite, *J. Natl. Cancer Inst.,* 50, 745, 1972.

108. **Mirvish, S. S., Jarlowski, K., Sams, J. P., and Arnold, S. D.,** Studies related to nitrosamide formation: nitrosation in solvent: water and solvent systems. Nitrosomethylurea formation in the rat stomach and analyses of a fish product for ureas, in *Environmental Aspects of N-Nitroso Compounds,* No. 19, World Health Organization and IARC Scientific Publications, Lyon, 1978, 161.

109. **Lijinsky, W.,** Reaction of drugs with nitrous acid as a source of carcinogenic nitrosamines, *Cancer Res.,* 34, 255, 1974.

110. **Tannenbaum, S. R., Archer, M. C., Wishnok, J. S., and Bishop, W. W.,** Nitrosamine formation in human saliva, *J. Natl. Cancer Inst.,* 60, 251, 1978.

111. **Sander, J. and Bürkle, G.,** Induktion maligner Tumoren bei Ratten durch gleichzeitige Verfutterung von Nitrit und sekundären Aminen, *Z. Krebsforsch,* 73, 54, 1969.

112. **Lijinsky, W. and Taylor, H. W.,** Nitrosamines and their precursors in food, in *Origins of Human Cancer,* Hiatt, H. H., Watson, J. D., and Winsten, J. A., Eds., Cold Spring Harbor Conf. on Cells Proliferation, Cold Spring Harbor Laboratory, Cold Spring Harbor, N.Y., 1977, 1579.

113. **Wogan, G. N., Paglialunga, S., Archer, M. C., and Tannenbaum, S. R.,** Carcinogenicity of nitrosation products of ephedrine, sarcosine folic acid and creatinine, *Cancer Res.,* 35, 1981, 1975.

114. **Mottram, D. S. and Wood, J. D.,** Some uses of chemicals in meat production: benefits and hazards, in *Chemistry and Agriculture,* Chem. Soc., London, 1979, 199.

115. **Gough, T. A., Goodhead, K., and Walters, C. L.,** Distribution of some volatile nitrosamines in cooked bacon, *J. Sci. Food Agric.,* 27, 181, 1976.

116. **Fine, D. H., Rounbehler, D. P., Fan, T., and Ross, R.,** Human exposure to *N*-nitroso compounds in the environment, in *Origins of Human Cancer,* Hiatt, H. H., Watson, J. D., and Winsten, J. A., Eds., Cold Spring Harbor Laboratory, Cold Spring Harbor, N.Y., 1977, 293.

117. **Lee, J. S., Libbey, L. M., Scanlan, R. A., and Barbour,** *N*-Nitroso-3-hydroxypyrrolidine in fried bacon and fried out fat, in *Environmental Aspects of N-nitroso compounds,* No. 19, World Health Organization and IARC Scientific Publications, Lyon, 1978, 325.

118. **Sen, N. P., Smith, D. C., Schwinghammer, L., and Marleau, J. J.,** Diethylnitrosamine and other *N*-nitrosamines in foods, *J. Assoc. Off. Anal. Chem.,* 52, 47, 1969.

119. **Singer, S. S., Lijinsky, W., and Singer, G. M.,** Transnitrosation: an important aspect of the chemistry of aliphatic nitrosamines, in *Environmental Aspects of N-Nitroso Compounds,* No. 19, World Health Organization and IARC Scientific Publications, 1978, 175.

120. **Linjinsky, W. and Shubik, P.,** Benzo(a)pyrene and polynuclear hydrocarbons in charcoal-broiled meat, *Science,* 145, 53, 1974.

121. **Schoental, R.,** Carcinogenic hazards to the suckling and to the very young due to milk from females exposed to carcinogenic or oestrogenic agents during lactation, in *Tumours of Early Life in Man and Animals,* Severi, L., Ed., Division of Cancer Research, University of Perugia, Italy 1978, 985.

122. **Richter, H. E.,** Beeinflussung der Milchqualität durch einheimische Pflanzen. II. Veränderung von Geschmack, Geruch und der Farbe, *Wien. Tierarztl. Monatsschr.,* 52, 635, 1965.

123. **Knowles, J. A.,** Excretion of drugs in milk, a review, *J. Pediatr.,* 66, 1068, 1966.

124. **D'Arcy, P. F.,** Drugs in milk, in *Iatrogenic Diseases,* 2nd ed., D'Arcy, P. F. and Griffin, J. P., Eds., Oxford University Press, Oxford, 1979, 425.

125. **Miller, R. W.,** Pollutants in breast milk, *J. Pediatr.,* 90, 510, 1977.

126. **Anon.,** Insecticides in breast milk, *Nutr. Rev.,* 35, 72, 1977.

127. **Nilsson, S., Nygren, K.-G., Johansson, E. D. M.,** d-Norgestrel concentration in maternal plasma, milk and child plasma during administration of oral contraceptives to nursing women, *Am. J. Obstet. Gynecol.,* 129, 178, 1977.

128. **Nilsson, S., Nygren, K. G., and Johansson, E. D. B.,** Megastrol acetate concentrations in plasma and milk during administration of an oral contraceptive containing 4 mg megastrol acetate to nursing women, *Contraception,* 16, 615, 1977.

129. **Schoental, R.,** Carcinogenicity as related to age, *Ann. Rev. Pharmacol.,* 14, 185, 1974.

130. **Schoental, R.,** Carcinogens in plants and microorganisms, *Am. Chem. Soc. Monogr.,* 173, 626, 1976.

131. **Schoental, R.,** Liver lesions in young rats suckled by mothers treated with the pyrrolizidine (Senecie) alkaloids, lasiocarpine and retrorsine, *J. Pathol. Bacteriol.,* 77, 485, 1959.

132. **Johnson, A. E.,** Changes in calves and rats consuming milk from cows fed chronic lethal doses of *Senecio Jacobaea* (Tansy ragwort), *Am. J. Vet. Res.,* 37, 107, 1976.

133. **Dickinson, J. O., Cooke, M. P., King, R. R., and Mohamed, P. A.,** Milk transfer of pyrrolizidine alkaloids in cattle, *J. Am. Vet. Med. Assoc.,* 169, 1192, 1976.

134. **Hakim, S. A. E., Kijovic, V., and Walker, J.,** Experimental transmission of sanguinarine in milk. Detection of a metabolic product, *Nature (London),* 189, 201, 1961.

135. **De Iongh, H., Vles, R. O., and van Pelt, J. G.,** Milk in mammals fed an aflatoxin-containing diet, *Nature (London),* 202, 466, 1964.

136. **Masri, M. S., Garcia, V. C., and Page, J. R.,** The aflatoxin M content of milk from cows fed known amounts of aflatoxin, *Vet. Rec.,* 84, 146, 1969.

137. **Masri, M. S., Ludin, R. E., Page, J. R., and Garcia, V. C.,** Crystalline aflatoxin M_1 from urine and milk, *Nature, (London),* 215, 753, 1967.

138. **Allcroft, R., Roberts, B. A., and Lloyd, M. K.,** Excretion of aflatoxin in lactating cows, *Food Cosmet. Toxicol.,* 6, 619, 1968.

139. **Kiermeier, F., Weiss, G., Behringer, G., Miller, M., and Ranfit, K.,** The presence and concentration of aflatoxin M_1 in milk shipped to a dairy plant, *Z. Lebensm. Unters. Forsch.,* 163, 171, 1977.

140. **Polzhofer, K.,** Determination of aflatoxin in milk and milk products, *Z. Lebensm. Unters. Forsch.,* 163, 175, 1977.

141. **Spatz, M. and Laqueur, G. L.,** Evidence for transplacental passage of the natural carcinogen cycasin and its aglycone, *Proc. Soc. Exp. Biol. Med.,* 127, 281, 1968.

142. **Lunaas, T.,** Transfer of oestradiol-17β to milk in cattle, *Nature (London),* 198, 288, 1963.

143. **Nilsson, S., Nygren, K., Johansson, E. D. B.,** Transfer of estradiol to human milk, *Am. J. Obstet. Gynecol.,* 132, 653, 1978.

144. **Evans, I. A., Jones, R. S., and Wainwaring-Burton, R.,** Passage of bracken-fern toxicity into milk, *Nature (London),* 237, 107, 1972.

145. **Pamukcu, A. M., Erturk, E., Yalciner, U. M., and Bryan, G.,** Carcinogenic and mutagenic action of milk from cows fed bracken, *Cancer Res.,* 38, 1556, 1978.

146. **Ribelin, W. E., Smalley, E. B., and Strong, F. M.,** Effect of Ochratoxin and Other Mycotoxins on Cattle, 2nd Int. Congr. Plant Pathol., Minneapolis, September 5, 1973.

147. **Robinson, T. S., Mirocha, C. J., Kurtz, H. J., Behrens, C. C., Chi, M. S., Weaver, G. A., and Nystrom, S. D.,** Transmission of T-2 toxin into bovine and porcine milk, *J. Dairy Sci.,* 62, 637, 1979.

147a. **Yoshizawa, T., Mirocha, C. J., Behrens, C. J., and Swanson, S. P.,** Metabolic fate of T-2 toxin in a lactating cow, *Food, Cosmet., Toxicol.,* 19, 31, 1981.

148. **Miller, J. K., Hacking- A., Harrison, J., and Gross, V. J.,** Stillbirth, neonatal mortality and small litters in pigs associated with ingestion of *Fusarium* toxin by pregnant sows, *Vet. Rec.,* 93, 555, 1973.

149. **Mirocha, C. J., Pathre, S. V., and Robinson, T. S.,** Comparative metabolism of zearalenone and transmission into bovine milk, *Food Cosmet. Toxicol.,* 19, 25, 1981.

150. **Shay, H., Friedmann, B., Gruenstein, M., and Weinhouse, S.,** Mammary excretion of 20-methylcholanthrene, *Cancer Res.,* 10, 797, 1950.

151. **Shay, H., Weinhouse, S., Gruenstein, M., Marx, H. E., and Friedman, B.,** Development of malignant lymphoma in some of the young rats suckled by mothers receiving methylcholanthrene by stomach tube only during the lactation period, *Cancer,* 3, 891, 1950.

152. **West, C. E. and Horton, B. J.,** Transfer of polycyclic hydrocarbons from diet to milk in rats, rabbits and sheep, *Life Sci.,* 19, 1543, 1976.

153. **De Benedictis, G., Maiorano, G., Chieco-Bianchi, L., and Flore-Donati, L.,** Lung carcinogenesis by urethane in newborn suckling and adult Swiss mice, *Br. J. Cancer,* 16, 686, 1962.

154. **Adenis, L., Vlaeminck, M. N., and Driessens, J.,** Pulmonary adenoma in urethane-treated mice. IX. Adenoma development in neonate mice nursed by urethane-treated mothers, *C. R. Soc. Biol.,* 164, 2526, 1971.

155. **Nomura, T.,** Carcinogenesis by urethan via mother's milk and its enhancement of transplacental carcinogenesis in mice, *Cancer Res.,* 33, 1677, 1973.

156. **Nomura, T.,** Tumor induction in the progeny of mice receiving 4-nitroquinoline 1-oxide and *N*-methyl-*N*-nitrosourethan during pregnancy or lactation, *Cancer Res.,* 34, 3373, 1974.

157. **Maekawa, A. and Odashima, S.,** Induction of tumors of the nervous system in the AC1/N rat with 1-butyl-1-nitrosourea administered transplacentally, neonatally, or via maternal milk, *Gann,* 66, 175, 1975.

158. **Spielhoff, R., Bresch, H., Hönig, M., and Mohr, U.,** Brief communication: milk as transport agent for diethylnitrosamine in Syrian Golden hamsters, *J. Natl. Cancer Inst.,* 53, 281, 1974.

159. **Schoental, R., Gough, T. A., and Webb, K. S.,** Carcinogens in rat milk. Transfer of ingested diethylnitrosamine into milk of lactating rats, *Br. J. Cancer,* 30, 238, 1974.

160. **Schoental, R.,** Multiple primary Tumours in Rats Treated with Certain "Natural" Carcinogens from Plants or Fungi, in Multiple Primary Tumours, Severi, L., Ed., 5th Perugia Quandrennial Int. Conf. Cancer, Perugia, 1974, 801.

161. **Mohr, U. and Althoff, J.,** Carcinogenic activity of aliphatic nitrosamines via the mother's milk in the offspring of Syrian golden hamsters, *Proc. Soc. Exp. Biol. Med.,* 136, 1007, 1971.

162. **Mohr, U., Althoff, J., Emminger, A., Bresch, H., and Spielhoff, R.,** Effect of nitrosamines on nursing Syrian Golden hamsters and their offspring, *Z. Krebsforsch,* 78, 73, 1972.

163. **Juszkiewicz, T. and Kowalski, B.,** Dietary nitrosamines, *Food Cosmet. Toxicol.,* 14, 653, 1976.

164. **Kraybill, H. F.,** Conceptual approaches to the assessment of non-occupational environmental cancer, in *Advances in Modern Toxicology,* Vol. 3, Kraybill, H. F. and Mehlman, M. A., Eds., John Wiley & Sons, New York, 1977, 22.

164a. **Kraybill, H. F.,** Evaluation of public health aspects of carcinogenic/mutagenic biofreractories in drinking water, *Prev. Med.,* 9, 212, 1980.

165. **Mussman, H. C.,** Drug and chemical residues in domestic animals, *Fed. Proc. Fed. Am. Soc. Exp. Med.,* 34, 197, 1975.

166. **Kimbrough, R. D., Squire, R. A., Linder, R. E., Strandberg, J. D., Montali, R. J., and Burse, V. W.,** Induction of liver tumors in Sherman strain female rats by polychlorinated biphenyl araclor 1260, *J. Natl. Cancer Inst.,* 55, 1453, 1975.

167. **Kimbrough, R. D.,** The carcinogenic and other chronic effects of persistent halogenated organic compounds, *Ann. N.Y. Acad. Sci.,* 320, 415, 1979.

168. **Allen, J. R. and Norback, D. H.,** Carcinogenic potential of the polychlorinated biphenyls, in *Origin of Human Cancer,* Vol. A, Hiatt, H. H., Watson, J. D., and Winsten, J. A., Eds, Cold Spring Harbor Laboratory, Cold Spring Harbor, N.Y., 1977, 173.

169. **Burchfield, H. P. and Storrs, E. C.,** Organohalogen carcinogens, in *Advances in Modern Toxicology,* Vol. 3, Kraybill, H. F. and Mehlman, M. A., Eds., John Wiley & Sons, New York, 1977, 319.

170. Evaluation of the carcinogenic risk of chemicals to man. Some fumigants, the herbicides 2,4-D and 2,4,5-T, chlorinated dibenzodioxins and miscellaneous industrial chemicals, *IARC Monogr.,* Vol. 18, Int. Agency Res. Cancer; Lyon, 1977.

171. **Kociba, R. J., Keyes, D. G., Beyer, J. E., Carreon, R. M., Wade, C. E., Dittenber, D. A., Kalnins, R. P., Franson, L. E., Park, C. N., Barnard, S. D., Hummel, R. A., and Humiston, C. G.,** Results of a two-year chronic toxicity and oncogenicity study of 2,3,7,8-tetrachlorodibenzo-*p*-dioxin (TCDD) in rats, *Toxicol. Appl. Pharmacol.,* 46, 279, 1978.

172. **Firestone, D., Clower, M., Jr., Borsetti, A. P., Teske, R. H., and Long, P. E.,** Polychlorodibenzo-*p*-dioxin and pentachlorophenol residues in milk and blood of cows fed technical pentachlorophenol, *J. Argric. Food Chem.,* 27, 1171, 1979.

173. **Poland, A. and Kende, A.,** The genetic expression of aryl hydrocarbon hydroxylase activity: evidence for a receptor mutation in non-responsive mice, in *Origin of Human Cancer,* Hiatt, H. H., Watson, J. D., and Winsten, J. A., Eds., Cold Spring Harbor Laboratory, Cold Spring Harbor, N.Y., 1977, 847.

174. **Boyland, E., Dukes, C. E., Grover, P. L., and Mitchley, B. C. V.,** The induction of renal tumours by feeding lead acetate to rats, *Br. J. Cancer,* 16, 283, 1962.
175. **Schoental, R. and Gibbard, S.,** Increased excretion of urinary porphyrins by white rats given intragastrically several types of chemical carcinogens: diethylnitrosamine, monocrotaline, T-2 toxin, and ethyl methane sulphonate, *Biochem. Soc. Trans.,* 7, 127, 1978.
176. **Poland, A. and Glover, E.,** An estimate of the maximum in vivo covalent binding of 2,3,7,8,-tetrachlorodibenzo-*p*-dioxin to rat liver protein, ribosomal RNA and DNA, *Cancer Res.,* 39, 3341, 1979.
177. **Allen, J. R., Barsotti, D. A., Lambrecht, L. K., and van Miller, J. P.,** Reproductive effects of halogenated aromatic hydrocarbons on nonhuman primates, *Ann. N.Y. Acad. Sci.,* 320, 419, 1979.
178. **Murray, F. J., Smith, F. A., Nitschke, K. D., Humiston, C. G., Kociba, R. J., and Schwetz, B. A.,** Three-generation reproduction study of rats given, 2,3,7,8-tetrachlorodibenzo-*p*-dioxin (TCDD) in the diet, *Toxicol. Appl. Pharmacol.,* 50, 241, 1979.
179. **Greig, J. B.,** The toxicology of 2,3,7,8-tetrachlorodibenzo-*p*-dioxin and its structural analogues, *Ann. Occup. Hyg.,* 22, 411, 1979.
180. **Olson, J. R., Holscher, M. A., and Neal, R. A.,** Toxicity of 2,3,7,8-tetrachlorodibenzo-*p*-dioxin in the golden hamster, *Toxicol. Appl. Pharmacol.,* 55, 67, 1980.
181. **Sparschau, G. L., Dunn, F. L., and Rowe, V. K.,** Study of the teratogenicity of 2,3,7,8-tetrachlorodibenzo-*p*-dioxin in the rat, *Food Cosmet. Toxicol.,* 9, 405, 1971.
182. **Smith, F. A., Schwetz, B. A., and Nitschke, K. D.,** Teratogenicity of 2,3,7,8-tetrachlorodibenzo-*p*-dioxin in CF-1 mice, *Toxicol. Appl. Pharmacol.,* 38, 517, 1976.
183. **Van Miller, J. P., Lalich, J. J., and Allen, J. R.,** Increased incidence of neoplasms in rats exposed to low levels of 2,3,7,8-tetrachlorodibenzo-*p*-dioxin, *Chemosphere,* 10, 625, 1977.
184. **Di Giovanni, J., Berry, D. L., Gleason, G. L., Kishore, G. S., and Slaga, T. J.,** Time-dependent inhibition by 2,3,7,8-tetrachlorodibenzo-*p*-dioxin of skin tumorigenesis with polycyclic hydrocarbons, *Cancer Res.,* 40, 1580, 1980.
185. **Kouri, R. E., Rude, T. H., Joglekar, R., Dansette, P. M., Jerina, D. M., Atlas, S. A., Owens, R. S., and Newbert, D. W.,** 2,3,7,8-Tetrachlorodibenzo-*p*-dioxin as co-carcinogen causing 3-methylcholanthrene-initiated subcutaneous tumors in mice genetically "nonresponsive" at *Ah* locus, *Cancer Res.,* 38, 2777, 1978.
186. **Hernberg, S.,** Incidence of cancer in population with exceptional exposure to metals, in *Origin of Human Cancer,* Hiatt, H. H., Watson, J. A., and Winsten, J. A., Eds., Cold Spring Harbor Laboratory, Cold Spring Harbor, N.Y. 1977, 147.
187. **Furst, A.,** Inorganic agents as carcinogens, in *Advances in Modern Toxicology,* Vol. 3, Kraybill, H. F. and Mehlman, M. A., Eds., John Wiley & Sons, New York, 1977, 209.
188. **Arcos, J. C. and Argus, M. F.,** *Chemical Induction of Cancer. Structural Bases and Biological Mechanism,* Vol. 2, Academic Press, New York, 1974.
189. **Dipple, A.,** Polynuclear aromatic carcinogens, in *Chemical Carcinogens,* Monogr. 173, Searle, C. E., Ed., American Chemical Society, Washington, D.C., 1976, 245.
190. **Doll, R.,** The pattern of disease in the post-infection era: national trends, *Proc. R. Soc. London B.,* 205, 47, 1979.
191. **Segi, M., Kurihara, M., and Matsuyama, T.,** Cancer Mortality for Selected Sites in 24 Countires, No. 5 (1964 to 1965), Deparatment Public Health, Tohohu University School of Medicine, Sendae, Japan, 1969.
192. **Schoental, R.,** If I had 2500 million pounds to spare on cancer. . . , *Int. J. Environ. Stud.,* 15, 65, 1980.
193. **Mann, G.,** Diet-heart: End of an era, *N. Engl. J. Med.,* 297, 644, 1977.
194. **Glueck, C. J., Mattson, F., and Bierman, E. L.,** Diet and coronary heart disease: another view, *N. Engl. J. Med.,* 298, 1471, 1978.
195. **McMichael, J.,** Fats and atheroma: an inquest, *Br. Med. J.,* i, 173, 1979.
196. **Mann, J. L.,** Fats and atheroma: a retrial, *Br. Med. J.,* i, 732, 1979.
197. **Ahrens, E. H.,** Dietary fats and coronary heart disease: unfinished business, *Lancet,* ii, 1345, 1979.
198. **Wynder, E. L. and Reddy, B. S.,** Dietary fat and colon cancer, *J. Natl. Cancer Inst.,* 54, 7, 1975.
199. **de Waard, F.,** Breast cancer incidence and nutritional status with particular reference to body weight and height, *Cancer Res.,* 35, 3351, 1975.
200. **Armstrong, B. and Doll, R.,** Environmental factors and cancer incidence and mortality in different countries, with special reference to dietary practices, *Int. J. Cancer,* 15, 617, 1975.
201. **Armstrong, B. K.,** The role of diet in human carcinogenesis with special reference to endometrial cancer, in *Origin of Human Cancer,* Hiatt, H. H., Watson, J. A., and Winsten, J. A., Eds., Cold Spring Harbor Laboratory, Cold Spring Harbor, N.Y., 1977, 557.
202. **Weisburger, J. H., Cohen, L. A., and Wynder, E. L.,** On the etiology and metabolic epidemiology of the main human cancers, in *Origin of Human Cancer,* Hiatt, H. H., Watson, J. A., and Winsten, J. A., Eds, Cold Spring Harbor Laboratory, Cold Spring Harbor, N.Y., 1977, 567.

203. **Pearce, M. L. and Dayton, S.,** Incidence of cancer in men on a diet high in polyunsaturated fat, *Lancet* i, 464, 1971.

204. **Hopkins, G. J. and West, C. E.,** Minireview: Possible roles of dietary fats in carcinogenesis, *Life Sci.,* 19, 1103, 1976.

205. **Enig, M. G., Munn, R. J., and Kenney, M.,** Dietary fat and cancer trends — a critique, *Fed. Proc. Fed. Am. Soc. Exp. Med.,* 37, 2215, 1978.

206. **Liv, K., Stammler, J., and Moss, D.,** Dietary cholesterol, fat and fibre and colon-cancer mortality, *Lancet* ii, 782, 1979.

207. **Gaskill, S. P., McGuire, W. L., Osborne, C. K., and Stern, M. P.,** Breast cancer mortality and diet in the United States, *Cancer Res.,* 39, 3628, 1979.

208. **Rogers, A. E.,** Variable effects of a lipotrope-deficient, high-fat diet on chemical carcinogenesis in rats, *Cancer Res.,* 35, 2469, 1975.

209. **Swern, D.,** Ed., *Bailey's Industrial Oil and Fat Products,* Vol. 1, 4th ed., John Wiley & Sons, Chichester, 1979.

210. **Campbell, T. C., Caedo, J. P., Jr., Bulato-Jayme, J., Salamat, L., and Engel, R. W.,** Aflatoxin M_1 in human urine, *Nature (London),* 227, 403, 1970.

211. **Parker, W. A. and Melnick, D.,** Absence of aflatoxin from refined vegetable oils, *J. Am, Oil Chem. Soc.,* 43, 635, 1966.

212. **Beebe, R. M. and Takahashi, D. M.,** Determination of aflatoxin M_1 by high pressure liquid chromatography using fluorescence detection, *J. Agric. Food Chem.,* 28, 481, 1980.

213. **Suzangar, M., Emami, A., and Barnett, R.,** Aflatoxin contamination of village milk in Isfahan, Iran, *Trop. Sci.,* 18, 155, 1976.

214. **Rodricks, J. V. and Stoloff, L.,** Aflatoxin residues from contaminated feed in edible tissues of food-producing animals, in *Mycotoxins in Human and Animal Health,* Rodricks, J. V., Hesseltine, C. W., and Mehlman, M. A., Eds., Pathotox Publ., Park Forest, Ill. 1977, 67.

215. **Grant, D. W. and Carlson, F. W.,** Partitioning behavior of aflatoxin M in dairy products, *Bull Environ. Contam. Toxicol.,* 6, 521, 1971.

216. **Hamsa, T. A. P. and Ayres, J. C.,** Factors affecting aflatoxin contamination of cottonseed. I. Contamination of cottonseeds with *Aspergillus flavus* at harvest and during storage, *J. Am. Oil Chem. Soc.,* 54, 219, 1977.

217. **Hendricks, J. D., Sinnhuber, R. O., Loveland, P. M., Pawlowski, N. E., and Nixon, J. E.,** Hepatocarcinogenicity of glandless cottonseeds and cottonseed oil to rainbow trout *(Salmo gairdnerii), Science,* 208, 309, 1980.

218. **Yahl, K. R., Watson, S. A., Smith, R. J., and Barabolok, R.,** Laboratory wet milling of corn containing high levels of aflatoxin, a survey of commercial wet milling products, *Cereal Chem.,* 48, 385, 1971.

219. **Brekke, O. L., Peplinski, A. J., Nelson, G. E. N., and Griffin, E. L. Jr.,** Pilot-plant dry milling of corn containing aflatoxin, *Cereal Chem.,* 52, 205, 1975.

220. **Bennett, G. A., Peplinski, A. J., Brekke, O. L., Jackson, L. K., and Wischer, W. R.,** Zearalenone: distribution in dry-milled fractions of contaminated corn, *Cereal Chem.,* 53, 299, 1976.

221. **Roe, D. A.,** *A plague of Corn — the Social History of Pellagra,* Cornell University Press, Ithaca, N.Y., 1973.

222. **Schoental, R.,** Pellagra and *Fusarium* mycotoxins, *Int. J. Environ.,* Stud., 13, 327, 1979.

223. **Ullola-Sosa, M. and Schroeder, H. W.,** Note on aflatoxin decomposition in the process of making tortillas from corn, *Cereal Chem.,* 46, 397, 1969.

224. **Kelsey, J. L.,** A review of research on effects of fiber intake on man, *Am. J. Clinic. Nutr.,* 31, 142, 1978.

225. **Graham, S. and Mettlin, C.,** Reviews and commentary. Diet and colon cancer, *Am. J. Epidemiol.,* 109, 1, 1979.

226. **Fleiszer, D., Murray D., MacFarlane, J., and Brown, R. A.,** Protective effect of dietary fibre against chemically induced bowel tumours in rats, *Lancet,* 2, 525, 1978.

227. **Freeman, H. J., Spiller, G. A., and Kim, Y. S.,** A double-blind study on the effect of purified cellulose dietary fiber on 1,2,-dimethylhydrazine-induced rat colonic neoplasia, *Cancer Res.,* 38, 2912, 1978.

228. **Bauer, H. G., Asp. N., Öste, R., Dahlqvist, A., and Fredlund, P. E.,** Effect of dietary fiber on the induction of colorectal tumors and fecal β-glucuronidase activity in the rat, *Cancer Res.,* 39, 3752, 1979.

229. **Hieger, I.,** Carcinogenesis by cholesterol, *Br. J. Cancer,* 13, 439, 1959.

230. **Olifson, L. E.,** The chemical nature of toxins isolated from over-wintered cereals, *Mendeleyev Chem. Soc. Monitor,* 7, 21, 1957.

231. **Mirocha, C. J. and Pathre, S.,** Identification of the toxic principle in a sample of poaefusarin, *Appl. Microbiol.,* 26, 719, 1973.

232. **Yagen, B., Joffe, A. Z., Horn, P., Mor, N., and Lutsky, I. I.,** Toxins from a strain involved in ATA, *Mycotoxins in Human and Animal Health,* Rodricks, J. V., Hesseltine, C. W., and Mehlman, M., Eds., Pathotox Publications, Ill. Park Forest, 1977, 329.

233. **Lutsky, I., Mor, N., Yagen, B., and Joffe, A. Z.,** The role of T-2 toxin in experimental alimentary toxic aleukia. A toxicity study in cats, *Toxicol. Appl. Pharmacol.,* 43, 111, 1978.
234. **Yagen, B., Horn, P., Joffe, A. Z., and Cox, R. H.,** Isolation and structural elucidation of a novel sterol metabolite of *Fusarium sporotrichioides,* 921, *J. Chem. Soc. Perkin Trans 1:* p. 2914, 1980.
235. **Schoental, R.,** Mycotoxins in food and the variations in tumor incidence in laboratory rodents, *Nutr. Cancer,* 1, 13, 1978.
236. **Schoental, R.,** Variations in the incidence of "spontaneous" tumours, *Br. J. Cancer,* 39, 101, 1979.
237. **Schoental, R.,** The role of *Fusarium* mycotoxins in the aetiology of tumours of the digestive tract and of certain other organs in man and animals, *Front. Gastrointestinal Res.,* 4, 17, 1979.
238. **Silverstone, H. and Tannenbaum, A.,** The effect of promotion of dietary fat on the rate of formation of mammary carcinoma in mice, *Cancer Res.,* 10, 448, 1950.
239. **Carroll, K. K. and Khor, H. T.,** Effects of dietary fat and dose level of 7,12-dimethylbenz(a)anthracene on mammary tumor incidence in rats, *Cancer Res.,* 30, 2260, 1970.
240. **Carroll, K. K.,** Experimental evidence of dietary factors and hormone dependent cancers, *Cancer Res.,* 35, 3374, 1975.
241. **Chan, P. C., Cohen, L. A., and Wynder, E. L.,** Increased yield of N-nitrosomethylurea-induced mammary tumors by dietary fat, *Proc. Am. Assoc. Cancer Res.,* 17, 133, 1976.
242. **Reddy, B. S., Narisawa, T., Vukusich, D., Weisburger, J. H., and Wynder, E. L.,** Effect of quality and quantity of dietary fat and dimethylhydrazine in colon carcinogenesis in rats, *Proc. Soc. Exp. Biol Med.,* 151, 237, 1976.
243. **Reddy, B. S., Cohen, L. A., McCoy, G. D., Hill, P., Weisburger, J. H., and Wynder, E. L.,** Nutrition and its relationship to cancer, *Adv. Cancer Res.,* 32, 237, 1980.
244. **Robinson, T. S., Mirocha, C. J., Kurtz, H. J., Behrens, J. C., Weaver, G. A., and Chi, M. S.,** Distribution of tritium-labeled T-2 toxin in swine, *J. Agric. Food. Chem.,* 27, 1411, 1979.
245. **Chi, M. S., Robinson, T. S., Mirocha, C. J., Swanson, S. P., and Shimoda, W.,** Excretion and tissue distribution of radioactivity from tritium labelled T-2 toxin in chicks, *Toxicol. Appl. Pharmacol.,* 45, 391, 1978.
246. **Chi, M. S., Robinson, T. S., Mirocha, C. J., Behrens, J. C., and Shimoda, W.,** Transmission of radioactivity into egg from laying hens *(Gallus domesticus)* administered tritium labeled T-2 toxin, *Poultry Sci.,* 57, 1234, 1978.
247. **Wyatt, R. D., Collwell, W. M., Hamilton, P. B., and Burmeister, H. R.,** Neural disturbances in chickens caused by dietary T-2 toxin, *Appl. Microbiol.,* 26, 757, 1973.
248. **Wyatt, R. D., Doerr, J. A., Hamilton, P. B., and Burmeister, H. R.,** Egg production, shell thickness and other physiological parameters of laying hens affected by T-2 toxin, *Appl. Microbiol.,* 29, 641, 1975.
249. **Wyatt, R. D., Hamilton, P. B., and Burmeister, H. R.,** Altered feathering of chicks caused by T-2 toxin, *Poultry Sci.,* 54, 1042, 1975.
250. **Joffe, A. Z. and Yagen, B.,** Intoxication produced by toxic fungi *Fusarium poae* and *F. sporotrichioides* on chicks, *Toxicon,* 16, 263, 1978.
250a. **Dailey, R. E., Reese, R. E., and Brouwer, E. A.,** Metabolism of [^{14}C] zearalenone in laying hens, *J. Agric. Food Chem.,* 28, 286, 1980.
251. **Szepsenwol, J.,** Carcinogenic effects of egg white, egg yolk and egg lipids in mice, *Proc. Soc. Exp. Biol. Med.,* 112, 1073, 1963.
252. **Szepsenwol, J.,** Intracranial tumors in mice of two definite strains maintained on fats enriched diet, *Eur. J. Cancer,* 7, 529, 1971.
253. **Szepsenwol, J.,** Gastrointestinal tumors in mice of three strains maintained on fat-enriched diets, *Oncology,* 35, 143, 1978.
254. **Szepsenwol, J.,** Carcinogenic effect of ether extract of whole egg, alcohol extract of egg yolk and powdered egg free of the ether extractable part in mice, *Proc. Soc. Exp. Biol. Med.,* 116, 1135, 1964.
255. **Ross, M. H. and Bras, G.,** Lasting influence of early caloric restriction on prevalence of neoplasms in the rat, *J. Natl. Cancer Inst.,* 47, 1095, 1971.
256. **Rodricks, J. V.,** Food hazards of natural origin, *Fed. Proc. Fed. Am. Soc. Exp. Med.,* 37, 2587, 1978.
257. **Schoental, R.,** unpublished results.

Chapter 9

AN ASSESSMENT OF THE HAZARD TO PUBLIC
HEALTH OF FUSARIAL TOXINS

P. M. D. Martin

TABLE OF CONTENTS

I. *FUSARIUM* TOXINS

The last few years have seen a dramatic increase in scientific knowledge of mycotoxins with respect to their involvement in chronic as well as acute diseases. In the case of aflatoxin, there was almost immediate realization of its role in carcinogenesis, whereas some time was to elapse before such a connection could be proven in the case of other mycotoxins. This is especially true of fusarial toxins, even though their role in animal poisoning clearly antedates the discovery of aflatoxin. In common with other mycotoxins, they appear to have a specific action on certain "target" tissues or organs, and it is this ability which has aroused curiosity about their mechanism of action and long term effects.

Fusarial toxins are comprised of three groups: the trichothecenes, moniliformin, and the estrogenic mycotoxins, which are nonsteroidal lactones differing in structure from the natural estrogens.

The main mycotoxins produced by various *Fusarium* species and some of their causal agents are given in Tables 1 and 2.

A. Trichothecenes

1. T_1 Toxin (Butenolide Lactone)

T_1 toxin and the next are known as the "fescue toxins" because they were originally isolated from fungi in moldy fescue grass. The fescue disease syndrome, including lameness of hind quarters and gangrene in tail and hooves of cattle,[1] was reproduced when the toxin was injected experimentally into the shoulders and thigh of a heifer intramuscularly.[2] In steers, similar diverse effects have been reported[3] including pericarditis, rumenitis, acute pneumonia, gastric lesions and edema of the tail.

2. T_2 Toxin and Other Trichothecenes

T_2 toxin, perhaps the best known of the trichothecenes, has been responsible for generalized toxicosis and high mortality rate in cattle.[4] Its effects on experimental animals resemble those of moldy corn toxicosis in cattle,[2] a fairly frequent disease characterized by severe gastrointestinal necrosis. The recent discovery that *F. sporotrichioides* is able to produce this toxin,[5] and the similarity of the acute lesions in experimental animals[6-8] makes it highly probable that it was the cause of the outbreak of Alimentary Toxic Aleukia (ATA) in the Orenburg district in the U.S.S.R.[9] On that occasion overwintered grain that had been eaten by the peasant population yielded several toxicogenic fungi, including *F. poae, F. sporotrichioides,* and *Cladosporium epiphyllum.* Likewise various epizootics in sheep and horses associated with *F. poae* are probably due to this toxin.[10,11]

Other symptoms due to T_2 toxin in experimental animals are very diverse including emesis, altered feathering, loss of weight, drop in temperature, diarrhea, paraplegia, anemia, tetanic spasm and various neural disturbances, leucopenia, prothrombinopenia, and mouth lesions.[35-49] There is also some evidence that T_2 toxin is a teratogen.[50,51]

Diacetoxyscirpenol appears to be the toxin responsible for the "hemorrhagic syndrome" reported in many cases of mycotoxicoses due to trichothecenesin farm animals. Swine fed experimentally with this toxin developed, *inter alia,* lymphoid necrosis, mucosal congestion of the small intestine, and hemorrhagic bowel lesions.[52,53] The effect of this toxin on poultry is similar to that of T_2 toxin and comprises various debilitative symptoms, including decline in weight and egg production associated with characteristic yellow oral lesions.

Trichothecenes commonly appear to cause hematuria and hemorrhagia,[54] but the capacity of T_2 toxin to do so alone is still disputed.[36,55] No evidence of clinical or subclinical hemorrhagic disease was observed after long-term feeding of calves with T_2 toxin at low doses (2 mg/kg of feed).

Table 1
THE MAIN TRICHOTHECENES PRODUCED BY VARIOUS *FUSARIUM* SPECIES

Produced by

T_1 toxin (butenolide lactone)	H[12], N[2]
T_2 toxin	A[13], B[13], C[13], E[13], F[14], H[15], I[16], J[17], K[18], L[13], N[19]
Monoacetoxyscirpenol	E[20], F[21]
Diacetoxyscirpenol	A[13], B[13], C[13], E[22-23], F[21], I[16], K[24], L[13], M[25], N[15]
HT₂ toxin	B[13], J[17], K[13], L[17], N[27]
Neosolaniol	A[13], B[13], C[13], E[13], J[17], K[24], L[17], N[13]
Nivalenol	D[13], F[18], H[26,27]
Monoacetylnivalenol (fusarenon X)	D[29], F[29], G[13,29], H[27,23], I[13]
Diacetylnivalenol	H[30], I[13]
Acetyldeoxynivalenol	B[34]
Deoxynivalenol (emetic principle, vomiting factor)	B[31-33], F[21,30]

Note: Species (classified according to Booth[285] and Nirenberg[286]) are the following:

A. *Fusarium avenaceum* (Corda ex fr.) Sacc.
B. *F. culmorum* (W.G. Smith) Sacc.
C. *F. decemcellylare* Brick (=*F. rigidius-culum* Berk & Br.)
D. *F. dimerum* Penzia (= *F. episphaeria* (Tode) Snyder & Hansen)
E. *F. equiseti* (Corda) Sacc. (= *F. scirpi* Lamb & Fautr.)
F. *F. Graminearum* Schwabe

G. *F. verticillioides* (Sacc.) Nirenberg (=*F. moniliforme* Sheldon)
H. *F. nivale* (Fr.) Ces
I. *F. oxysporum* Schlect.
J. *F. poae* (Peck) Wr.
K. *F. solani* (Mart.) Sacc.
L. *F. sporotrichioides* Sherb.
M. *F. sulphureum* Schlect.
N. *F. tricinctum* (Corda) Sacc.

Table 2
ESTROGENIC COMPOUNDS PRODUCED BY VARIOUS *FUSARIUM* SPECIES

Toxin	**Produced by**
Zearalenone (F₂)	A[102], B[102], C[102], D[103], E[104], F[105], G[105], G[105], I[106], J[17], K[102]
F₃	D[99], E[99,104]
F₄	L[106]
Zearalenol (zearanol)	C[107], H[107]
Hydroxyzearalenone	C[107], H[108]

Note: Species are the following:

A. *Fusarium avenaceum* (Corda ex Fr.) Sacc.
B. *F. culmorum* (W.G. Smith) Sacc.
C. *F. equiseti* (F. gibbosum) (Corda) Sacc. (=*F. gibbasum* Wr.)
D. *F. graminearum* Schwabe
E. *F. moniliforme* (Sacc.) Nirenberg (= *F. moniliforme* Sheld.)
F. *F. nivale* (Fr.) Ces.

G. *F. sambucinum* Fuckel
H. *F. semitectum* Berk. & Rav.
I. *F. solani* (Mart) Sacc.
J. *F. sporotrichioides* Sherb.
K. *F. tricinctum* (Corda) Sacc.
L. *F. spp.*

Other important toxins, HT₂ toxin, monoacetyl nivalenol (fusarenon X), diacetyl nivalenol, nivalenol, and neosolaniol, cause comparable and diverse toxic symptoms in experimental animals, but, except for the last two, have not yet been associated with toxicoses in nature.

At the cellular level the general effect of trichothecenes is to cause necrosis and karyorrhexis of actively dividing cells, especially those of the gastrointestinal tract and the germ centers of the lymph follicles, spleen, lymph nodes, thymus, bone marrow, ovary, and testis.[56,57] They have a destructive effect on eggs and semen.[7,58] Most have an irritating or necrotizing effect when applied experimentally to the skin.[30,59] This effect can be severe and potentially extremely dangerous for humans.[27]

Various feeding experiments with chickens have established that the main chronic effect of T_2 toxin is to increase the prothrombin time[60] and to depress leucocyte formation.[48,61] This is associated with reduction in size of the thymus gland, typical of the atrophy attributable to other factors such as malnutrition, cortisone, radiomimetic drugs, or systemic infectious disease. An immunosuppressive effect by T_2 toxin, as well as by diacetoxyscirpenol, has also been observed in mice,[62] in cats,[63] in sheep,[64] and in humans.[65] In horses the crude toxins produced by bean hull poisoning resulted in cellular degradation and karyorrhexis in actively dividing cells of various hemopoietic tissues.[18] Crude extracts from cultures of *F. poae* and *F. sporotrichioides* also resulted in depletion of the lymphoid tissues of mice and rats followed by various widespread infections.[66] These effects on the immune system may have important implications in terms of neoplastic development which will be discussed later on.

Trichothecenes appear to affect the synthesis of certain specific enzymes and proteins inhibiting some and enhancing others.[67,68] Toxins from *F. sporotrichioides*, for example, reduced the activity of blood cholinesterase in rabbits and hens.[69] A general effect of trichothecenes seems to be the inhibition of leucine uptake in reticulocytes.[30,70,71,56] This is accompanied by cellular degeneration and karyorrhexis of actively dividing cells. Experiments with labelled T_2 toxin and fusarenon-X revealed that these toxins bind to and disaggregate polysomes and ribosomes within affected cells.[53]

The effect of neosolaniol, nivalenol, and fusarenon-X on tissue is similar to that of T_2 toxin but is less powerful.[72,63] Nivalenol also inhibits polypeptide synthesis by ribosomes.[73] The primary effect of fusarenon-X is a rapid and complete disaggregation of polyribosomes into monomers.[30] Trichothecenes also inhibit DNA synthesis in Ehrlich ascites tumor cells, in a protozoan, *Tetrahymena pyriformis,* and in He La cells.[63]

B. Moniliformin

This toxin is produced by *F. verticillioides*[74] (Sacc.) Nir., *F. sacchari* (Butl.) Gams *V. subglutinans*[75] (Wr. and Reink) Nir.,[76] *F. fusarioides*[77] (Frag. and Cif.) Booth, and F. avenaceum and *F. oxysporum.*[284] As a cyclobutane it is distinct in chemical structure, but lesions in 1-day-old chicks were similar to the usual trichothecene pattern: ascites with edema of the mesenteries and small hemorrhages in the proventriculus, gizzard, small and large intestine, and skin. At the molecular level the toxin has been found to inhibit oxidation of pyruvate and α-ketoglutarate in rat liver mitochondria.[77]

F. verticilliodes was probably responsible for producing the same toxin in another experiment involving older chickens[78] which developed severe ricketts with widening of the growth plates, insufficient cartilage formation, demineralization of the spongiosa and compacta, and production of fibrous bone marrow and granulomatous proliferation of osteoclasts. Administration of vitamin D had a rapid favorable effect. *F. verticillioides* has also been implicated in leukoencephalomalacia of horses.[79,80] In addition to brain lesions, experimental animals developed severe cardiac hemorrhages, petechiae and ecchymoses in various organs, edema, icterus, and liver damage. Toxin produced by *F. verticillioides* has also caused paralysis in pigs and poultry[81] and various degenerative disorders.

C. Estrogenic Agents (Zearalenone)

The estrogenic toxins belong to the general group known as resorcylic acid lactones and include zearalenone and related compounds[82] (Table 2).

The symptoms of toxicosis due to zearalenone are well-known, comprising vulvova-ginitis, tumefaction and edema of the vulva, enlargement of the mammary glands, and the increase in the size and weight of the uterus in pigs[83-93] and in rats.[94] Consumption of a moldy corn diet led to abortion in sheep[95] and to reduction in litter size and live pigs born per litter, and to increased fetal mummification.[96] This has been confirmed exper-imentally by Miller et al.[97] who showed that zearalenone is responsible for reduced litter size and "splayleg" in piglets. Although most cattle can be affected by zearalenone, pigs appear to be especially susceptible. Several outbreaks of toxicosis in these and other animals due to zearalenone have been reported since 1928, when it was first described by McNutt. Most of these have occurred in continental North America and in the U.S.S.R. where there is a swing from a hot summer to a cold winter.[98]

F_3 toxin is similar to zearalenone and is known to cause abortion and/or infertility in dairy cattle.[99] Zearanol, a derivative from zearalenone,[100] does not appear to have a toxic effect and is used as a growth promotion for cattle under the name "Ralgro". When administered to mice, however, above a concentration of 300 mg/kg daily, zearanol has a fetotoxic and teratogenic effect.[101]

On smaller animals than cattle, reports of the effect of zearalenone are contradictory. In some it is reported to reduce gain in weight or result in weight loss and also to affect fertility. Hens and chickens fed zearalenone in their basal ration decreased in weight and failed to lay eggs, or laid eggs with poor quality shell, whereas chicks showed an increase in total weight, weight of comb, and ovary length.[108,109] Young turkeys and chickens eating contaminated shelled maize suffered loss of weight, some dying as well.[110] The turkeys exhibited swollen vents, prolapsed cloacae, and enlarged bursae of Fabricius. On the other hand, in other experiments there was no fall-off in weight gain of chickens when fed corn infested with *Fusarium graminearum,* though rats were severely af-fected.[111,112] Diets containing either *Fusarium*-infected maize supplying 25 and 100 ppm of zearalenone or of the pure substance also did not adversely influence the reproductive performance of laying hens,[113] and egg production was in fact superior to that of non-treated controls.

The fact that zearalenone acts as a true estrogen is indicated by studies in which rats were exposed to concentrations in the feed of 0.1, 1.0, and 3.0 mg/kg day.[114] Exfoliative cytology suggested a prolongation of estrus cycles in females receiving the highest dosage, whereas a decrease in body weight gain, also dose dependent, was observed in these rats and also in the male rats. On young male chickens, zearalenone administered at the rate of 40 ppm in the food for 10 days had little effect on weight gain or effective food conversion, but caused a significant increase in the weight of the testes and comb.[115] A detailed study of young female Minnesota dwarf piglets[89] exposed to the toxin over 10 to 12 days indicated that zearalenone could stimulate estrus and formation of the corpus luteum in the ovary in a manner similar to the follicle stimulatory hormone (FSH). On post-mortem examination the uterus and cervix of each gilt was found to be greatly hypertrophied owing to proliferation of smooth muscle. In the cervix there was also hyperplasia of the epithelium and connective tissue elements as well. Other effects of zearalone are the inhibition of spermatogenesis in carp, cockerels, ganders, and pigs[93,116,118,119] and teratogenicity in rats.[120]

Microscopic changes due to feeding pigs with zearalenone comprise edema and hy-perplasia of the uterus due to thickening of the myometrium and endometrium, duct proliferation, degeneration of endometrial cells, and squamous metaplasia of the cervix and vagina and follicular atresia.[88,119] This is accompanied by karyopyknosis and kar-yorrhexis.[93] Likewise, cellular proliferation and mitosis have also been observed in the uterine muscle cells of the rat.[94] A comparative study of the effects on gilts of estradiol, zearalenone, and maize inoculated with *F. graminearum*[121] showed that they had basically the same effect — squamous cell metaplasia and loss of the normal epithelium of the vagina and cervix.

The biological and metabolic effects of zearalenone are currently receiving much attention. They appear to be basically similar to those of estradiol, a natural estrogen, which accelerates the synthesis of RNA and increases the permeability of uterine cells. Administration of zearalenone to ovariectomized mice induced an increase in the contents of uterine RNA, protein, and DNA. In vitro incubation of uterine tissue taken from mice pretreated with zearalenone resulted in a temporary increase in cellular permeability of the uterine cells to α-aminobutyric acid and 3-0 methyl glucose.[122] This is accompanied by increased incorporation of ^{14}C-leucine into protein. In comparison with diethylstilbestrol, it stimulates nitrogen retention in cells,[123] hence its use as a growth promoter in cattle and sheep. Zearalenone also inhibits synthesis and secretion of pituitary gonadotrophins as expected for estrogens, and can reduce blood lipids in rats, including blood cholesterol.

The action of zearalenone on small laboratory animals is complemented by a recent investigation on monkeys,[124] showing that there is a similarity in action between zearalenone, diethylstilbestrol (DES), and estradiol-17B upon the level of gonadotrophin for some time after injection. The action of zearalenone on the hypothalamus and pituitary was also similar to that of other estrogens. While zearalenone was only slightly less potent than estradiol or DES when given in a subcutaneous injection, its potency is, however, significantly reduced when administered orally. It is also interesting that zearalenone and its derivative dihydrozearalenol bind competitively with estradiol binding sites in uteri or mammary glands,[125,126] and zearalenol in turn has ten times the strength of zearalenone[127] and DES about a hundred times.[128]

Zearalenone may also have effects that are not related to its estrogenic action and which could have important implications if these had the same influence on humans as on experimental animals. For example, its capacity to inhibit proteolysis in phagolysosomes[129] would result in impairment of natural resistance to disease. It is interesting to note that moniliformin and T_2 toxin do not have this effect.

D. Other Important Metabolites of *Fusarium*

If the effects of various species of *Fusarium* are synergistic, then the formation of substances which are not strictly toxins could be significant. One of these is thiaminase,[130] produced by *F. verticillioides,* that caused a noticeable deficiency in chicks that was only relieved by adding thiamine to the diet or by injection of thiamine hydrochloride.

Two substances, sporofusarin and poaefusarin, attributed to *F. sporotrichioides* and *F. poae* respectively, are discounted today as having real importance.[131] The toxic principles produced by these fungi are in all probability trichothecenes. It has been recently established[5] that *F. sporotrichioides* can produce T_2 toxin that is by itself able to produce all of the signs, symptoms, and pathological symptoms of ATA for which sporofusarin was originally thought responsible.

Recently, *F. verticillioides, F. "roseum"* (=? *graminearum,*)[285] and *F. solani* have been implicated in an epizootic in cattle of a typical interstitial pneumonia caused by ingestion of moldy sweet potatoes.[132] The metabolites are still under investigation.[133]

II. CHRONIC EFFECTS OF *FUSARIUM* TOXINS

In contrast to aflatoxin, where evidence of carcinogenicity in animals and man was not long in coming after its discovery, unequivocal proof of long term effects due to *Fusarium* toxins has been difficult to obtain. Part of this difficulty has been due to the lack of consistency of experimental results with laboratory animals, and to the low rate of malignancies obtained in positive experiments which could be attributed to other causes than the mycotoxins.

A number of tests have been developed in recent years using tissue culture cells or protozoal or bacterial cell cultures to demonstrate the effect of a potential toxin on the nuclei. An adverse effect is nearly always related to toxicity in animals. Similarly mutagenic effects are often correlated with carcinogenicity.

In the simplest test, the He La test involving cell cultures, a good though not complete correlation has been demonstrated[134] between the cytotoxicity of culture filtrates and mycelium extracts towards the cells and general toxicity to DDD mice for 133 species from 24 genera of assorted fungi, including *Aspergillus, Chaetomium, Cladosporium, Fusarium* and *Penicillium*. The fungi were originally collected from two localities in Japan, where the mortality rate of cerebro-vascular diseases and that of hepatic diseases was high. As an initial mass screening test, therefore, to find out which fungi might be of significance, this method was thought to be reliable. Unfortunately, only two strains of *Fusarium* were used (one identified as *F. nivale*), and both were negative. Thus, it is not possible to compare this genus as a whole with the others which had considerably more representatives. In a study restricted to seven mycotoxins,[135] all related chemically and collectively termed as "aglycoside macrolide antibiotics", zearalenone was found to have a relatively low degree of cytotoxicity. Cyanein and monorden were approximately 20 times more effective than three cytochalasins, and these again were on average 70 to 200 times more effective than zearalenone and curvularin. Likewise, in another study of the effects of aflatoxinB_1, penicillic acid, patulin, luteoskyrin, rubratoxin B, and fusarenon-X on the DNA of He La cells, the last three toxins exhibited only minor breakage.[136] Thus it seems clear that fusarial mycotoxins cannot be regarded as strongly cytotoxic on the basis of this test.

On the other hand, extracts of many species of *Fusarium* were toxic when applied directly to rabbit skin,[59,137] including *F. poae, F. tricinctum* and *F. fusarioides*. Pure T_2 toxin induced pyknosis and karyorrhexis in pig kidney epithelial cell cultures,[138] and the sensitivity was reckoned to be even higher than that for the skin test. Severe cytotoxicity for plant and mammalian cells was caused by diacetoxyscirpenol.[139] Zearalenone also produces cytopathic effects in testis cell cultures.[140,141]

The *Salmonella* test was devised by Ames et al.[142,143] to detect mutagenic toxins. Strains of the bacteria are used which require histidine for growth and which also lack the enzymes required for repair of damage to DNA, since these strains are much more sensitive to killing and mutation. The effect of the mutagen is to convert a proportion of the histidine deficient bacteria to the prototropic form. The value of the test lies in its relationship to the hypothesis that most chemical carcinogens are converted by enzymes in living tissue to chemically reactive molecules[144,145] that react with the DNA or RNA in the cell in such a way that a carcinogenic transformation may result.

So far it has been shown that aflatoxin B was not toxic to *Salmonella* alone, but was so when mixed with rat liver enzymes.[146] The toxicity was lost when heat denatured enzymes were used. Therefore, aflatoxin B has to be changed into a specific metabolite, possibly an epoxide, for acting on DNA. Aflatoxins, therefore, do require metabolic activation and do not act directly as was thought originally. The *Salmonella* test is not restricted by animal species specificity, while being able to discriminate well between chemical compounds, even those highly related like the carcinogenic aflatoxin B_1 and the noncarcinogenic aflatoxin B_2.

As far as *Fusarium* toxins are concerned, none of these are mutagenic according to the *Salmonella* test.[147-149] Out of 17 mycotoxins and their derivatives, only aflatoxin B and sterigmatocystin were found to be mutagenic after enzymatic activation.[150] On the other hand, fusarenon-X and sterigmatocystin were found to be mutagenic to yeast cells,[57] and zearalenone and diacetoscirpenol were highly toxic to *Chlorella pyrenoidosa* cells,[151] which despite the variability of the reaction against the four strains tested, compared well with that observed for aflatoxin B. Zearalenone has also been found toxic to *Bacillus thuringiensis* and to induce the formation of atypical cells.[152]

When the extracts of various fungi were tested rather than specific known mycotoxins, *F. verticillioides* along with *Alternaria tenuis* and five species of *Aspergillus* were found to be highly mutagenic.[153] Negative reactions were obtained for *F. oxysporum, F. solani* and *F. tricinctum.*

Another test of DNA interference compares the relative growth of a normal and mutant strain of *Bacillus subtilis* that is unable to recombine DNA following exposure to a mutagen.[154] This "rec-effect" was tested for 30 mycotoxins and 5 derivatives, of which 13 were found positive,[155] including zearalenone and its derivative zearalenol-B, 6 *Penicillium* toxins, and 5 *Aspergillus* toxins. Eight of these toxins were previously known to be carcinogenic to animals. The addition of zearalenone to this list, in spite of its negative result on the *Salmonella* test,[156] is a puzzling feature. On the other hand, 5 trichothecene *Fusarium* toxins, T_1 toxin, fusarenon-X, fusaric acid, moniliformin, and T_2 toxin, were negative, though fusaric acid had a toxic effect.

In overall terms, then, the evidence for mutagenic behavior of *Fusarium* is not as convincing as it is for *Aspergillus,* since the results of the tests are equivocal. It is important to remember though, that in spite of the high correlation between carcinogenicity and mutagenicity of known mammalian carcinogens to *Salmonella,*[157] there may be good reasons why not all carcinogens will be detected. It is reasonable to assume that bacteria may have developed defense mechanisms against fungi, since they often develop in close proximity, and there are also major differences in metabolism between mammalian and bacterial cells.[158]

III. EPIDEMIOLOGY

The linkage of a mycotoxin to a chronic pathological condition in humans and animals is a difficult task, especially since the microbial agent may have a short duration and the substance itself is often difficult to identify, or at least may not be ascribed to a known compound. In addition, there are the four postulates by Oettlé[159] which ought to be satisfied before any factor can be seriously considered as implicated in the etiology of a disease:

1. In the presence of the suspected etiologic factor there should be an increased risk of contacting the disease.
2. The risk should vary with the dosage.
3. The site affected should be shown to have been exposed to the etiological factor.
4. The factor should be capable of inducing the disease in the same or comparable site in experimental animals.

In the case of aflatoxins all four postulates can be considered satisfied with respect to acute and chronic disease.[98] With respect to fusarial toxins the position is much less certain.

It is clear that trichothecenes have great potential danger for human health, but the effects of long-term dosage are unknown.

The best documented account of toxicity in humans due to *Fusarium* is that of alimentary toxic aleukia mentioned above, but there are at least two further ones recorded in Tokyo.[30,70] Symptoms included vomiting, nausea, and drowsiness after eating rice contaminated by *F. nivale* and other species. *F. sporotrichioides* has also been implicated in endemic arthritis in certain river valleys in the Transbaikal area of Siberia.[160] As in

ATA, evidence suggested that the disease was caused by ingesting locally grown cereals contaminated by the fungus.

Some evidence for carcinogenicity due to trichothecenes is available from several animal experiments. A low rate of tumor formation was observed in mice and rats fed rice cultures of *F. nivale* and *F. graminearum*[161,162] and in rats injected with or fed fusarenon-X.

Ingestion of grain infested with *F. sporotrichioides* also caused a significant increase in lung adenomas in male rats and of adenocarcinomas in female rats.[163] However, long term feeding of rainbow trout, rats, and mice with T_2 toxin did not cause neoplasia or hyperplasia.[164]

The best evidence for trichothecene involvement in neoplasia is that of Schoental et al.[165] Intermittent dosages of rats with T_2 toxin over 9 months resulted in immediate development of typical acute symptoms followed by depletion of lymphoid elements in spleen and lymph glands, and involution and necrosis of the thymus. Chronic lesions developing after 22 months comprised cardiovascular lesions, adenocarcinomata of stomach and pituitary, neuroblastomata of the brain, and tumors in the pancreas. The next step is to determine whether the tumors occur due to other causes as a result of immunosuppression, or whether they are direct or secondary effect after the acute necrotic primary reaction.

It is the first three postulates that still constitute a problem. It is tempting to wonder whether trichothecenes could be implicated in man in tumors of the stomach and colon in eastern Europe and the U.S.S.R.,[166] and of the esophagus in the Transkei in southern Africa,[167,287,288] and also in leukemia in "moldy" houses.[168,169] At present there is only circumstantial evidence, based on the marked occurrence of trichothecenes in local foodstuffs or of a peculiarly large number of fungi, including *Fusarium,* in the environment of the people concerned. More accurate determination of the exposure to mycotoxins is required. In assessing the situation one must remember that the technique for the isolation of mycotoxins have been developed relatively recently and have not been employed on a wide scale.

Trichothecenes in foodstuffs have been reliably reported in North America, Japan, and Yugoslavia,[170,171] and from southern Africa.[167,287,288] The incidence of zearalenone seems to be more universal covering North America, Mexico, Finland, U.K., France, Italy, eastern Europe, Japan, and southern Africa.

There are relatively few comparative surveys of mycotoxins in foodstuffs. Recent papers by Shotwell et al.[172-175] and Funnell,[176] however, indicate that aflatoxins, zearalenone, and trichothecenes usually occur in that order of concentration. These reports, together with other reports of sporadic isolates of mycotoxins in foodstuffs, also show that trichothecenes, while present in maize, are more commonly found in various small grain cereals such as barley[177] and brewer's grain,[178] while zearalenone is prevalent in maize, though it has been detected also in sorghum, wheat, hay, and barley. Both kinds of toxin have been primarily isolated from animal feeds, but also from maize intended for export and domestic use. Zearalenone has also been detected in silos,[179] in freshly harvested corn,[167,180-183] in cribs,[184] in market wheat,[185,175] and from mixed feeds containing barley, wheat, rye, oats and maize.[186,187] The quantities of zearalenone recorded are very variable but can be quite high, up to 2909 ppm.[87]

Appendices 1 and 2 list some of the more important epizootics caused by mycotoxins in man and animals. It is obvious that there is ample opportunity for the mycotoxin levels that occasionally build up in foodstuffs to present a health hazard to birds and animals, but is this true for humans also? If fusarial toxins are of significance, then there must be a reasonable possibility of their being transmitted through common foodstuffs. Our knowledge is still very imperfect concerning the metabolism of mycotoxins within farm animals and birds. The fact that aflatoxin can be transmitted from animal tissues is well-known,[188] so it is probable that fusarial toxins can be as well. Chicken livers and edible portions of the carcasses have been found to contain residues of T_2 toxin, the latter up to 28 and 48 hr after feeding.[189,190] Animals fed maize contaminated with *F. culmorum* and *F. graminearum* similarly contained zearalenone (F_2) and F_4 toxins in the gastric contents, liver, and testicles.[191] Perhaps the best proof of the indirect action of zearalenone come from a study of pregnant sows given feed contaminated with *F. graminearum* for 15 days before farrowing, which then produced piglets with characteristic toxic symptoms.[192]

Zearalenone may be consumed directly in processed food in developed countries, since it has been recently isolated from cornflakes in Canada.[193] It would be interesting to conduct a further study along the lines of a previous survey of retail stores and processing plants, also in Canada, where the discovery of tiny quantities of aflatoxins was linked to reported causes of illness in households and complaints of the reception of moldy bread by consumers.[194] It might also be extremely revealing to conduct a survey of chronic disease in relation to a recent distribution map of zearalenone incidence in Ontario (Figure 1) in which it was found that high numbers of toxic feed samples and high concentrations of zearalenone occurred where the annual rainfall exceeded 60 mm,[195] and where the soils were predominately clay and inadequately drained, rather than coarse and sandy[196] (Figure 1).

A similar problem awaits further investigation in southern Africa. Relatively high zearalenone levels have been determined 0.1 to 4.6 ppm in maize beer in Zambia, 0.3 to 53 ppm in sorghum and maize beers in Lesotho, 8 to 17 ppm in sour fermented porridges in Swaziland, and 6.4 to 12.8 ppm in recently harvested maize in South Africa.[182,197,198]

Indigenous beer and "sour drinks" in southern Africa are commonly brewed by a village brewer. Various proportions of malted sorghum, maize meal, flour, hops, sugar, and water are brewed in a large pot, usually after the addition of yeast. The fermentation period lasts from 3 days to a week, mainly according to temperature, and the mixture is then boiled before use. "Sour porridge" is prepared by adding maize meal to warm water and setting it aside to ferment naturally under a cover. The resulting product is a thick gruel. The beverages also contain proportion of solid or suspended material, at least enough to render the mixture turbid.

Mycological examination of sorghum malt, beer and beer residues, and maize and maize derivatives has shown that *F. verticillioides* is present at all stages in the making of beer and sour porridge. It is clear that there is ample opportunity for zearalenone to be produced, although it is not yet known at which stage[199] (Figure 2).

Mycological examination of grain has also shown that *F. verticillioides* is common through southern Africa, although *F. graminearum* and *F. tricinctum* have also been recorded.[198,200,201] *F. verticillioides* is dominant both in recently harvested maize[202] where 46% of the grains were found to be infested, and to a lesser extent in stored maize,[203] where 22% of the grain from underground pits and from various containers above ground was infested.[204] Other species such as *F. fusarioides, F. sporotrichioides,* and *F. semitectum* also occur in grain to lesser but significant extent.

These findings could be significant in the light of the cancer spectrum in southern Africa. Cancer of the cervix has a fairly high general incidence in southern Africa,[205] and detailed studies in Botswana, Swaziland, and Lesotho have shown that it is the major cancer affecting women, accounting for nearly 40% of all cancer registrations.[206-208]

In a recent prospective study of the cancer spectrum in Lesotho,[209] data concerning background, habits, and customs were gathered by means of questionnaires. When the results were compared with those for a group of control patients, it appeared that while

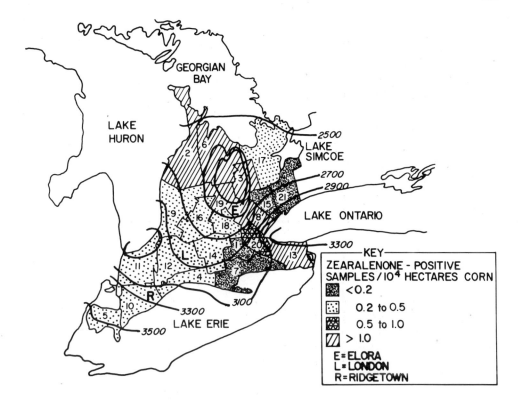

FIGURE 1. Map of southern Ontario showing difference in incidence of zearalenone — positive samples. (From Sutton, J. C., Baliko, W., and Funnell, H. S., *Can. J. Plant Sci.,* 60, 149, 1980. With permission.)

cancer patients as a whole were more underprivileged than the rest of the community, cervical cancer patients in particular were so, especially in respect to occupation, literacy, school attainment, and availability of clean water. There was a marked difference between cervix patients and controls in the use of drugs, tobacco, and fermented drinks that persisted even when a proportion of the cervical cancer patients were carefully matched to controls in terms of age, number of children, and home area. (Figures 3 and 4)

If the occurrence of zearalenone is widespread as the results seem to suggest, then the conclusion that cervical cancer patients are more exposed to these and possibly other toxins is inescapable. The actual intake is difficult to assess since both solid food and drink are involved, and the latter is taken less regularly than the meals which can be assessed according to the food from the plate method. Nevertheless, the reported quantities of zearalenone in various substrates fall within the range known to cause changes in experimental animals, and the cumulative effect over a long period of time may be decisive in inducing a malignant cell change.

Davies[210,211] has commented on the differences in estrogen levels between whites and blacks in southern Africa that could be related to the high rates of liver and cervical cancer in the latter. Obviously the estrogen could have an endogenous as well as an exogenous source, but this cannot always be identified. Schoental[212,213] has also made out a strong case for the long-term involvement of estrogens in the development of cancers in laboratory animals and in humans. Natural estrogens as well as contraceptive steroids (e.g. Enovid) and diethylstilbestrol have been implicated.[214-218]

There appear to be two difficulties, however, in interpreting the results obtained from experimental animals and humans known to be exposed to estrogens. In the first place,

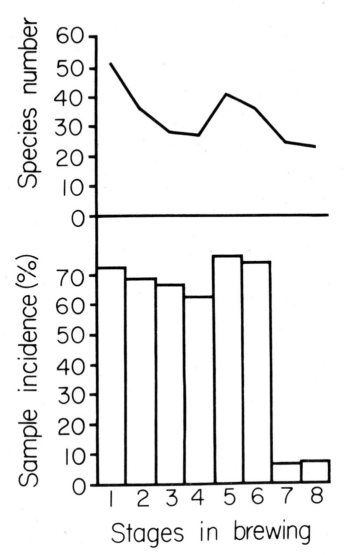

FIGURE 2.   The graph represents the total number of fungus species cultured from each of 8 stages in the indigenous brewing process in Swaziland and Lesotho. The histograms represent the equivalent % incidence of *Fusarium verticillioides* in collected samples of material in each stage. Stages are (1) harvested whole sorghum grain, (2) sorghum in storage prior to beer making, (3) sorghum after 2 days immersion in water, (4) germinating malted sorghum, (5) dried malted sorghum, (6) malted sorghum powder, (7) beer and beer residue during fermentation, and (8) beer and beer residue in material for sale.

various organs are attacked in experimental animals — breast, uterus, vagina, anterior pituitary gland, adrenal and thyroid — whereas in humans neoplasia seems to be restricted to the vagina, cervix, uterus, and liver. In the second place, whereas the evidence for a causal association between exogenous estrogens and human cancer is very strong,[219-221] it is the endometrium rather than the cervix which is affected and adenocarcinomas rather than squamous cancers are developed. The majority of cancers which occur in the human female genital system are, however, squamous cell carcinomas of the cervix. The possible link between estrogens and cervical neoplasia in humans is

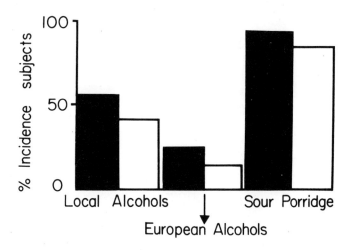

FIGURE 3. Difference in consumption patterns of 257 pairs of cervical cancer patients and controls matched in terms of age, number of children, and area. The histograms represent the percentage incidences of patients and controls taking local alcohols, European wine and spirits, and local sour fermented porridges. Black = cervix patients; white = controls.

thus regarded by Thomas as still requiring confirmation, but it is important to note that various experiments with mice[222] indicate that the type of cancer may depend on the time of administration in the life cycle, since endometrial cancers were obtained with early treatment and cervical cancers with delayed treatment. Estrogens may also induce breast cancer, but most of the differences between cases and controls in studies reviewed by Thomas are not significant. The most striking observation is that oral contraceptives predispose women with benign breast disease to breast cancer. Finally, there is strong evidence that oral contraceptives are the cause of liver adenomas, although studies of the problem have not been completed.[223] Malignant tumors of the liver may also be caused by treatment with male hormones.[224] Four patients with aplastic anemia developed hepatocellular carcinoma after long term therapy with androgenic anabolic steroids. Christopherson and Mays[225] have found that 13% of the liver tumors in women on the pill were of the primary hepatocellular type.

The consideration of the "mechanism" of cancer induction also has an important bearing on epidemiology. It is possible that estrogens may be responsible for malignant transformation of cells directly, since it is well-known that they interact with the nucleic acids through hormone receptors.[226,227] It is also possible, however, that they could interact with carcinogenic viruses. Estrogens normally fulfill a protective role against virus diseases.[228-230] In the majority of cases such viruses are nontumorigenic, and the immediate effect would be a reduction in the severity of the disease. In the case of a tumorigenic virus such as *Herpes simplex* type II, however, the effect of an estrogen might be similar to that of light and photoreactive dyes,[231] or to that of a tumor promoter TPA,[232] in that the virus may be inactivated while releasing that portion of the viral genome containing the gene responsible for transforming host cells into cancer cells. At present there is little published evidence to support this view. However, it is known that the antigen Ag 4 represents the *Herpes* virus in a latent state within cervical cancer cells[233-235] and that *Herpes simplex* is almost certainly involved in the induction of this cancer.[233,234,236-238] While the *Herpes* virus appears to be widely distributed, cancer of the cervix is not, and it is interesting to speculate whether exogenous or endogenous estrogens could play a

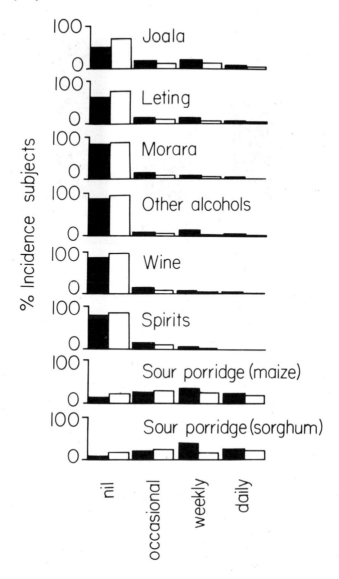

FIGURE 4. Difference in frequency of drinking patterns of matched cervical cancer patients and controls. Histograms represent percentages of patients falling into four arbitrary categories. Black = cervix patients; white = controls.

synergistic role. The possibility of such an association between zearalenone and a virus such as *Herpes* is an exciting topic for future research.

ACKNOWLEDGMENTS

It is a pleasure to acknowledge the ICRETT grant awarded by the International Union Against Cancer which made it possible for the writer to visit several laboratories and obtain information first-hand. The writer is also grateful for the comments and advice of Dr. Paul Keen in the preparation of this paper.

Appendix 1

Some Epizootics Associated With: *Fusarium Graminearum*

Place	Species	Symptoms/remarks	Ref.
Iowa	Pigs	Hyperestrogenism (swelling, reddening, and edema/necrosis of vulva)	239
Iowa	Pigs	Hyperestrogenism	240
Minn., Iowa, Ind., Ill.	Pigs	Hyperestrogenism	241
Minn.	Pigs	Vomiting, toxicity, death	242
Victoria, Australia	Pigs	Vomiting, toxicity, death	243
Iowa	Pigs	Vomiting, toxicity, death	244
Ireland	Pigs	Vomiting, toxicity, death	245
Ind.	Pigs	Vomiting, toxicity, death	103
Russia	Pigs	Vomiting, diarrhea, death, abortion in ewes	246
Italy	Pigs	Hyperestrogenism	247
Yugoslavia	Pigs	Hyperestrogenism	248
Kirov, U.S.S.R.	Cattle	GIT disturbances, arrhythmia, restlessness	249
Minn.	Pigs	Hyperestrogenism	250
Rumania	Cows	Toxicosis	251
Rumania	Pigs	Hyperestrogenism	252
Denmark	Pigs	Hyperestrogenism	253
Minn.	Cattle	Hyperestrogenism	99
England	Cattle	Hyperestrogenism	254
Japan	Human	Toxicosis	255
Hungary	Pigs	Hyperestrogenism	256
Rumania	Horses	Loss of appetite, fever, hematological changes	257
Minn.	Poultry	Swollen vents, prolapsed cloacae, enlarged bursae	110
Yugoslavia	Pigs	Hyperestrogenism	258, 259
Finland	Cows	Hyperestrogenism	260
Russia	Cattle	Loss of reflexes, vision, staggering, and paresis	261
Canada	Pigs	Hyperestrogenism	383
Hungary	Pigs	Death	262
Korea	Humans and animals	Toxicosis	263
Wis.	Pigs	Feed refusal, probably trichothecenes and zearalenone were both involved	264
Miss.	Pigs	Emesis and feed refusal	265

F. moniliforme

Place	Species	Symptoms/remarks	Ref.
South Africa	Horses	Leukoencephalomalacia	79
France	Pigs and chickens	Bone dystrophy, nervousness, paraplegia, and osteomalacia	81
Buenos Aires, Argentina	Pigs	Toxicosis	266
Germany	Broiler chickens	Rickets	267
U.S.A.	Horses	Reviews history of leukoencephalomalacia	268

Appendix 1 (continued)

Some Epizootics Associated With: *Fusarium Graminearum*

Place	Species	Symptoms/remarks	Ref.
		F. sporotrichioides	
Orenburg, U.S.S.R.	Humans, cattle	"Scalding" of mouth and stomach, destruction of bone marrow, hemorrhage, necrosis, and drop in leucocyte count	9
Russia	Pigs	Pyrexia, inflammation of mucous membranes of nose and throat, swelling of inflammation of lymph nodes, inflammation of lungs and intestines	269
Russia	Pigs	General inflammation, edema of eye lids, neck, and jaw, dyspnea; several deaths	270
Russia	Sheep	Toxicosis, *F. poae* and *F. sporotrichiodes* isolated from fodder and pasturage	10
Western Ukraine	Cattle	Mass disease with high rate of death, loss of appetite, drop in milk yield, nasal discharge, salivation, high temperature	271
Siberia, U.S.S.R.	Humans	Premature generalized osteorthritis (circumstantial evidence only)	160
Russia	Sheep	GIT disorders, functional disturbance of CNS and cardiovascular systems, abortion in ewes, loss of hair, death	272
Russia	Horses	Toxicosis and death	273

Appendix 2

Some Epizootics Associated With: Fusarial Toxins

Place	Species	Symptoms/Remarks	Ref.
		Zearlalenone	
Yugoslavia	Pigs	Vulvovaginitis and estrogenism, *F. graminearum* and *F. moniliforme* present	274
Yugoslavia	Pigs, calves, chickens	Feed refusal, loss of body weight present, *F. graminearum* present	275
Hungary	Cows	Loss of appetite, fall in milk production, vulval swelling, zearalenone: 5-7 ppm	276
France	Sheep	Prostration, paraplegia, and death	95
Czechoslovakia	Cattle	Vulvovaginal edema, prolapse, modification of mammary glands; *F. graminearum,* *F. poae,* *F. moniliforme,* *F. culmorum* present; zearalenone at 1-12 mg/kg	86
Scotland	Pigs	22 cases described	277
		Deoxynivalenol	
Ind.	Pigs	Vomiting	31
Ind.	Pigs	Vomiting and feed refusal	278

Appendix 2 (continued)

Some Epizootics Associated With: Fusarial Toxins

Place	Species	Symptoms/Remarks	Ref.
		T₂ Toxin	
Wis.	Cows	Toxicosis and death, T_2 toxin at 2 ppm	4
Portugal	Poultry	Hemorrhage, renal hypertrophy and acute enteritis; prevalent over several years	279
U.S.A.	Cattle	Toxicosis and death	280
N.C.	Hens	Oral lesions, decreased egg production, and thin fragile shells	281
B.C., Canada	Ducks, geese horses and pigs	Necrosis of esophagus and death; barley yielded *F. graminearum* and T_2 toxin at 25 ppm	14
Scotland	Cattle	Toxicosis and death	178
		Assorted Trichothecenes	
U.S.A.	Cattle	Lameness of headquarters, gangrene in tail and hooves, fever	1
Japan	Humans and farm animals	Toxicosis: "akakabi" (red mold) poisoning	29
Tokyo, Japan	Humans	Nausea, vomiting and drowsiness, *F. nivale* present	70
Hokkaido, Japan	Horses	Toxicosis, *F. solani* and *F. roseum* (? = *F. graminearum*), 6 further horse intoxications listed	24
U.S.A.	Chickens	Summary of various outbreaks, T_2 toxin, diacetoxyscirpenol and solaniol recovered from *F. solani*	282
Tokyo, Japan	Humans	Toxicosis, *F. nivale, F. solani, F. roseum* *Trichothecium roseum* present (? = *graminearum*	30
Scotland	Cows	Hemorrhage, leucopenia, thrombocytopenia, and death; circumstantial evidence in accordance with trichothecene poisoning	283
Scotland	Pigs	6 occurrences of the hemorrhagic syndrome, suggestive of trichothecenes	277

REFERENCES

1. **Keyl, A. C., Lewis, J. C., Ellis, J. J., Yates, S. G., and Tookey, H. L.,** Toxic fungi isolated from tall fescue, *Mycopathology Mycol. Appl.,* 31, 327, 1967.
2. **Grove, M. D., Yates, S. G., and Tallent, W. H.,** Mycotoxins produced by *Fusarium tricinctum* as possible causes of cattle disease, *J. Agric. Food Chem.,*18, 734, 1970.
3. **Tookey, H. L., Yates, S. G., Ellis, J. J., Grove, M. D., and Nichols, R. E.,** Toxic effects of a butenolide mycotoxin and of *Fusarium tricinctum* cultures in cattle, *J. Am. Vet. Med. Assoc.,* 160, 1522, 1972.
4. **Hsu, H. S., Smalley, E. B., Strong, F. M., and Ribelin, W. R.,** Identification of T_2 toxin in mouldy corn associated with a lethal toxicosis in dairy cattle, *Appl. Microbiol.,* 24, 684, 1972.
5. **Lutsky, I., Mor, N., Yagen, B., and Joffe, A. Z.,** The role of T_2 toxin in experimental alimentary toxic aleukia, *Toxicol. Appl. Pharmacol.,* 43, 111, 1978.
6. **Joffe, A. Z. and Yagen, B.,** Intoxication produced by toxic fungi, *Toxicon,* 16, 263, 1978.
7. **Palyusik, M.,** Experimental fusariotoxicosis of geese, *Byull. Vses. Inst. Eksp. Vet.,* 25, 83, 1976; *Vet. Bull.,* 48, 503, 1978.

8. **Wyatt, R. D., Weeks, B. A., Hamilton, P. B., and Burmeister, H. R.,** Severe oral lesions in chickens caused by ingestion of dietary fusariotoxin T_2, *Appl. Microbiol.*, 24, 251, 1972.

9. **Mayer, G. F.,** Endemic panmyelotoxicosis in the Russian grain belt, *Mil. Surgeon*, 113, 295, 1953.

10. **Kurmanov, I. A.,** Fusariotoxicosis of sheep in the Stavropol area, *Veterinariya*, 38, 30, 1961; *Rev. Med. Vet. Mycol. (RMVM);* 4, 239, 1962.

11. **Spesivtseva, N. A.,** Fusariotoxicosis in horses, *Trudy Vses. Inst. Vet. Sanit.*, 28, 11, 1967; *RMVM*, 6, 545, 1969.

12. **Yates, S. G., Tookey, H. L., Ellis, J. J., and Burkhardt, H. J.,** Mycotoxins produced by *Fusarium nivale* isolated from tall fescue, *Phytochemistry*, 7, 139, 1968.

13. **Ueno, Y., Saito, N., Ishii, K., Sakai, K., Tsunoda, H., and Enomoto, M.,** Biological and chemical detection of trichothecene mycotoxins of *Fusarium* species, *Appl. Microbiol.*, 25, 669, 1973.

14. **Greenway, J. A. and Puls, R.,** Fusariotoxicosis from barley in British Columbia. I. Natural occurrence and diagnosis, *Can. J. Comp. Med.*, 40, 12, 1976.

15. **Bamburg, J. R., Marasas, W. F., Riggs, N. W., Smalley, E. B., and Strong, F. M.** Toxic spiroepoxy compounds from fusaria and other hyphomycetes, *Biotechnol. Bioeng.*, 10, 445, 1968.

16. **Ghosal, S., Chakrabarti, D. K., and Chaudhary, C. K. B.,** The occurrence of 12,13-epoxytrichothecenes in seeds of safflower infected with *Fusarium oxysporum* f.sp. *carthami.*, *Experientia*, 33, 574, 1977.

17. **Szathmary, C. I., Mirocha, C. J., Palyusik, M., and Pathre, S. V.,** Identification of mycotoxins produced by species of *Fusarium* and *Stachybotrys* obtained from eastern Europe, *Appl. Environ. Microbiol.*, 32, 579, 1976.

18. **Ueno, Y., Ishii, K., Sakai, K., Kanaeda, S., Tsunoda, H., Tanaka, T., and Enomoto, M.,** Toxicological approaches to the metabolites of Fusaria IV, *Jpn. J. Exp. Med.*, 42, 187, 1972.

19. **Gilgan, M. W., Smalley, E. B., and Strong, F. M.,** Isolation and partial characterization of a toxin from *Fusarium tricinctum* on mouldy corn, *Arch. Biochem. Biophys.*, 114, 1, 1966.

20. **Pathre, S. V., Mirocha, C. J., Christensen, C. M., and Behrens, J.,** Monoacetoxyscirpenol. A new mycotoxin produced by *Fusarium roseum gibbosum*, *J. Agric. Food Chem.*, 24, 97, 1976.

21. **Mirocha, C. J., Pathre, S. V., Schauerhamer, B., and Christensen, C.,** Natural occurrence of *Fusarium* toxins in feedstuff, *Appl. Environ. Microbiol.*, 32, 553, 1976.

22. **Brian, P. W.,** Phytotoxic compounds produced from *Fusarium equiseti*, *J. Exp. Bot.*, 12, 1, 1971.

23. **Bamburg, J. R., Riggs, N. W., and Strong, F. M.,** The structure of toxins from two strains of *Fusarium tricinctum*, *Tetrahedron*, 24, 3329, 1968.

24. **Ishii, K., Sakai, K., Ueno, V., Tsunoda, H., and Enomoto, M.,** Solaniol, a toxic metabolite of *Fusarium solani*, *Appl. Microbiol.*, 22, 718, 1971.

25. **Steyn, P. S., Vleggar, R., Rabie, C. J., Kriek, N. P., and Harington, J. S.,** Trichothecene mycotoxins from *Fusarium sulphureum*, *Phytochemistry*, 17, 949, 1974.

26. **Tatsuno, T.,** Toxicologic research on substances from *Fusarium nivale*, *Cancer Res.*, 28, 2393, 1968.

27. **Bamburg, J. R. and Strong, F. N.,** 12,13-Epoxytrichothecenes, in *Microbial Toxins*, Ajl, S. J., Ed., Academic Press, New York, 1971.

28. **Tatsuno, T., Saito, M., Enomoto, M., and Tsunoda, H.,** Nivalenol, a toxic principle of *Fusarium nivale*, *Chem. Pharm. Bull*, 16, 2519,1968.

29. **Ueno, Y., Ishikawa, Y., Nakajima, M., Sakai, K., Ishi, K.,Tsunoda, H., Saito, M., Enomoto, M., Ohtsubo, K., and Umeda, M.,** Toxicological approaches to the metabolites of Fusaria I. Screening of toxic strains, *Jpn. J. Exp. Med.*, 41, 257, 1971.

30. **Tatsuno, T., Ohtsubo, M. K., and Saito, M.,** Chemical and biological detection of 12, 13-epoxytrichothecenes isolated from *Fusarium* species, *Pure Appl. Chem.*, 35, 309, 1973.

31. **Vesonder, R. F., Ciegler, A., and Jensen, A. H.,** Isolation of the emetic principle from *Fusarium* infected corn, *Appl. Microbiol.*, 26, 1008, 1973.

32. **Vesonder, R. F., Ciegler, A., and Jensen, A. H.,** Production of refusal factors by *Fusarium* strains on grains, *Appl. Environ. Microbiol.*, 34, 105, 1977.

33. **Vesonder, R. F., Ciegler, A., Jensen, A. H., Rohwedder, W. K., and Weisleder, D.,** Co-identity of the refusal and emetic principle from *Fusarium* infected corn, *Appl. Environ. Microbiol.*, 31, 280, 1976.

34. **Birbin, S. S.,** Fusariotoxicosis in ducks, *Veterinariya*, 43, 54, 1966.

35. **Burdelev, T. E. and Akulin, N. A.,** Fusariotoxicosis in swine, *Izv. timiryazev. Selkhoz. Akad.*, 143, 1966; *RMVM*, 5, 433, 1966,. *Vet. Bull*, 36, 634, 1966.

36. **Chi, M. S., Mirocha, C. J., Kurtz, H. J., Weaver, G., Bates, F., and Shimoda, V. W.,** Subacute toxicity of T_2 toxin in broiler chicks, *Poultry Sci.*, 56, 306, 1977.

37. **Chi, M. S., Mirocha, C. J., Kurtz, H. J., Weaver, G., Bates, F., and Shimoda,V. W.,** Effects of T_2 toxin on reproductive performance and health of laying hens, *Poultry Sci.*, 56, 628, 1977.

38. **Chi, M. S., Mirocha, C. J., Kurtz, H. J., Weaver, G., Bates, F., Shimoda, W., and Burmeister, H. R.,** Acute toxicity of T_2 toxin in broiler chicks and laying hens, *Poultry Sci.*, 56, 103, 1977.

39. **Ellison, R. A. and Kotsonis, F. N.,** T_2 toxin as an emetic factor in mouldy corn, *Appl. Microbiol.*, 26, 540, 1973.

40. **Hamilton, P. B., Wyatt, R. D., and Burmeister, H.,** Effect of fusariotoxin T₂ in chickens, *Poultry Sci.,* 50, 1583, 1971.

41. **Kosuri, N. R.,** *Fusarium tricinctum* in rats and cattle, *Diss. Abstr.,* 318, 835, 1970; *RMVM,* 7, 515, 1972.

42. **Kosuri, N. R., Smalley, E. B., and Nichols, R. E.,** Toxicologic studies of *Fusarium tricinctum* (Corda) Snyder & Hansen from mouldy corn, *Am. J. Vet. Res.,* 32, 1843, 1971.

43. **Kurmanov, I. A.,** Fusariotoxicosis in fowls, *Veterinariya,* 37, 62, 1960; *Vet. Bull,* 31, 63, 1961.

44. **Kurmanov, I. A.,** Experimental fusariotoxicosis in pigs, *Tr. Vses. Nauchi-Issled Inst. Vet. Sanit.,* 22, 206, 1963; *RMVM,* 5, 345, 1966.

45. **Marchenko, G. G.,** Experimental fusariotoxicosis in sheep, *Veterinariya,* 40, 46, 1963; *Vet. Bull.,* 33, 552, 1963.

46. **Wyatt, R. D., Colwell, W. M., Hamilton, P. B., and Burmeister, H. R.,** Neural disturbances in chickens caused by dietary T₂ toxin, *Appl. Microbiol.,* 26, 757, 1973.

47. **Wyatt, R. D., Hamilton, P. B., and Burmeister, A. R.,** The effects of T₂ toxin in broiler chickens, *Poultry Sci.,* 52, 1853, 1973.

48. **Wyatt, R. D., Doerr, J. A., Hamilton, P. B., and Burmeister, H. R.,** Egg production, shell thickness and other physiological parameters of laying hens affected by T₂ toxin, *Appl. Microbiol.,* 29, 641, 1975.

49. **Wyatt, R. D., Hamilton, P. B.,and Burmeister, H.,** Altered feathering of chicks caused by T₂ toxin, *Poultry Sci.,* 54, 1042, 1975.

50. **Hayes, A. W.,** Mycotoxin teratogenicity, *Toxicon,* 17, Suppl.1, 739, 1978.

51. **Weaver, G. A., Kurtz, H. J., Mirocha, C. J., Bates, F. V., Behrens, J. C., Robinson, T. S., and Gipp, W. F.,** Mycotoxin-induced abortions in swine, *Can. Vet. J.,* 19, 72, 1978.

52. **Kurtz, H. J., Mirocha, C. J., and Meade, R.,** The Association of the Mycotoxin Diacetoxyscirpenol (DAS) with Hemorrhagic Bowel Syndrome, in Int. Pig Soc. Proc. 4th Int. Congr., Ames, June 22, 1976.

53. **Mirocha, C. J.,** Fusarium Toxins and Their Effects on Farm Animals, Proc. 15th Annu. Conf. Feed Manuf., University of Guelph, Ontario, April 24, 1979.

54. **Korpinen, E. L. and Uoti, J.,** The variation in toxic effect of five *Fusarium* species on rats, *Ann. Agric.Fenn.,* 13, 34, 1974.

55. **Matthews, J. G., Patterson, D. S. P., Roberts, B. A., and Shreeve, B. J.,** The T₂ toxin and haemorrhagic syndromes of cattle, *Vet. Rec.,* 101, 391, 1977.

56. **Ueno, Y., Ueno, I., Tatsuno, T., Ohtsubo, K., and Tsunoda, H.,** Fusarenon X, a toxic principle of *Fusarium nivale* culture filtrate, *Experientia,* 25, 1062, 1969.

57. **Ueno, Y., Ueno, I., Iitoi, Y., Tsunoda, H., Enomoto, M., and Ohtsubo, K.,** Toxicological approaches to the metabolites of Fusaria III, *Jpn. J. Exp. Med.,* 41, 521, 1971.

58. **Palyusik, M. and Koplikne-Kovacs, E.,** Effect of food containing T₂ and F-2 toxins on laying geese, *Magy. Allatorv. Lapja,* 30, 842, 1975; *RMVM,* 12, 113, 1977.

59. **Joffe, A. A.,** Growth and toxigenicity of fusaria of the sporotrichiella section as related to environmental factors and culture substrates, *Mycophathol. Mycol. Appl.,* 54, 35, 1974.

60. **Doerr, J. A., Hugg, W. E., Tung, H. T., Wyatt, R. D., and Hamilton, P. B.,** A survey of T₂ toxin, ochratoxin and aflatoxin for their effects on the coagulation of blood in young broiled chickens, *Poultry Sci.,* 53, 1728, 1974.

61. **Richard, J. L., Cysewski, S. J., Pier, A. C.,and Booth, G. D.,** Comparison of effects of dietary T₂ toxin on growth, immunogenic organs, antibody formation and pathologic changes in turkeys and chickens, *Am. J. Vet. Res.,* 39, 1674, 1978.

62. **Lafarge-Frayssinet, C., Lespinats, G., Lafont, P., Loisillier, F., Rosenstein, Y., and Frayssinet, C.,** Immunosuppressive effects of *Fusarium* extracts and trichothecenes, *Proc. Soc. Exp. Biol. Med.,* 160, 302, 1979.

63. **Ueno, Y., Sato, N., Ishii, K., Shimada, N., Tokita, K., Enomoto, M., Saito, M., Ohtsubo, K., and Ueno, I.,** Subacute toxicity of trichothece mycotoxins of *Fusarium* to cats and mice, *Jpn. J. Pharmacol.,* 23, 133, 1973; *RMVM,*11, 10, 1976.

64. **Rosenstein, N., Lafarge-Frayssinet, C., Lespinats, G., Loisillier, F., Lafont, P., and Frayssinet, C.,** Immunosuppressive activity of *Fusarium* toxins, *Immunology,* 36, 111, 1979.

65. **Goodwin, W., Haas, C. D., Fabian, C., Heller-Bettinger, I., and Hoogstraten, B.,** Phase I evaluation of anguidine, *Cancer,* 42, 23, 1978.

66. **Schoental, R. and Joffe, A. Z.,** Lesions induced in rodents by extracts from cultures of *Fusarium poae* and *F. sporotrichioides, J. Pathol.,* 112, 37, 1974.

67. **Pearson, A. W.,** Biochemical changes produced by *Fusarium* T₂ toxin in the chicken, *Res. Vet. Sci.,* 24, 92, 1978.

68. **Sawhney, D. S.,** Changes in plasma proteins of ducklings from dietary fusariotoxins, *Toxicol. Appl. Pharmacol.,*41, 168, 1978.

69. **Khmelevski, B. N.,** Activity of blood cholinesterases during fusariotoxicosis, *Tr. Vses. Nauchi-Issled Inst.Vet. Sanit.,* 37, 67, 1970; *RMVM,* 7, 660, 1972.

70. **Ueno, Y., and Fukushima, K.,** Inhibition of protein and DNA synthesis in Ehrlich ascites tumour by nivalenol, *Experientia,* 24, 1032, 1968.
71. **Ueno, Y., Hosoya, M., and Ishikawa, Y.,** Inhibitory effects of mycotoxins on the protein synthesis in rabbit reticulocytes, *J. Biochem.,* 66, 419, 1969.
72. **Ueno,Y., Ishikawa, Y., Amakai, K., Nakajima, M., Saito, M., Enomoto, M., and Ohtsubo, K.,** Comparative study on skin necrotizing effect of scirpene metabolites of Fusaria, *Jpn. J. Exp. Med.,* 40, 33, 1970.
73. **Ueno, Y., Hosoya, M., Morita, Y., Ueno, I., and Tatsuno, T.,** Inhibition of protein synthesis in rabbit reticulocytes by nivalenol, *J. Biochem.,* 64, 479, 1968.
74. **Cole, R. J., Kirksey, J. W., Cutler, H. G., Doupnik, B. L., and Peckham, J. C.,** Toxin from *Fusarium moniliforme:* effects on plants and animals, *Science,* 179, 1324, 1973.
75. **Kriek, N. P. J., Marasas, W. F. O., Steyn, P. S., Van Rensburg, S. J., and Steyn, M.,** Toxicity of a moniliformin producing strain of *Fusarium moniliforme* var. *subglutinans* isolated from maize, *Food Cosmet. Toxicol.,* 15, 579, 1977.
76. **Rabie, C. J., Lubben, A., Louw, A. I., Rathbone, E. B., Steyn, P. S., and Vleggaar, R.,** Moniliformin, a mycotoxin from *Fusarium fusarioides, J. Agric. Food Chem.,* 26, 275, 1978.
77. **Thiel, P. G.,** A molecular mechanism for the toxic action of moniliformin, a mycotoxin produced by *Fusarium moniliforme, Biochem. Pharmacol.,* 27, 483, 1978.
78. **Kohler, B., Huttner, B., Vielitz, E., Kahlau, D. I., Gedek, B.,** Ricketts in broilers by food contamination with *Fusarium moniliforme* Sheldon, *Zent. fur Veterinaermed.,* B25, 89, 1978: *RMVM,* 13, 231, 1978.
79. **Kellerman, T. S., Marasas, W. F. O., Pienaar, J. G., and Naude, T. W.,** A mycotoxicosis of Equidae caused by *Fusarium moniliforme, Onderstepoort J. Vet. Res.,* 30, 205, 1972.
80. **Marasas, W. F. O., Kellerman, T. S., Pienaar, J. G.,and Naude, T. W.,** Leukoencephalomalacia: a mycotoxicosis of Equidae caused by *Fusarium moniliforme* Sheldon, *Onderstepoort J. Vet. Res.,* 43, 113, 1976.
81. **Moreau, C.,** Trois cas de paralysis chez des porcs et des volailles vraisemblablement lies a une action toxique du *Fusarium moniliforme* Sheld., *Bull. Trimest. Soc. Myc. Fr.,* 90, 201, 1974.
82. **Shipchandler, M. T.,** Chemistry of zearalenone and some of its derivatives, *Heterocycles,* 3, 471, 1975.
83. **Bristol, F. M., and Djurickovic S.,** Hyperoestrogenism in female swine as the result of feeding mouldy corn, *Can. Vet. J.,* 12, 132, 1971.
84. **Cottereau, P., Laval, A., Bastien, G., and Magnan, G.,** Une mycotoxicose oestrogenique chez le porc, *Rev. Med. Vet. (Toulouse),* 125, 1095, 1974.
85. **Cuturic, S., Marzan, B., Pavlicek, A., Hajsig, M., Riznar, S., Sertic, V., and Bencevic, K.,** Mycotoxicoses in pigs. II. Changes in the genital organs and their behaviour after feeding mouldy foodstuffs, *Vet. Arh.,* 42, 126, 1972; *Vet. Bull.,* 43, 86, 1973.
86. **Grigore, C., Mitrou, P., Sofletea, I., and Arvanitopol, N.,** Oestrogenic syndrome of a mycotic nature in cattle, *Revista de Cresterea Animalelor,* 25, 59, 1975; *RMVM,* 12, 96, 1977.
87. **Mirocha, C. J. and Christensen, C. M.,** Oestrogenic mycotoxins synthesized by *Fusarium,* in *Mycotoxins,* Purchase, I. F. H., Ed., Elsevier, Amsterdam, 1974, 129.
88. **Nelson, G. H.,** Effect of *Fusarium* invaded feed and F$_2$ on swine, 2nd Int. Congr. Plant Pathol. Minn., 866 (Abstr.), 1973.
89. **Palyusik, M.,** Experimental oedema of the porcine vagina: fusariotoxicosis caused by *Fusarium graminearum, Magyar Allatorv. Lapja,* 28, 297, 1973; *RMVM,* 9, 1186, 1974; *Vet. Bull.,* 44, 91, 1974.
90. **Palyusik, K.,** Experimental fusariotoxicosis in swine, *Prog. Anim. Hyg. (Budapest),* 1975, 303; RMVM, 13, 231, 1978.
91. **Simonella, P.,** Oestrogenic mycotoxicosis. I. Outbreak of hyperoestrogenisim in sows and rabbits fed mouldy maize, *Att. Soc. Ital. Sci. Vet.,* 26, 436, 1972.
92. **Stankushev, K., Duparinova, M., Vranska, T., and Tikhova, D.,** Parasitic *Fusarium* strains on maize and experiments to isolate their phyto-oestrogens, *Vet. Nauki,* 14, 33, 1977; *RMVM,* 13, 166, 1978.
93. **Vanyi, A.,** The Effect of F$_2$ Fusariotoxin, Zearalenone on the Reproductive Process of Swine, Proc. 3rd Int. Pig Vet. Soc. Congr., Int. Pig Vet. Soc. Sect. G 33, 1974; *RMVM,* 12, 114, 1977.
94. **Ueno, Y., Shimada, N., Yagasaki, S. S., and Enomoto, M.,** Toxicological approaches to the metabolites of Fusaria VII. Effects of zearalenone on the uteri of mice and rats, *Chem. Pharm. Bull.,* 22, 2830, 1974.
95. **Mitton, A., Collet, J. C., Szymansi, J., and Gousse, R.,** Avortements dan unélevage ovin et presence de zéaralénone dans l'alimentation, *Rev. Med. Vet. (Toulouse),* 126, 813, 1975.
96. **Sharma, V. D., Wilson, R. F., and Williams, L. E.,** Reproductive performance of female swine fed corn naturally molded or inoculated with *Fusarium roseum, J. Anim. Sci.,* 38, 598, 1974.
97. **Miller, J. K., Hacking, A., and Gross, V. J.,** Still births, neonatal mortality and small litters in pigs associated with the ingestion of *Fusarium* toxin by pregnant sows, *Vet. Rec.,* 93,555, 1973.
98. **Martin, P. M. D. and Gilman, G.,** A consideration of the mycotoxin hypothesis, *Trop. Prod. Rep.,* G105, London, 1976.
99. **Mirocha, C. J., Christensen, C. M., and Nelson, G. H.,** Physiologic activity of some fungal oestrogens produced by *Fusarium, Cancer Res.,* 28, 2319, 1968.

100. **Bennett, G., Beaumont, W. H., and Brown, P. R. M.,** Use of the anabolic agent zearanol (resorcylic acid lactone) as a growth promoter for cattle, *Vet. Rec.,* 98, 235, 1974.

101. **Davis, G. J., MacLachlan, J. A., and Lucier, G. W.,** Fetotoxicity and teratogenicity of zearanol in mice, *Toxicol. Appl. Pharmacol.,* 41, 138, 1977.

102. **Ishii, K., Sawano, M., Ueno, Y., and Tsunoda, H.,** Distribution of zearalenone producing *Fusarium* species in Japan, *Appl. Microbiol.,* 27, 625, 1974.

103. **Stob, M., Baldwin, R. S., Tuite, J., Andrew, F. N., and Gillette, K. G.,** Isolation of an anabolic uterotrophic compound from corn infected with *Gibberella zeae, Nature (London),* 196, 1318, 1962.

104. **Mirocha, C. J., Christensen, C. M., and Nelson, G. N.,** Biosynthesis of the fungal oestrogen F_2 and a naturally occurring derivative F_3 by *Fusarium moniliforme, Appl. Microbiol.,* 17, 482, 1969.

105. **Hacking, A., Rosser, W. R., and Dervish, M. T. D.,** Zearalenone producing strains of *Fusarium* on barley seeds, *Ann. Appl. Biol.,* 84, 7, 1976.

106. **Lasztity, R., Tamas, K., and Woller, L.,** Occurrence of *Fusarium* mycotoxins in some Hungarian corn crops, *Ann. Nutr. Alimentation,* 31, 495, 1977.

107. **Stipanovic, R. D. and Schroeder, H. W.,** Zearalenone and 8' hydroxyzearalenone from *Fusarium roseum. Mycopathol. Mycol. Appl.,* 57, 77, 1975.

108. **Harrison, J.,** Moulds in Agriculture and Food, in Symp. Mycotoxicosis, Natural Institute of Environmental Sciences, U.K., October 17, 1974.

109. **Speers, G. M., Meronuck, R. A., Barnes, D. M., and Mirocha, C. J.,** Effect of feeding *Fusarium roseum* f.sp. *graminearum* contaminated corn and the mycotoxin F-2 on growing chick and laying hen, *Poultry Sci.,* 50, 627, 1971.

110. **Meronuck, R. A., Garren, K. H., Christensen, C. M., Nelson, G. H., and Bates, F.,** Effect on turkey poults and chicks of rations containing corn invaded by *Penicillium* and *Fusarium, J. Vet. Res.,* 31, 551, 1970.

111. **Featherston, W. R.,** Utilization of *Gibberella* infected corn by chicks and rats, *Poultry Sci.,* 52, 2334, 1973.

112. **Korpinen, E. L., Kallela, K., and Ylimaki, A.,** Oestrogenic activity of *Fusarium graminearum* on rats in experimental conditions, *Nord. Veterinaermed.,* 21, 62, 1972.

113. **Marks, H. L. and Bacon, C. W.,** Influence of *Fusarium* infected corn and F_2 on laying hens, *Poultry Sci.,* 55, 1864, 1976.

114. **Gallo, M. A., Bailey, D. E., Babish, J. G., Cox, G. E., and Taylor, J. M.,** Observations on the toxicity of zearalenone in the rat, *Toxicol. Appl. Pharm.* 41, 133, 1977.

115. **Sherwood, R. F. and Peberdy, J. F.,** Effects of zearalenone on the developing male chick, *Br. Poultry Sci.,* 14, 127, 1973.

116. **Palyusik, M., Nagy, G., and Zoldag, L.,** Effect of different *Fusarium* species on spermatogenesis in ganders, *Magyar Allatorvosok Lapja,* 29, 551, 1974; *RMVM,* 10, 291, 1975.

117. **Vanyi, A., Danko, G., Aldasy, P., Eros, I., and Szigeti, D. G.,** Fusariotoxicoses I. Studies on the oestrogenic effect of *Fusarium* strains, *Magy. Allatorv. Lapja,* 28, 303, 1973.

118. **Vanyi, A., Buza, L., and Szeky, A.,** Fusariotoxicoses IV. Effect of F_2 toxin (zearalenone) on spermiogenesis of carp, *Magy. Allatorv. Lapja,* 29, 457, 1974; *RMVM,* 10, 291, 1975.

119. **Vanyi, A., Szeky, A., and Szailer, E. R.,** Fusariotoxicoses V. Effect of F_2 toxin on reproduction in female swine, *Magy. Allatorv. Lapja,* 29, 723, 1974; *Vet. Bull.,* 45, 346, 1975; *RMVM,* 11, 211, 1976.

120. **Ruddick, J. A., Scott, P. M., and Harwig, J.,** Teralogical evaluation of zearalenone administered orally to the rat, *Bull. Env. Contam. Toxicol.,* 15, 678, 1976.

121. **Kurtz, H. J., Nainn, M. E., Nelson, G. H., Christensen, C. M., and Mirocha, C. J.,** Histological changes in the genital tracts of swine fed oestrogenic mycotoxin, *Am. J. Vet. Res.,* 30, 551, 1969.

122. **Ueno, Y. and Yagasaki, S.,** Toxicological approaches to the metabolites fusaria X. Accelerating effect of zearalenone on RNA and protein synthesis in the uterus of ovariectomized mice, *Jpn. J. Exp. Med.,* 45, 199, 1975.

123. **Hidy, P. H., Baldwin, R. S., Greasham, R. L., Keith, C. L., and McMullen, J. R.,** Zearalenone and some derivatives: production and biological activities, *Adv. Appl. Microbiol.,* 22, 59, 1977.

124. **Hobson, W., Bailey, J., and Fuller, G. B.,** Cytotoxic activity of macrocyclic metabolites from fungi, *Neoplasme,* 24, 21, 1977.

125. **Boyd, P. A. and Wittliff, J. L.,** Mechanism of *Fusarium* mycotoxin action in mammary gland, *J. Toxicol. Env. Health,* 4, 1, 1978.

126. **Greenman, D. L.** Interaction of *Fusarium* Mycotoxins with oestradiol binding sites in target tissues, *J. Toxicol. Env. Health,* 3, 348, 1977.

127. **Ingerowski, G. H. and Stan, H. J.,** In vitro metabolism of the anabolic drug zearanol, *J. Env. Pathol. Toxicol.,* 2, 1173, 1979.

128. **Karg, H.,** Lebensmittel hygienische Aspekte bein Einsatz von Ostrogenen in der Nutziermast *Arch. Lebensmittlehyg.,* 4, 77, 1973.

129. **Farb, R. M., Mego, J. L., and Hayes, A. W.,** Effect of mycotoxins on uptake and degradation of albumin in mouse liver and kidney lysosomes, *J. Toxicol. Environ. Health,* 1, 985, 1976.

130. **Fritz, J. C., Mislivec, P. B., Pla, G. W., Harrison, B. N., Weeks, C., and Dantzman, J. G.,** Toxigenicity of mouldy feed for young chicks, *Poultry Sci.,* 52, 1523, 1973.

131. **Mirocha, C. J. and Pathre, S. V.,** Identification of the toxic principle in a sample of poaefusarin, *Appl. Microbiol.,* 26, 719, 1974.

132. **Doupnik, B., Jones, O. H., and Peckham, J. C.,** Toxic fusaria isolated from mouldy potatoes involved in an epizootic of atypical interstitial pneumonia in cattle, *Phytopathology,* 6, 890, 1971.

133. **Peckham, J. C., Mitchell, F. E., Jones, O. H., and Doupnik, B.,** A typical interstitial pneumonia in cattle fed mouldy sweet potatoes, *J. Am. Vet. Med. Assoc.,* 160, 169, 1972.

134. **Saito, M., Ohtsubo, K., Umeda, M., Enomoto, M., Kurata, H., Ndagawa, S., Sakebe, F., and Ichinoe, M.,** Screening tests using He La cells and mice for detection of mycotoxin producing fungi isolated from foodstuffs, *Jpn. J. Exp. Med.,* 41, 1, 1971.

135. **Horakova, K. and Betina, V.,** Cytotoxic activity of macrocyclic metabolites from fungi, *Neoplasma,* 24, 21, 1977.

136. **Umeda, M., Yamamoto, T., and Saito, M.,** DNA strand breakage of He La cells induced by several mycotoxins, *Jpn. J. Exp. Med.,* 42, 527, 1972.

137. **Joffe, A. Z. and Palti, J.,** Relations between harmful effects on plants and on animals of toxins produced by species of *Fusarium, Mycopath. Mycol. Appl.,* 52, 209, 1974.

138. **Bodon, L. and Zoldag, L.,** Cytotoxicity tests on T_2 fusariotoxin, *Acta Vet. Acad. Sci. Hung.,* 24, 451, 1974; *RMVM,* 11, 326, 1976.

139. **Grove, J. F. and Mortimer, P. H.,** The cytoxicity of some transformation products of diacetoxyscirpenol, *Biochem. Pharmacol.,* 18, 1473, 1969.

140. **Vanyi, A. and Szailer, E.,** Investigation of the cytotoxic effect of F_2 toxin (zearalenone) in various monolayer cultures, *Acta Vet. Acad. Sci. Hung.,* 24, 407, 1974; *Vet. Bull.,* 45, 739, 1975; *RMVM,* 2, 326, 1976.

141. **Vanyi, A. and Szailer, E. R.,** Fusariotoxicoses. III. Cytotoxic effect of F_2 toxin (zearalenone) in monolayer tissue cultures, *Magy. Allatorv. Lapja,* 29, 191, 1974; *Vet. Bull.,* 44, 481, *RMVM,* 10, 96, 1975.

142. **Ames, B. N., Durston, W. E., Yamasaki, E., and Lee, F. D.,** Carcinogens are mutagens: a simple test system combining liver homogenates for activation and bacteria for detection, *Proc. Natl. Acad. Sci. U.S.A.,* 70, 2281, 1973.

143. **Ames, B. N., Lee, F. D., and Durston, W. E.,** An improved bacterial test system for the detection and classification of mutagens and carcinogens, *Proc. Natl. Acad. Sci. U.S.A.,* 70, 728, 1973.

144. **Miller, E. C. and Miller, J. A.,** *Chemical Mutagens,* Hollaender, A., Ed., Plenum Press, New York, 1971, 83.

145. **Miller, J. A. and Miller, E. C.,** Carcinogens occurring naturally in foods, *Fed. Proc. Fed. Am. Soc. Exp. Med.,* 35, 1316, 1976.

146. **Ames, B. N., McCann, J., and Yamasaki Y.,** Methods for detecting carcinogens and mutagens with the *Salmonella* mammalian microsome mutagenicity test, *Mutation Res.,* 31, 347, 1975.

147. **Kuczuk, M. H., Benson, P. M., Heath, H., and Hayes, A. W.,** Evaluation of the mutagenic potential of mycotoxins using *Salmonella typhimurium* and *Saccharomyces cerevisiae, Mutation Res.,* 53, 11, 1978.

148. **Wehner, F. C., Marasas, W. F. C., and Thiel, P. G.,** Lack of mutagenicity to *Salmonella typhimurium* of some *Fusarium* mycotoxins, *Appl. Environ. Microbiol.,* 35, 659, 1978.

149. **Nagao, M., Honda, M., Hamasaki, T., Natori, S., Ueno, Y., Yamasaki, M., Yahagi, Y., and Sugimura, T.,** Mutagenicity of mycotoxins on *Salmonella, Proc. Jpn. Assoc. Mycotoxicol.,* 314, 41, 1976.

150. **Ueno, Y., Kubota, K., and Nakamura, Y.,** Mutagenicity of carcinogenic mycotoxins in *Salmonella typhimurium, Cancer Res.,* 38 536, 1978.

151. **Sullivan, J. D. and Ikawa, M.,** Variation in inhibition of frowth of five *Chlorella* strains by mycotoxins and other toxic substances, *J. Agric. Food Chem.,* 20, 921, 1972.

152. **Boutibonnes, P.,** A propos de L'activité antibactérienne de la zearalenone, *Can. J. Microbiol.,* 25, 421, 1979.

153. **Bjeldanes, L. F., Chang, G. W., and Thomson, S. V.,** Detection of mutagens produced by fungi with the *Salmonella typhimurium* assay, *Appl. Environ. Microbiol.,* 35, 1150, 1978.

154. **Kada, K., Tsuchikawa, K., and Sadie, V.,** In vitro and host mediated "rec-essay" procedures for screening chemical mutagens and phloxine mutagenic red dye detected, *Mutation Res.,* 16, 165, 1972.

155. **Ueno, Y., Kubota, K. K.,** DNA-attacking ability of carcinogenic mycotoxins in recombination deficient mutant cells of *Bacillus subtilis, Cancer Res.,* 36, 445, 1976.

156. **Boutibonnes, P. and Loquet, C.,** Antibacterial activity, DNA attacking ability and mutagenic ability of the mycotoxin zearalenone, *Pharmacology,* 7, 204, 1979.

157. **McCann, J., Choi, E., Yamasaki, E., and Ames, B. N.,** Detection of carcinogens as mutagens in the *Salmonella* microsome test: assay of 300 chemicals, *Proc. Natl. Acad. Sci. U.S.A.,* 72, 5135, 1975; *Proc. Natl. Acad. Sci. U.S.A.,* 73, 950, 1976.

158. **Rowland, I. R.,** Mutagenicity testing with bacteria, *Food Cosmet. Toxicol.,* 13, 465, 1975.

159. **Oettlé, A. G.,** Cigarette smoking as the major cause of lung cancer, *S. Afr. Med. J.,* 37, 935, 1963.

160. **Anon.,** a fungus in osteoarthritis, *Br. Med. J.,* 1, 999, 1964.
161. **Enomoto, M. and Saito, J.,** Carcinogens produced by fungi, *Ann. Rev. Microbiol.,* 26, 279, 1972.
162. **Saito, M. and Ohtsubo, K.,** Trichothecene toxins of *Fusarium* species, in *Mycotoxins,* Purchase, I. F. H., Ed., Elsevier, Amsterdam, 1974, 263.
163. **Akhmeteli, M. A., Linnik, A. B., Cernov, K. S., Voronin, V. M., Hesina, A. J. A., Guseva, N. A., and Sabad, L. M.,** Study of toxins isolated from grain infected with *Fusarium sporotrichioides, Pure Appl. Chem.,* 35, 209, 1973.
164. **Marasas, W. F. O., Bamburg, J. R., Smalley, E. B., Strong, F. M., Ragland, W. L., and Degurse, P. E.,** Toxic effects on trouts, rats, and mice of T_2 toxin produced by the fungus *Fusarium tricinctum* (Cd) Synd & Hans, *Toxicol. Appl. Pharmacol.,* 15, 471, 1969.
165. **Schoental, R., Joffe, A. Z., and Yagen, B.,** Cardiovascular lesions and various tumours found in rats given T_2 toxin, a trichothecene metabolite of *Fusarium, Cancer Res.,* 39, 2179, 1979.
166. **Schoental,** The role of *Fusarium* mycotoxins in the aetiology of tumors of the digestive tract and of certain other organs in man and animals, *Front. Gast. Res.,* 4, 17, 1978.
167. **Marasas, W. F. O.,** Natural Occurrence of *Fusarium* Toxins in Southern African Maize, Int. Conf.: Mycotoxins, Munich, August 14, 1978.
168. **Aleksandrowicz, J. and Smyk, B.,** The association of neoplastic diseases and mycotoxins in the environment, *Tex. Rep. Biol. Med.,* 31, 715, 1973.
169. **Wray, B. B. and O'Steen, K. G.,** Mycotoxins producing fungi from horse associated with leukaemia, *Arch. Environ. Health,* 30, 571, 1975.
170. **Scott, P. M.,** Mycotoxins in feeds and ingredients and their origin, *J. Food Prot.,* 41, 385, 1978.
171. **Schiefer, H. B. and Hayes, M. A.,** Are Trichothecene Mycotoxins a Threat to the Canadian Livestock Industry?, Proc. 15th Ann. Nutr. Conf. Feed Manuf., Guelph, Ontario, April 24, 1979.
172. **Shotwell, O. L., Hesseltine, C. W., Goulden, M. L., and Vandergraft, E. E.,** Survey of corn for aflatoxin, zearalenone and ochratoxin, *Cereal Chem.,* 47, 700, 1970.
173. **Shotwell, O. L., Hesseltine, C. W., Vandergraft, E. E., and Goulden, M. L.,** Survey of corn from different regions for aflatoxin, ochratoxin and zearalenone, *Cereal Sci. Today,* 16, 266, 1971.
174. **Shotwell, O. L., Goulden, M. L., Bothast, R. J., and Hesseltine, C. W.,** Mycotoxins in hot spots in grains. I, *Cereal Chem.,* 52, 687, 1975.
175. **Shotwell, O. L., Goulden, M. L., Bennett, G. A., Plattner, R. D., and Hesseltine, C. W.,** Survey of 1975 wheat and soybeans for aflatoxin zearalenone and ochratoxin, *J.Assoc. Off. Agric. Chem.,* 60, 778, 1977.
176. **Funnell, H. S.,** The Occurrence of Mycotoxins in Ontario, Proc. 15th Ann. Nutr. Conf. Feed Manuf., Toronto, Ontario, April 24, 1979.
177. **Puls, R. and Greenway, J. A.,** Fusariotoxicosis from barley in British Columbia. II, *Can. J. Comp. Med.,* 40, 16, 1976.
178. **Petrie, L., Robb, J., and Stewart, A. F.,** The identification of T_2 toxin and its association with a haemorrhagic syndrome in cattle, *Vet. Rec.,* 101, 326, 1977.
179. **Bottalico, A.,** La presenza di *Fusarium moniliforme* Sheldon nelle cariossidi del granturico (*Zeamays* L), *Phytophathol. Med.,* 15, 54,1976.
180. **Caldwell, R. W. and Tuite, J. F.,** Zearalenone production in field corn in Indiana, *Phytopathology,* 60, 1696, 1970.
181. **Caldwell, R. W., and Tuite, J. F.,** Zearalenone in freshly harvested corn, *Phytopathology,* 64, 752, 1974.
182. **Martin, P. M. D. and Keen, P.,** The occurrence of zearalenone in raw and fermented products from Swaziland and Lesotho, *Sabouraudia,* 16, 15, 1978.
183. **Stoloff, L., Henry, S., and Francis, O. J.,** Survey for aflatoxins and zearalenone in 1973, *J. Assoc. Off. Agric. Chem.,* 59, 118, 1976.
184. **Collet, J. C., Regnier, J. M., and Marechal, J.,** Contamination par mycotoxines de mais conservés en cribs et visiblement altérés, *Ann. Nutr. Aliment.,* 31, 403, 1977.
185. **Hesseltine, C. W., Rogers, R. F., and Shotwell, O.,** Fungi, especially *Gibberella zeae* and zearalenone occurrence in wheat, *Mycologia,* 70, 14, 1978.
186. **Juskiewicz, T. and Piskorska-Pliszczynska, J.,** Aflatoxin B,B$_2$,G, and G$_2$, ochratoxin A and B, sterigmatocystin and zearalenone content in cereals, *Med. Weter.,* 32, 617, 1976,. *RMVM,* 13, 59, 1978.
187. **Juskiewicz, T. and Piskorska-Pliszczynska, J.,** Mycotoxins in grain for animal feeds, *Ann. Nutr. Aliment.,* 31, 489, 1977.
188. **Leistner, L.,** Mycotoxin Residues in Food of Animal Origin, Abst. Int. Conf.: Mycotoxins, Munich, August 14 to 15, 1978.
189. **Mirocha, C. J., Robison, T. S., and Chi, M.,** Metabolism and Distribution of T_2 Toxin in Animal Tissue, Abst. Int. Conf.: Mycotoxins, Munich, August 14 to 15, 1978.
190. **Hofman, G. and Leistner, L.,** Carry over of *Fusarium* toxins in children, Abst.Int. Conf.: Mycotoxins, Munich, August 14 to 15, 1978.
191. **Lasztity, R. and Woller, L.,** Investigation of the effect of zearalenone toxin produced by *Fusarium* fungi and its derivatives on animal organisms fed with infested fodder, I.U.P.A.C., p. 193, 1974.

192. **Loncarevic, A., Jovanovic, M., Ljesevic, Z., Stankov, Z., Tosevski, J., and Bogetic, V.,** Vulvovaginitis in newborn piglets, *Praxis Vet.,* 25, 299, 1977, *Vet. Bull.,* 48, 599, 1978.

193. **Scott, P. M., Panalaks, T., Kannere, S., and Miles, W. F.,** Determination of zearalenone in cornflakes and other corn based foods, *J. Assoc. Off. Anal. Chem.,* 61, 593, 1978.

194. **Van Walbeek, W., Scott, P. M., and Thatcher, F. S.,** Mycotoxins from foodborne fungi, *Can. J. Microbiol.,* 14, 131, 1968.

195. **Sutton, J. C., Baliko, W., and Funnell, H. S.,** Relation of weather variables to incidence of zearalenone in corn in southern Ontario, *Can. J.Plant Sci.,* 60, 149, 1980.

196. **Sutton, J. C.,** personal communication, 1979.

197. **Lovelace, C. E. A. and Nyathi, C. B.,** Estimation of the fungal toxins zearalenone and aflatoxininating opaque maize beer in Zambia, *J. Sci. Food Agric.,* 28, 288, 1977.

198. **Marasas, W. F. O., Kriek, N. P. J., Van Rensburg, S. J., Steyn, M., and Van Schalkwyk, G. C.,** Occurrence of zearalenone and deoxynivalenol, *S. Am. J. Sci.,* 73, 346, 1977.

199. **Martin, P. M. D.,** Unpublished work on the incidence of fungi in maize in southern Africa, 1979.

200. **Marasas, W. F. O. and Smalley,E. B.,** Mycoflora, toxicity and nutritive value of mouldy maize, *Onderstepoort J. Vet. Res.,* 39, 1, 1972.

201. **Marasas, W. F. O., Kriek, N. P. J., Steyn, M., Van Rensburg, S. J., and Van Schalkwyk, D. J.,** Mycotoxicological investigations on Zambian maize, *Food Cosmet.Toxicol.,* 16, 39, 1978.

202. **Martin, P. M. D.,** Annual report of the Malkerns Research Station, Swaziland, 1977 to 1978.

203. **Martin, P. M. D., Gilman, G., and Keen, P.,** The incidence of fungi in foodstuffs and their significance, based on a survey in the eastern Transvaal and Swaziland, in *Symposium on Mycotoxins in Human Health,* Purchase, I. F. H., Ed., Macmillan, London, 1971, 281.

204. **Gilman, G. A.,** Report of a Survey of Food Storage and Handling Techniques Used in Eastern Transvaal and Swaziland, *Trop. Prod. Inst.,* Report R397, London, 1974.

205. **Harington, J. S.,** Cancer of the uterine cervix, *S. Afr. J. Hosp. Med.,* 1977, 34, 1977.

206. **Johnson, R. H.,** The cases of cancer seen at a Botswana Hospital, 1968-1972, *Cent. Afr. J. Med.,* 21, 260, 1975.

207. **Macrae, S. M. and Cook, B. V.,** A retrospective study of cancer patients among hospital inpatients in Botswana, 1960-1972, *Br. J. Cancer,* 32, 121, 1975.

208. **Martin, P. M. D. and Keen, P.,** The cancer spectrum in Lesotho 1970–1974, *S. Afr. J. Sci.,* 75, 501, 1979.

209. **Martin, P. M. D., Perry, J. W. B., and Keen, P.,**The cancer spectrum in Lesotho; 1950–1969, *S. Afr. J. Sci.,* 72, 168,1976.

210. **Davies, J. N. P.,** Sex hormone upset in Africans, *Br. Med. J.,* 2, 676, 1949.

211. **Davies, J. N. P.,** Liver tumours and steroid hormones, *Lancet,* 1, 516, 1974.

212. **Schoental, R.,** Carcinogenicity as related to age, *Ann. Rev. Pharmacol.,* 14, 185, 1974.

213. **Schoental, R.,** Carcinogens in plants and microorganisms, in *Chemical Carcinogens,* Searle, E. A., Ed., ACS Monograph, 173, 626, 1976.

214. **Allen, E. and Gardner, W. U.,** Cancer of the cervix of the uterus in hybrid mice following long continued administration of oestrogen, *Cancer Res.,*1, 359, 1941.

215. **Dunn, T. B.,** Carcinogenic action of oestrogens, *N. Engl. J. Med.,* 284, 1147, 1971.

216. **Gardner, W. W.,** Carcinoma of the uterine cervix and upper vagina: induction under experimental conditions in mice, *Ann. N.Y. Acad. Sci.,* 75, 543, 1959.

217. **Greenwald, P., Barlow, J. J., and Nasca, P. C.,** Vaginal cancer after maternal treatment with synthetic oestrogens, *N. Engl. J. Med.,* 285, 390, 1971.

218. **O'Grady, W. P. and McDivitt, R. W.,** Breast cancer in a man treated with diethylstilbestrol, *Arch. Pathol.,* 88, 162, 1969.

219. **Herbst, A. L., Robboy, S. J., Scully, R. E., and Poskanzer, D. C.,** Clear cell adenocarcinoma of the vagina and cervix in girls, *Am. J. Obstet. Gynecol.,* 119, 713, 1974.

220. **Herbst, A. L., Ulfelder, H., and Poskanzer, D. C.,** Adenocarcinoma of the vagina, *N. Engl. J. Med.,* 284, 878, 1971.

221. **Thomas, D. B.,** Role of exogenous female hormones in altering the risk of benign and malignant neoplasms in humans, *Cancer Res.,* 38, 3991, 1978.

222. **Dunn, T. B.,** Cancer of the uterine cervix in mice fed a liquid diet containing an antifertility drug, *J. Natl. Cancer Inst.,* 43, 671, 1969.

223. **Anon.,** Liver tumours and the pill, *Br. Med. J.,* 6083, 345, 1977.

224. **Johnson, F. L., Feagler, J. R., Lerner, K. G., Majerus, P. W., Siegel, M., Hartmann, J. R., and Thomas, E. D.,** Association of androgenic anabolic steroid therapy with development of hepatocellular carcinoma, *Lancet,* 2, 1273, 1972.

225. **Christopherson, W. M. and Mays, E. T.,** *J. Natl. Cancer Inst.,* 56, 167, 1977.

226. **Hamilton, T.,** Control by oestrogen of genetic transcription and translation, *Science,* 161, 649, 1968.

227. **O'Malley, B. W. and Schrader, W. T.,** The receptors of steroid hormones, *Sci. Am.,* 234, 32, 1976.

228. **Anderson, J. A. and Bolin, V.,** The influence of various hormones on the resistance of Swiss mice to adapted poliomyelitis virus, *J. Clin. Endocrinol.,* 6, 466, 1946.
229. **Foley, G. E. and Aycock, W. L.,** Alterations in the autarceologic susceptibility of the mouse to experimental poliomyelitis by oestrogenic substances, *Endocrinology,* 37, 245, 1945.
230. **Sprunt, D. H. and McDearman, S.,** Studies on the relationship of sex hormones to infection. III, *J. Immunol.,* 38, 81, 1940.
231. **Rapp, F. and Kemeny, B. A.,** Oncogenic potential of *Herpes simplex* virus in mammalian cells following photodynamic inactivation, *Photochem. Photobiol.,* 24, 335, 1976.
232. **Yamamoto, N. and Zur Hausen, H.,** Tumour promoter TPA enhances transformation of human leukocytes by Epstein-Barr virus, *Nature (London),* 280, 244, 1979.
233. **Aurelian, L.,** Antibody to HSV induced tumour specific antigens in serums from patients with cervical carcinoma, *Science,* 181, 161, 1973.
234. **Aurelian, L.,** The "viruses of love" and cancer, *Am. Med. Tech.,* 40, 496, 1974.
235. **Aurelian, L.,** Persistence and expression of the *Herpes simplex* virus type 2 genome in cervical tumour cells, *Cancer Res.,* 34, 1126, 1974.
236. **Aurelian, L.,** Sexually transmitted cancers? The case for genital *Herpes, J. Am. Vener. Dis. Assoc.,* 2, 10, 1976.
237. **Aurelian, L., Royston, I., and Davis, H. J.,** Antibody to genital *Herpes simplex* virus. Association with cervical atypia and carcinoma *in situ, J. Natl. Cancer Inst.,* 45, 455, 1970.
238. **Kessler, I. I., Kulczar, Z., Rawls, W. E., et al.,** Cervical cancer in Yugoslavia. I, *J. Natl. Cancer Inst.,* 52, 359, 1974.
239. **Buxton, E. A.,** *Vet. Med.,* 22, 451, 1927.
240. **Legenhausen, A. H.,** Probably a cryptogam poisoning due to mould on the corn. *Vet. Med.,* 23, 29, 1928.
241. **McNutt, S. H., Purwin, P., and Murray, C. J.,** Vulvovaginitis in swine, *J. Am. Vet. Med. Assoc.,* 73, 484, 1928.
242. **Christensen, J. J. and Kernkamp, H. C. H.,** *Minn. Agric. Exp. Stn. Tech. Bull.,* 113, 28, 1963.
243. **Pullar, E. M. and Lerew, W. M.,** Vulvovaginitis of swine, *Aust. Vet. J.,* 13, 28, 1973.
244. **Koen, J. S. and Smith, H. C.,** An unusual case of genital involvement in swine associated with eating mouldy corn, *Vet. Med.,* 40, 131, 1945.
245. **McErlean, B. A.,** Vulvovaginitis of swine, *Vet. Rec.,* 64, 539, 1952.
246. **Kyurtov, N.,** Poisoning of pigs with barley contaminated by *Fusarium, Vet. Sbir. Sofia,* 1962, 19, 1962.
247. **Christensen, C. M., Nelson, G. H., and Mirocha, C. J.,** *Microbial Toxins,* Vol. 7, Ajl, S. J., Ed., Academic Press, New York, 1971.
248. **Stamatovic S., Ljesevic, Z., and Durickovic, S.,** Vulvovaginitis in sows associated with alimentary mycotic intoxication, *Vet. Glas.,* 17, 507, 1963; *Vet. Bull.,* 34, 327, 1964.
249. **Demakov, G. P.,** On fusariotoxicosis in cattle, *Veterinariya,* 41, 59, 1964; *RMVM,* 5, 233, 1965.
250. **Christensen, C. M., Nelson, G. H., and Mirocha, C. J.,** Effects on the white rat uterus of a toxic substance isolated from *Fusarium, Appl. Microbiol.,* 13, 653, 1965.
251. **Mitroiu, P., Ungareanu, Minciuna, V., Grigore, C., Sirbu, Z., and Ripeanu, M.,** Contributions a l'étude de la flore mycotique des fourrages et observations sur, certains foyers de mycotoxicosis et de botulisme en Roumane, *Archiva Vet.,* 3, 69, 1966; *RMVM,* 6, 497, 1969.
252. **Bugeac, T. and Berbinschi, C.,** Observations and investigations on vulvovaginitis of sows, *Revta Zootec. Med. Vet. Bucuresti,* 17, 56, 1967; *RMVM,* 6, 447, 1969.
253. **Eriksen, E.,** Oestrogene faktorer i nuggent korn Vulvovaginitis hos svin, *Nord. Veterinaermed.,* 20, 396, 1969.
254. **Mirocha, C. J., Harrison, J., Nichols, A. A., and McClintock, M.,** Detection of a fungal oestrogen (F_2) in hay associated with infertility in cattle, *Appl. Microbiol.,* 16, 797, 1968.
255. **Kurata, W.,** A mycological examination for the presence of mycotoxin producers on 1954-1967 stored rice grains, *Bull. Natl. Inst. Hyg. Sci. (Tokyo),* 86, 183, 1968.
256. **Danko, G. and Aldasy, P.,** *Magyar Allatorv. Lapja,* 24, 517, 1969.
257. **Jivoin, P. et al.,** Research into Fusarial toxicosis in horses, *Lucr. Inst. Cercet. Vet. Bioprep. Pasteur,* 8, 281, 1970; *RMVM,* 8, 94, 1973.
258. **Ozegovic, L.,** Mouldy maize poisoning in pigs, *Veterinaria (Sarajevo),* 19, 525, 1970; *RMVM,* 7, 592, 1972.
259. **Ozegovic, L. and Vukovic, V.,** Vulvovaginitis mycotoca bei schweinen durch Verfutterung von Verschimmelten Mais, *Mykosen,* 14, 545, 1971.
260. **Roine, K., Korpinen, E. L., and Kallela, K.,** Mycotoxicosis as a probable cause of infertility in dairy cows, *Nord. Veterinaermed.,* 23, 628, 1971; *RMVM,* 7, 658, 1972.
261. **Boltushkin, A. N., Koval's Skaya, M. G., Inpardina, K. N., and Stupnikov, V. D.,** Fusariotoxicosis of dairy cattle, *Mikol Fitopatol.,* 5, 75, 1971; *RMVM,* 7, 372, 1971.
262. **Debrezceni, I. and Borda, I.,** Losses due to fusarial toxicosis on a pig fattening farm, *Magyar Allatorv. Lapja,* 27, 109, 1972; *RMVM,* 8, 94, 1973.

263. **Chung, H. S.,** Cereal scab causing mycotoxicoses in Korea and present status of mycotoxin researches, *Korean J. Mycol.,* 3, 31, 1975; *RMVM,* 2, 414, 1976.

264. **Kotsonis, F. N., Smalley, E. B., Ellison, R. A., and Gale, C. M.,** Feed refusal factors in pure cultures of *Fusarium roseum "graminearum",* Appl. Microbiol., 30, 362, 1975.

265. **Futrell, M. C., Scott, G. E., and Vaughn, G. F.,** Problems created by fungus infected corn shipped to swine feeders in the southern United States, *Econ. Bot.,* 30, 291, 1976.

266. **Vallejo, L. C. and Gemetro, L.,** Fusariotoxicosis en cerdos, *Gaceta Vet.,* 38, 14, 1976; *RMVM,* 12, 427, 1977.

267. **Gedek, B., Huttner, B., Kahlan, D. I., Kohler, N., and Vielitz, E.,** Rachitis bei Mastflugel duck Kontamination des Futters mit *Fusarium moniliforme* Sheldon I, *Zentralbl. Veterinaermed.,* 258, 29, 1978.

268. **Wilson, B. J., Maronpot, R. R., and Hildebrandt, P. K.,** Equine leukoencephalomalacia, *J. Am. Vet. Med. Assoc.,* 163, 1293, 1974.

269. **Loginov, V. P.,** Acute fusariotoxicosis in piglets, *Veterinariya,* 35, 68, 1958; *RMVM,* 3, 97, 1958.

270. **Marchenko, G. F. and Renyanskaya, E. V.,** Fusariotoxicosis of pigs in the Stavropol territory, *Veterinariya,* 36, 70, 1959; *Vet. Bull.,* 30, 992, 1960.

271. **Izmailov, I. H. et al.,** Mycotoxicosis of cattle in western Ukraine, *Izri Noukovi Pratsi,* 11, 151, 1961.

272. **Kalmykov, S. T., Kochetov, V. I., Penkov, A. I., and Ponomareva, T. M.,** Fusariotoxicosis in sheep, *Veterinariya,* 43, 65, 1967; *RMVM,* 5, 590, 1967.

273. **Kokhtyuk, F. P., Tsimbal, I. K., Ivanova, L. G., and Dashkerich, P. D.,** Mycotoxicosis induced in horses by toxic strains of *Fusarium sporotrichioides, Byull. Vses. Inst. Eksp. Vet.,* 25, 80, 1976; *RMVM,* 13, 232, 1978.

274. **Ozegovic, L. and Vukovic, V.,** Zearalenone (F_2) *Fusarium* toxicosis of pigs in Yugoslavia, *Mykosen,* 15, 171, 1972; *RMVM,* 10, 96, 1975.

275. **Stojanovic, Z., Zivkovic, S., Sayed, M. El., Sijacki, N., et al.,** Effect of the use of mouldy maize harvested in 1972 on the fattening of pigs, poultry and cattle, *Poljoprivedna Znantstvena Smotra,* 31, 521, 1974; *RMVM,* 12, 412, 1977.

276. **Vanyi, A., Szemeredi, G., Quarini, L, and Szailer, E. R.,** Fusariotoxicosis on a dairy farm, *Magyar Allatorvosok Lapja,* 29, 544, 1974; *RMVM,* 10, 291, 1975.

277. **Miller, J. K.,** Suspected mycotoxic diseases of pigs in Scotland, in *Second Meeting on Mycotoxins in Animal Disease,* Patterson, D. S. P., Pepin, G. A., and Shreeve, B. J., Eds., MAFF Publications, U.K., 1977.

278. **Forsyth, D. M., Yoshizawa, T., Morooka, N., and Tuite, J.,** Emetic and refusal activity of deoxynivalenol to swine, *Appl. Environ. Microbiol.,* 34, 547, 1977.

279. **Lage, M. C. D., Dias, M. C. S., and Barrets, M. L. M.,** Algunas consideracoes sobre micotoxicoses em patologia aviaria, *Rep. Trabal. Lab. Nac. Inv. Vet.,* 8, 19, 1976; *Vet. Bull.,* 48, 852, 1978.

280. **Smalley, E. B.,** T_2 toxin, *J. Am. Vet. Med. Assoc.,* 163, 1278, 1973.

281. **Wyatt, R. D. and Hamilton, P. B.,** Some case reports of T_2 toxicosis and aflatoxicosis in chickens, *Poultry Sci.,* 54, 1830, 1975.

282. **Wyatt, R. D., Harris, J. R., Hamilton, P. B., and Burmeister, H. R.,** Possible outbreaks of fusariotoxicosis in avians, *Avian Dis.,* 16, 1123, 1972.

283. **Dyson, D. A.,** Haemorrhagic syndrome of cattle of suspected mycotoxic origin, *Vet. Rec.,* 100, 400, 1977.

284. **Marasas, W. F. O., Leistner, L., Hofman, G., and Eckhardt, C.,** Occurrence of toxigenic strains of *Fusarium* in maize and barley in Germany, *Eur. J. Appl. Microbiol.,* 7, 289, 1979.

285. **Booth, C.,** *The Genus Fusarium,* Commonwealth Mycological Inst., Kew, Surrey, 1971.

286. **Nirenberg, H.,** Untersuchungen uber die morphologische und biologische Differenzierungin der Fusarium Sektion Liseola, *Mitt. Biol. Bundesanst. Land Forstwirtsch. Berlin-Dahlem,* 169, 1, 1976.

287. **Marasas, W. F. O., Van Rensburg, S. J., and Mirocha, C. J.,** Incidence of *Fusarium* species and the mycotoxins deoxynivalenol and zearalenone in corn produced in esohageal cancer areas in the Transkei, *Agric. Fd. Chem.,* 27, 1108, 1979.

288. **Marasas, W. F. O.,** Occurence of toxic fungi and mycotoxins in food, in *Environmental Associations with Oesophageal Cancer in Trnanskei,* National Research Institute for Nutritional Diseases, Tygerberg, South Africa, 1979, chap. 2.

289. **Marasas, W. F. O., Kriek, N. P. T., Wiggins, V. M., Steyn, P. S., Towers, D. K., and Hastie, T. J.,** Incidence, geographic distribution and toxigenicity of *fusarium* species in South African corn, *Phytopathology,* 69, 1181, 1979.

Chapter 10

MUTACARCINOGENS IN ORDINARILY COOKED FOODS

Minako Nagao and Takashi Sugimura

TABLE OF CONTENTS

I. INTRODUCTION

Chemical carcinogens in our environment play important roles in development of human cancers. Chemical carcinogens are categorized by their sources into occupational hazards (microenvironmental hazards), general pollutants (macroenvironmental hazards), iatrogenic substances, and carcinogens in tobacco smoke and foods.

Human cancers due to industrial chemicals sometimes have a very clear and simple cause-result relationship, as exemplified by hemoangioendotheliosarcomas in the liver of people exposed to vinyl chloride monomer under occupational conditions, and by squamous cell carcinomas in the trachea and bronchi of people exposed to sulfur mustard in factories during the war. Thus scientists have paid much attention to occupational cancers. On the contrary, the contributions of carcinogenic substances and especially naturally occurring carcinogens in foods have been underestimated. Epidemiological data on human cancers due to carcinogens in the normal environment appear to be very complicated. However, as demonstrated by investigations on stomach cancer in Japanese immigrants to Hawaii and California and also by epidemiological studies in Columbia, some human cancers are directly related to the diet.[1,2] Moreover, the incidence of cancer of the colon is generally thought to be influenced by dietary and nutritional conditions. Another reason why carcinogens in foods have received little attention is that human beings have eaten the same cooked foods for many generations, and they have the blind and unscientific belief that foods that have been eaten for many generations are "safe". Is it true? Carcinogenesis experiments on usual cooked foods by in vivo long-term animal experiments were not started until 10 years ago, because scientists were naturally reluctant to carry out this sort of experiment, especially unless it promised to yield worthwhile results.

However, the situation has changed very rapidly in the last few years, especially after the introduction of mutagenicity tests using microbes for screening environmental carcinogens. These tests are valuable because the process of carcinogenesis consists at least of two steps, namely initiation and promotion, and the initiation step has been shown to be closely related to mutation, namely alteration of DNA. Most carcinogens can modify nucleic acid bases, and these modifications may result in mutations. Some carcinogens can act directly on DNA, but most carcinogens (procarcinogen) must be activated to ultimate form through proximate forms by a metabolic activation system in mammalian cells before interaction with DNA. Exceptionally, some carcinogens such as 4-nitroquinoline 1-oxide and nitrofuran derivatives are activated to their ultimate forms by microbial enzymes as well as by mammalian enzymes. Among the many methods using microbes developed for assay of mutagens, the method developed by Ames and his associates using uv-repair deficient and surface lipopolysaccharide-barrier deficient mutants of *Salmonella typhimurium* and a microsomal and supernatant fraction designated as S-9 from the liver of rats treated with polychlorinated biphenyls have been most widely adopted.[3]

The overlapping of in vivo carcinogenicity of compounds with these mutagenicities demonstrated in Ames system has been well documented, and now most carcinogens have been found to be mutagens, although there are several exceptional cases, such as asbestos and hormones.[4-9] Mutagenic carcinogens could be called genotoxic carcinogens or muta-carcinogens. Most carcinogens may also have some promoting activity; for instance, asbestos and hormones may induce conditions that are favorable for promotion of initiated cells to malignant cells.

This review is mainly on recent findings about muta-carcinogens in cooked foods, principally based on microbial mutation tests. However, it also includes relevant data obtained in in vivo long-term animal experiments and short-term tests, other than microbial tests — namely, tests on transformation, sister chromatid exchanges, and chromosomal aberrations of cultured mammalian cells.

As described previously, among descendants of Japanese immigrants to California and Hawaii, the incidence of stomach cancer has decreased, while the incidence of colon cancer has increased significantly, reaching almost the incidence in white Americans. These changes may be closely related to changes in diet with consequent changes in the intakes of various types of muta-carcinogens. However, the effects of other factors than muta-carcinogens present in cooked foods should be considered in explaining this change. A high content of sodium chloride in Japanese diet may produce chronic gastritis, which favors promotion of initiated cells in the stomach. Intake of more meat and fat may result in change in the intestinal flora and consequent change in the rate of formation of endogenous muta-carcinogens and/or promoters, especially in the large intestine. Changes may also occur in the metabolisms of cholesterol and bile acids.[10] These factors may actually be more important in carcinogenesis than the muta-carcinogens present in foods. However, in this review these factors are only mentioned briefly in the "Discussion."

II. BROILED FOODS

A. Charred Surface of Fish and Meat

From ancient times fish and meat have often been cooked over an open fire. For instance, beefsteak broiled over charcoal has long been regarded as a special luxury all over the world, and in Japan salted and dried fishes have been eaten broiled for many generations. At present they are usually broiled on a gas range.

Beefsteak and broiled fish were suspected to be causes for human cancers.[11] Their contents of benzo[a] pyrene or other polycyclic aromatic hydrocarbons were not sufficiently high to be significantly carcinogenic; the actual amount of benzo[a] pyrene in broiled fish was reported to be 1.25 µg/kg original wet weight by Masuda et al.[12] and that in broiled steak to be 8 to 50 µg/kg by Lijinsky and Shubik.[13] However, we found that the charred parts of beefsteak and fish were mutagenic to S. typhimurium TA98 with Ames system, and that the mutagenicity was enhanced by the presence of a mammalian microsomal enzyme system.[14,15] We found that when a fresh sardine, weighing 100 g, was broiled in the normal way, 2 g of charred surface was equivalent in mutagenicity on S. typhimurium TA 98 to about 360 µg benzo[a] pyrene. Similarly, when a piece of beefsteak weighing 190 g was broiled, 5.2 g of charred material contained mutagenic activity equivalent to that of about 860 µg benzo[a] pyrene.

The correlation between the temperature of broiling, namely of pyrolysis, and the formation of mutagenic activity was studied using a temperature-controlled electric furnace.[16] As shown in Table 1, the water content in foods and the temperature are both important factors. In general, foods with low water contents yield most mutagens on heating at 300°C, whereas foods with high water contents yielded most mutagens at 400°C.

Vegetables, such as garlic and onion, were also mutagenic after pyrolysis. Both garlic and onion contain alliin and garlic also contains allicin. Pyrolysates of pure alliin and allicin were also mutagenic.[17]

B. Amino Acid and Protein Pyrolysates

Pyrolysis products of various amino acids have been found to be strongly mutagenic. The specific activities of pyrolysates of various amino acids were described elsewhere.[18-21] Very strongly mutagenic substances were isolated from a tryptophan pyrolysate and identified as the γ-carboline derivatives 3-amino-1,4-dimethyl-5H-pyrido[4,3-

Table 1
MUTAGENIC ACTIVITIES OF PYROLYSIS PRODUCTS OF FOODS[16]

Food	Water content (%)	Revertants/g pyrolysed food[a]		
		Temperature of pyrolysis (°C)		
		250	300	400
Sea weed	5.3	0	2,600	30,400
Soybean, raw	11.0	0	15,270	68,100
Skipjak, dried	18.0	12,200	243,000	62,000
Squid, dried	21.8	2,690	80,000	44,800
Chicken	64.4	0	6,610	151,200
Beef	67.2	0	1,780	114,000
Hairtail, fresh	72.8	0	8,490	123,200
Pork	72.9	0	2,490	97,250
Jack mackerel, fresh	73.0	0	2,250	82,350
Egg	74.5	0	1,210	47,500

[a] *S. typhimurium* TA 98 was used with S-9 mix prepared from the liver of rats treated with polychlorinated biphenyls.

b]indole (I) and 3-amino-1-methyl-5*H*-pyrido[4,3-*b*]indole (II), with the chemical structures shown in Figure 1. These compounds are abbreviated as Trp-P-1 and Trp-P-2, respectively, where Trp stands for typtophan and P for pyrolysis. Trp-P-1and Trp-P-2 are very strong mutagens inducing 40,000 revertants/μg and100,000 revertants/μg, respectively, of TA 98 in the presence of S-9 mix. They were synthesized by Akimoto *et al.*[22] and Takeda et al.,[23] and many of their biological characters were investigated. Both compounds induced sister chromatid exchanges in EBV-transformed human lymphocytes in the presence of rat liver S-9 mix[24] (Figure 2) and chromosomal aberrations in Chinese hamster cells.[25] They also induced transformation of Syrian hamster cells in Pienta's system.[26] These transformed colonies were shown to be composed of malignant cells by transplanting them into the cheek pouches of nonimmunosuppressed 4-week-old male hamsters.[27] Subcutaneous injection of 0.5 mg/0.1 mℓ olive oil suspension of Trp-P-1·CH_3COOH into hamsters produced fibrosarcomas locally as shown in Figure 3.[28] In a preliminary experiment the incidence of tumors after its injection was 60%. Analogues of Trp-P-1 and Trp-P-2 with various alkyl chains were synthesized, but mutagenicity tests showed that Trp-P-2 was the strongest mutagen to TA 98.

Pyrolysis of glutamic acid also produces a strong mutagen.[18-21] The mutagenic compounds Glu-P-1 and Glu-P-2 were isolated and identified as 2-amino-6-methyldipyrido–[1,2-*a*:3′,2′-*d*]imidazole (III) and 2-aminodipyrido[1,2-*a*:3′,2′-*d*]imidazole (IV), respectively. These compounds were also synthesized chemically.[29] Pyrolysis of lysine yielded Lys-P-1, 3,4-cyclopentenopyrido[3,2-*a*]carbazole (V) as a mutagenic compound, and its structure was confirmed by chemical synthesis.[30]

Various fungicidal compounds have been isolated from pyrolysates of fat-free soybean and identified. Among these, benzo[*f*]quinoline (VI) and phenanthridine (VII) were found to be mutagenic.[20] The α-carboline derivatives 2-amino-α-carboline (VIII) and 2-amino-3-methyl-α-carboline (IX) were identified as mutagenic principles in a pyrolysate of soybean globulin.[31]

Since proteins consist of 17 kinds of amino acids, many mutagenic compounds are probably present in the pyrolysates of proteins and charred proteinous foods. It is now possible to study these, and various compounds have already been characterized and can be used as standards. However, the yields of mutagenic activities of substances probably

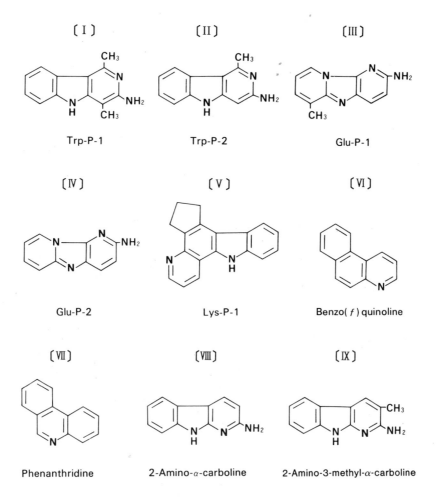

FIGURE 1. Structures of mutagenic compounds isolated from pyrolysates of amino acids and proteins.

depend on other factors besides the protein composition of the foods, and indeed it has been found that the presence of sugar depresses the formation of mutagenic principles from proteins.

C. Sugar Pyrolysates

Sugar pyrolysate also contains mutagens. Unlike pyrolysates of proteins or amino acids, sugar pyrolysates induced mutation in TA 100 without mammalian microsomal enzymes.[18,19] Pyrolysates of glucose, arabinose, fructose, and sorbitol induced 3000 to 6000 revertants per milligram of pyrolysate.[18,19] On the other hand, a glucosamine pyrolysate required microsomal enzymes to exhibit mutagenicity and, like an amino acid pyrolysate, it was more mutagenic to TA 98 than to TA 100. Setliff and Mower also reported the mutagenicity of a sugar pyrolysate.[32] Caramel, which is widely used as a food coloring and flavoring, is weakly mutagenic to TA 100.

As mentioned before, the presence of glucose with tryptophan during heating reduced the production of frame-shift mutagen tested with TA 98 to about 1/100th of that of a pyrolysate of tryptophan alone. Production of a base-pair change mutagen tested with TA 100 was also reduced by tryptophan to about 1/20th of that in a pyrolysate of glucose alone, as shown in Table 2.

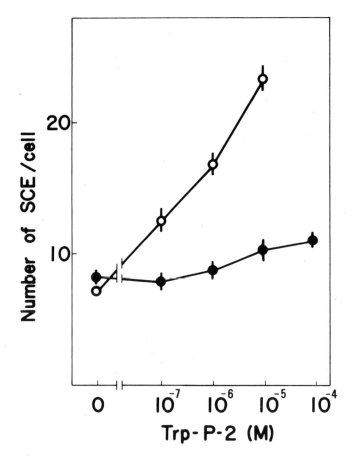

FIGURE 2.   Sister chromatid exchanges of EBV-transformed human lymphocytes[24] induced by Trp-P-2. O—O with S-9 mix, ●—● without S-9 mix.

III. FRIED AND BOILED FOODS

Commoner and his associates detected mutagens in boiled beef extracts.[33] An extract of lean ground beef with boiling water did not contain appreciable mutagens, but when the extract was reduced to 5% of its original volume by boiling for 10 hr, the mutagenicity was greatly increased, indicating that mutagens were not present either in the beef tissue or the beef extract, but were produced during prolonged boiling. The mutagens in the extract were soluble in methylenechloride, required metabolic activation, and were active toward TA 98 but not TA 100.

Similarly lean ground beef heated in a domestic hamburger cooker yielded mutagens that required metabolic activation. Prolonged cooking (well done) yielded more mutagens than brief cooking (rare). The mutagenic potency was 945 revertants per plate per 5 g dry weight of well done hamburger. They prepared a fraction with mutagenic activity and subject it to thin layer chromatographic fractionation on Gelman ITLC-SG sheets. The mutagen, which has not yet been identified, differed in mobility from benzo[a]–pyrene with hexane-acetone (50:50, v/v) as solvent. They found that the minimum specific mutagenic activity was about 350 revertants per microgram, and from this value they calculated the mutagen content as 1 to 14 μg/100 g of lean beef hamburger (0.01 to 0.14 ppm). Further work is required to identify the active principles.

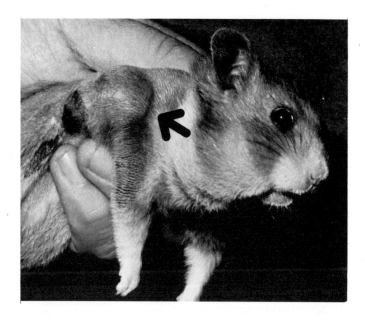

FIGURE 3A.   Tumor of hamster produced by Trp-P-1. Trp-P-1 was suspended in olive oil at the rate of 0.5 mg/0.1 mℓ and injected subcutaneously once a week for 5 months (macroscopic finding).

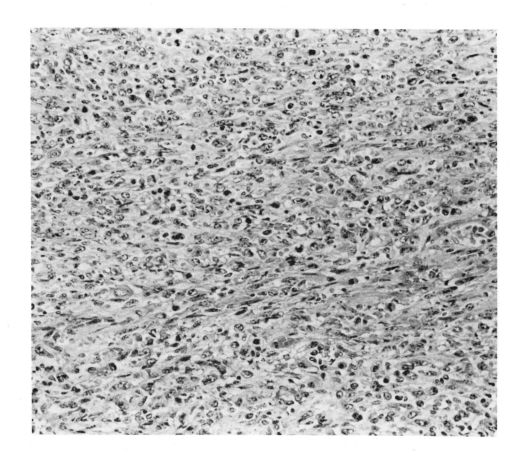

FIGURE 3B.   Fibrosarcoma of pleomorphic spindle cells with many mitotic cells (histological finding).

Table 2
REDUCTION OF MUTAGEN PRODUCTION BY THE PRESENCE OF
GLUCOSE AND TRYPTOPHAN DURING PYROLYSIS

	Amount (mg)	Revertants/total pyrolysate			
		TA 100		TA 98	
		+S-9 mix	−S-9 mix	+S-9 mix	−S-9 mix
Tryptophan	12.5	16,100	0	168,000	0
Glucose	50	11,800	216,000	0	0
Tryptophan	12.5	4,070	11,800	1,850	0
+ Glucose	50				

Note: Materials were heated in a flask over a gas burner.

IV. PICKLES

Linhsien county in China has a high incidence of esophageal cancer. From an epidemiological study, the pickles which are a specialty of Linhsien county were suspected as a cause of this esophageal cancer.[34] The mutagenicity of a methanol extract of these pickles was tested in our laboratory.[34,35] The extract was mutagenic to TA 100 with S-9 mix and to TA 98 with or without S-9 mix, but the mutagenic principle has not yet been isolated. These pickles, a traditional food in Linhsien, are heavily contaminated with the fungus *Geotrichum candidum,* Link, which was found to produce various nitrosamines.[36]

A kind of Japanese pickles with a very similar smell to Linhsein pickles was also subjected to the mutagenicity test. The mutagenicity of these pickles was about one tenth that of the Linhsien pickles. Starting with 100 g of pickles (45 g dry weight) 3000-fold purification of mutagens was achieved by Sephadex LH-20 and silica gel column chromatographies. Using high pressure liquid chromatography and mass spectrography, major mutagenic component of these pickles was identified as kaempherol, and a minor mutagenic component as isorhamnetin.[35]

V. SPICES

Preference for spices varies in different countries and tribes. Nagao et al. tested the mutagenicities of methanol extracts of 17 spices that are commercially available in Japan and the U.S. finding that seven were mutagenic to *S. typhimurium* TA 100 and/or TA 98, as shown in Table 3. The spices that were not mutagenic were turmeric, chili powder, cumim seeds, lavender flowers, poppy seeds, rose petals, lampong, mustard, sage, and rosemary. Almost all the spices had lethal effects on *S. typhimurium,* in the absence of S-9 mix. This was to be expected, because this antibacterial effect is one of the reasons why spices are used. Seino et al. purified an active component from a methanol extract of sumac, the seeds of the genus *Rhus* by chromatographies on Sephadex LH-20 and silica gel and identified it as the flavonoid quercetin.[37]

Nagao et al. also tested the mutagenicities of methanol extracts of 12 spices obtained from Thailand, finding that of these only cardamon seeds and fennel seeds were mutagenic.[38]

It should be pointed out, however, that the contribution of spices to the overall mutagenicity of ordinary foods is probably low, because very small amounts of spices are actually used and their specific mutagenic activities are low.

Table 3
MUTAGENICITIES OF SPICES

	Revertants/mg original spices			
	TA 100		TA 98	
Spice	+S-9 mix	−S-9 mix	+S-9 mix	−S-9 mix
Dill weed	3.2	0	2.4	0
Sumac	0	0	0.8	0
Thyme	8.0	0	1.2	0
Potpourri	2.0	0	2.0	0
Oregano	4.0	0	2.4	0
Bay leaves	0	0	1.2	0
Marjoram	2.0	0	0	0

Note: Methanol extracts were prepared, evaporated to dryness, dissolved in dimethylsulfoxide, and tested for mutagenicity.

VI. BEVERAGES

A. Nonalcoholic Beverages

Most people drink several cups of various kinds of beverages, such as coffee and tea, every day. However, tests have shown that these beverages have some mutagenicity.[38a]

Samples prepared in the ordinary way from two kinds of roasted coffee beans exhibited mutagenicity to TA 100 without metabolic activation. Addition of S-9 mix abolished the mutagenicities of the samples.

A cup of coffee, extracted from 20 g of roasted coffee beans, produced 1.4 to 4.6 × 10^5 revertants under standard conditions. Two brands of instant coffee were mutagenic to TA 100 without S-9 mix, addition of S-9 mix reducing the number of revertants. A cup of instant coffee containing 1 g of instant coffee powder yielded 5.5 to 5.8 × 10^4 revertants of TA 100 without S-9 mix. Caffein-free instant coffee also induced a similar number of revertants per gram.

A boiling water extract of 5 g of a certain brand of tea yielded 4 × 10^4 revertants of TA 100 without metabolic activation and as with coffee, addition of S-9 mix reduced the number of revertants. A hot water extract of Japanese green tea also induced mutation to TA 100 without metabolic activation, and addition of S-9 mix reduced the number of revertants in this case, too. Mutagenicity of green tea has also been reported by Uyeta et al.[39] Except for coffee, these beverages were not, or only slightly, mutagenic to TA 98, but after hydrolysis by a crude enzyme preparation, "crude hesperidinase," from *Aspergillus niger,* green tea and roasted tea were mutagenic to TA 98 with S-9 mix, as shown in Table 4. Intestinal microbes are known to hydrolize various glycosides and therefore, some bacterial enzyme(s) in the intestine may hydrolize the glycosides present in tea. An acid hydrolysate of green tea was also reported to be mutagenic to TA 98 with S-9 mix;[39] the mutagenicity in an acid hydrolysate of green tea was partly accounted for by its flavonoids, such as quercetin, kaempferol, and myricetin.[39]

A dimethylsulfoxide extract of coffee substitute, composed of chicory, roasted barley, rye, and shredded beet roots, was mutagenic. A dimethylsulfoxide extract of tea was also mutagenic to TA 100 without S-9 mix but a similar extract of linden flower tea was not mutagenic to TA 98 or TA 100 with or without S-9 mix.[41]

B. Alcoholic Beverages

Epidemiological studies have suggested a correlation between esophageal cancer and alcoholic intake.[42]

Table 4
MUTAGENICITIES OF NONALCOHOLIC BEVERAGES

	Revertants/mℓ beverage			
	TA 100		TA 98	
	+S-9 mix	−S-9 mix	+S-9 mix	−S-9 mix
Instant coffee	120	370	0	0
	49[a]	201[a]	0	0[a]
Instant coffee, caffein free	0	360	0	0
Coffee	0	1200	0	270
Tea	0	260	0	0
Green tea	0	250	0	0
	0[a]	0[a]	450[a]	0[a]
Japanese	0	190	0	0
roasted tea	100[a]	30[a]	440[a]	0[a]

Note: 200 mℓ of coffee was obtained by extracting 20 g of ground roasted coffee beans with 250 mℓ of boiling water. 175 mℓ of tea was obtained by extracting 5 g of tea leaves with 200 mℓ of boiling water. 590 mℓ each of green tea and Japanese roasted tea were obtained by extracting 7 g of tea leaves three times with 200 mℓ volumes of hot water. The resulting extracts were then lyophylized or evaporated and the residues were dissolved in dimethylsulfoxide for tests. Instant coffee was dissolved directly in dimethylsufoxide, the solution being equivalent to 1 g coffee powder per 200 mℓ water.

[a] Hesperidinase treatment was performed as described elsewhere.[38a]

Nagao et al. tested the mutagenicities of several kinds of whiskey and several kinds of brandy, finding that most of the samples induced mutation of TA 100 without a mammalian microsomal metabolic activation system.[38b] In addition, one kind of brandy was mutagenic to TA 100 and TA 98 with S-9 mix, 50 mℓ of brandy inducing from about 1200 to 10,000 revertants of *Salmonella typhimurium* TA 100 or TA 98 with or without S-9 mix. The red wine was not mutagenic to TA 98 without S-9 mix, and its mutagenicity was enhanced by fecalase.[42a]

VII. FLAVONOIDS IN VEGETABLES

During studies on the mutagen-carcinogens in bracken fern, which is eaten in some parts of the world including Japan, Wang et al.[43] found that flavonoids, such as quercetin and kaempferol, were mutagenic. Independently, Sugimura et al.[44] also observed the mutagenicity of kaempferol, when working on the mutagens in extracts of bracken. Subsequently, there have been several reports on the mutagenicities of flavonoids.[45-47]

For mutagenicity flavonoids require a double bond at the 2,3-position and hydroxy groups at the 3 and 5 positions. Mutagenicity of naturally occurring flavonol derivatives are shown in Table 5. Quercetin does not require metabolic activation by a mammalian microsomal enzyme, but its mutagenicity is enhanced by adding S-9 mix, and this enhancing activity is due to a factor(s) in the cytosol fraction.[48,49] Quercetin also induced frameshift mutation in *Escherichia coli* and gene conversion in *Saccharomyces cerevisiae*.[46] Kaempferol requires activation by a microsomal enzyme(s) to exhibit mutagenicity, and it is converted to quercetin by a microsomal enzymes.[49]

Quercetin, but not kaempferol, induced in vitro transformation of cryopreserved hamster embryo cells in Pienta's system.[50] It also induced sister chromatid exchanges in human lymphoblast cells[51] and chromosomal aberrations in hamster embryo cells.[51,52]

Table 5
MUTAGENICITY OF FLAVONOL DERIVATIVES

Compound	Substitution	Mutagenicity[a] (revertants/nmol)
3-Hydroxflavone	—	0.0
Fisetin	7, 3′, 4′-hydroxy	0.12
Galangin	5, 7-hydroxy	3.8
Kaempferol	5, 7, 4′-hydroxy	9.55
Kaempferid	5, 7-hydroxy, 4′-methoxy	2.42
Morin	5, 7, 2′, 4′-hydroxy	0.62
Quercetin	5, 7, 3′, 4′-hydroxy	19.0
Rhamnetin	5, 3′, 4′-hydroxy, 7-methoxy	12.7
Isorhamnetin	5, 7, 4′-hydroxy, 3′-methoxy	1.8
Myricetin	5, 7, 3′, 4′, 5′-hydroxy	0.11

[a] TA 98 was used in the presence of S-9 mix.

Eleven of 22 flavone derivatives with no hydroxy group at the three-position tested were slightly mutagenic — with TA 100 and TA 98 woogonin, 5,7-dihydroxy-8-methoxyflavone, induced 9.8 and 0.68 revertants per nano mole, respectively, but the other 10 derivatives induced one or less revertants of TA 100 per nano mole.[53]

In plants, most flavonoids are present as glycosides and these were not mutagenic even with S-9 mix. However, Nagao et al. found that on pretreatment with a crude hesperidinase preparation from *Aspergillus niger,* flavonol glycoside became mutagenic, as shown in Table 6, and Brown and Dietrich[49] reported that intestinal flora hydrolyse flavonol glycosides.

The contents of quercetin and kaempferol in vegetables have been documented by Herrmann.[54] Many vegetables were found to contain about 1 mg/kg fresh weight, but smaller amounts were found in carrots, radishes, beets, white asparagus without the tips or with white tips, cabbage without the outer leaves (white, red, Savoy cabbage), cauliflower, chicory, peas, cucumber, egg plants, and potatoes. On the other hand, the leaves of many root vegetables, potatoes, and asparagus contain concentrations of more than 1000 mg/kg. Moreover, the outer leaves of lettuce (Valentine) contain 462 mg quercetin per kilogram, although the inner leaves contain 7.6 mg/kg, and lettuce grown in a glasshouse contains less. Similarly the outer leaves of endives contain 258 mg/kg of kaempferol and the inner leaves contain 5.7 mg/kg.

The noncarcinogenicities of quercetin and quercitrin were reported about 30 years ago,[55] but these compounds are now being reexamined in animal tests under a program sponsored by the Ministry of Health and Welfare, Japan. Recent controversial results are available.[55a,55b]

VIII. ALKALOIDS AND OTHER COMPOUNDS IN PLANTS

A. Pyrrolizidines

More than 100 pyrrolizidine alkaloids have been isolated from plants and insects, and they are present in many plants used as herbal remedies. Some pyrrolizidine alkaloids were found to be carcinogenic to experimental animals[56,57] and to be mutagenic to *Drosophila,*[58] *Aspergillus,*[59] and *Salmonella typhimurium,*[14] but with the standard Ames' procedure they showed no detectable mutagenicity. Recently some pyrrolizidine alkaloids

Table 6
MUTAGENICITY OF FLAVONOL GLYCOSIDES

Compound	Structure	Mutagenicity (revertant/nmol)
Rutin	Quercetin-3-O-Glc-Rha	7.7
Isoquercitrin	Quercetin-3-O-Glc	5.7
Tiliroside	Kaempferol-3 (6-p-coumaroyl)-Glc	5.7
Astragalin	Kaempferol-3-O-Glc	9.3
Hyperin	Quercetin-3-O-Gal	8.5
Kaempferitrin	Kaempferol-3-O-Rha-7-O-Rha	8.7

Note: Flavonol glycosides were treated with hesperidinase at pH 4.0, neutralized, and subjected to test for mutagenicity. TA 98 was used in the presence of S-9 mix. Without hesperidinase treatment, all these glycosides did not induce revertant.

were found to be mutagenic to *S. typhimurium* strain TA 100, but not to the other strains of *Salmonella*, TA 1535, TA 92, *his*G 46, TA 1537, and TA 98.[60] Heliotrine and lasiocarpine, which contain heliotridine as the necine base and are carcinogenic, were mutagenic to TA 100 in the presence of S-9 from the liver of a PCB-treated rat. The mutagenicity of pyrrolizidine alkaloids could be detected only when these compounds were incubated with bacteria and S-9 mix in liquid medium. Fukinotoxin[61] (petasitenine[62]) from the flowerstalks of coltsfoot, *Petasites japonicus*, used as a herbal remedy and food, was found to be mutagenic to TA 100,[60] and coltsfoot and petasitenine (fukinotoxin) were both carcinogenic in rats.[63,64] Petasitenine (fukinotoxin) has otonecine as its necine base. Three other alkaloids, senkirkine, clivorine, and ligularidine, were all mutagenic to TA 100 after preincubation with S-9 mix. The carcinogenicity of plant containing senkirkine has also been reported.[56] However, the carcinogenicity suspected compounds lycopsamine,[65] seneciphylline,[56] and carcinogenic monocrotalline,[56] which have retronecine as their necine base, were not mutagenic by our method. Pyrrolizidines with retronecine were mutagenic to *Drosophila*.[66]

B. Hydrazine

Hydrazine is present in tobacco and tobacco smoke,[67] and one cigarette was reported to contain 30 ng of hydrazine.[67] Hydrazine is mutagenic to the *S. typhimurium* base-pair change mutants TA 1535, *his*G 46 and TA 100. Hydrazine induced 1.56 revertants/ μg of TA 100 in the presence of S-9 mix.[68]

Hydrazine derivatives were also found in mushrooms. *Agaricus bisporus*, the most commonly eaten commercial mushroom, contains agaritine, B-N[γ-L(+)-glutamyl]-4-hydroxyphenylhydrazine.[69] γ-Glutamyltransferase, present in mushroom, hydrolyzes agaritin to L-glutamate and 4-hydroxyphenylhydrazine, but the mutagenicity of 4-hydroxyphenylhydrazine is unknown, although phenylhydrazine is mutagenic to TA 100 with S-9 mix, inducing 0.1 revertants per microgram.[68] *Gyromitra esculenta*, a wild edible mushroom, contains ethyliden gyromitrin (acetaldehyde formylmethylhydrazone), N-methyl-N-formylhydrazine and methylhydrazine.[70] The last two compounds seem to be produced during cooking from ethylidene gyromitrin. Ethylidene gyromitrin was not mutagenic to *Escherichia coli*,[71] but its hydrolysis product, methylhydrazine, was mutagenic to *E. coli*,[71] *S. typhimurium his*G 46 and TA 92.[68] The annual consumption of *A. bisporus* in the U.S. was estimated to be 3 × 10⁸ lb. Fresh mushrooms contain 1.2 to 1.6 g/kg of ethylidene gyromitrin. One gram of methylhydrazine produced 1.7 × 10⁵ revertants of *S. typhimurium* TA 92.[68]

[X]

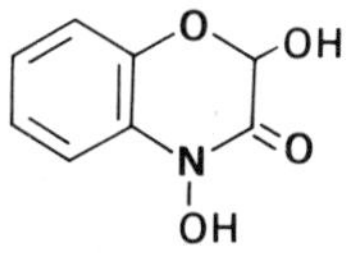

2,4-Dihydroxy-1,4-benzoxazinone

[XI]

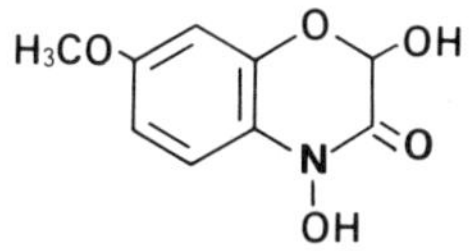

2,4-Dihydroxy-7-methoxy-1,4-benzoxazinone

FIGURE 4. Structures of naturally occurring mutagens in maize.

C. Benzoxazinone

Cereal plants, such as maize, wheat, and rye, contain the benzoxazinone derivatives 2,4-dihydroxy-1,4-benzoxazinone (X) and 2,4-dihydroxy-7-methyoxy-1,4-benzoxazinone (XI),[72,73] with the structures shown in Figure 4, which have been identified as insecticides and antifungal substances[74] and have recently been found to be mutagenic to *S. typhimurium* TA100 and TA 98.[75] 2,4-Dihydroxy-1,4-benzoxazinone was mutagenic to TA 100 without S-9 mix, although its activity was enhanced by S-9 mix. It is unknown whether these compounds are actual constituents of the grains.

D. Azoxymethanol

Methylazoxymethanol is present in cycad nuts as the glycoside cycasin. Until about 20 years ago, washed starch from cycad nuts was eaten on islands in the Pacific Ocean, including the islands southwest of Japan. Cycasin induces colon cancer in rodents.[76] It is hydrolyzed to methylazoxymethanol by intestinal microflora. Methylazoxymethanol induced base-change mutations of *S. typhimurium his*G 46[77] and TA 100, activity being increased by addition of S-9 mix.[78] Cycasin itself was not mutagenic, but it became mutagenic when hydrolyzed by β-glucosidase.[79]

XI. DISCUSSION — FACTORS MODIFYING MUTAGENICITY

As mentioned previously, this review is mainly on mutagenic substances in ordinarily cooked foods. There is now sufficient evidence for the overlapping of mutagens and carcinogens to suspect that most of these mutagens are probably carcinogenic. The level of mutagens in foods should be considered in evaluating their significance in carcinogenesis. Unlike the hazards of occupational carcinogens, those of mutagens and carcinogens in foods are hard to assess epidemiologically. However, the continuous intakes of minute amounts of mutagens in foods over a very long period may be a significant hazard.

Although it is impossible to evaluate this hazard exactly at present, several factors are known that must be taken into consideration in this evaluation. Various substances in food have comutagenic actions. Typical examples are harman and norharman, present in Japanese sake, mushrooms, charred parts of foods, and tobacco tar. They are β-carbolines and are nonmutagenic towards TA 100 or TA 98 with and without metabolic activation. However, norharman evokes fairly strong mutagenicity on TA 98 when incubated with S-9 mix and nonmutagenic aniline, *o*-toluidine, or the azo dye yellow OB.[80] Harman also has similar activity. The intercalation of norharman between base-pairs of double-stranded DNA and its interference with metabolic processes have been reported.[81,82]

The composition of the diet may alter the metabolism of carcinogens in vivo. For example, intake of charred material was found to induce activity for metabolizing aromatic hydrocarbons in the liver.[83]

In addition to the comutagenic actions of certain food constituents, desmutagenic actions must also be considered. Incubation with extracts of various vegetables and fruits resulted in inactivation of the mutagenicities of tryptophan pyrolysates.[84] A proteinous fraction responsible for this effect has been isolated from cabbage,[85] and a fraction from bean sprouts that interfered with the metabolic activation of aromatic hydrocarbons and decreased their mutagenicity has also been described.[86]

Nitrite ions inactivate Trp-P-1 under acidic conditions,[87,87a] although nitrite is considered to be hazardous in producing carcinogenic nitrosoamines.

Synthetic benzoflavones are known to interfere with metabolic activation, and naturally occurring flavonoids, which are themselves mutagenic, can also depress the mutagenicity of aromatic hydrocarbons by interfering with their metabolism. Tetramethylflavone derivatives are not mutagenic but depress the mutagenicity of aromatic hydrocarbons.[88]

Foods may be contaminated with mycotoxins such as aflatoxin, especially in regions with a hot, humid climate. There are also many mycotoxins which are known to be mutagenic, but which have not yet been tested for carcinogenicity.[89] Microbial products may also reduce mutagenicity. Some strains of *Actinomyces* produce protease inhibitors such as chymostatin and elastatinal, which inhibit chymotrypsin-like protease and elastase-like protease. Chymostatin and elastatinal are known to inhibit mutagenic processes[90,91] in microbes, and elastatinal also inhibits sister chromatid exchanges in cultured mammalian cells induced by mutagens.[92]

Thus, as described above, there are many interactions of food constituents which may have either positive or negative effects on mutagenesis. In addition, some components of foods may provide conditions favorable for promotion. However, little is known about this subject at present and it requires further investigation.

REFERENCES

1. **Doll, R.,** Strategy for detection of cancer hazards to man, *Nature (London),* 265, 589, 1977.
2. **Wynder, E. L. and Gori, G. B.,** Contribution of environment to cancer incidence; an epidemiologic exercise, *J. Natl. Cancer Inst.,* 58, 825, 1977.
3. **Ames, B. N., McCann, J., and Yamasaki, E.,** Methods for detecting carcinogens and mutagens with *Salmonella*/mammalian microsome mutagenicity test, *Mutation Res.,* 31, 347, 1975.
4. **McCann, J., Choi, E., Yamasaki, E., and Ames, B. N.,** Detection of carcinogens as mutagens in the *Salmonella*/microsome test: assay of 300 chemicals, *Proc. Natl. Acad. Sci. U.S.A.,* 72, 5135, 1975.
5. **McCann, J. and Ames, B. N.,** Detection of carcinogens as mutagens in the *Salmonella*/microsome test: assay of 300 chemicals: discussion, *Proc. Natl. Acad. Sci. U.S.A.,* 73, 950, 1976.
6. **Sugimura, T., Sato, S., Nagao, M., Yahagi, T., Matsushima, T., Seino, Y., Takeuchi, M., and Kawachi, T.,** Overlapping of carcinogens and mutagens, in *Fundamentals in Cancer Prevention,* Magee, P. N., Takayama, S., Sugimura, T., and Matsushima, T., Eds., University Park Press, Baltimore, 1976, 191.
7. **Nagao, M., Sugimura, T., and Matsushima, T.,** Environmental mutagens and carcinogens, *Ann. Rev. Genet.,* 12, 117, 1978.
8. **Ames, B. N. and McCann, J.,** Carcinogens are mutagens: a simple test system, *IARC Sci. Publ.,* No. 12, 493, 1976.
9. **Purchase, I. F. M., Longstaff, E., Ashby, J., Styles, J. A., Anderson, D., Lefevre, P. A., and Westwood, F. R.,** Evaluation of six short term tests for detecting organic chemical carcinogens and recommendations for their use, *Nature (London),* 264, 624, 1976.

10. **Reddy, B. S., Narisawa, T., Maronpot, R., Weisburger, J. H. and Wynder, E. L.,** Animal model for the study of dietary factors and cancer of the large bowel, *Cancer Res.,* 35, 3421, 1976.

11. **Grasso, P. and O'Hare, C.,** Carcinogens in food, in *Chemical Carcinogens,* Searle, C. E., Ed., American Chemical Society, Washington, D.C., 1976, 701.

12. **Masuda, Y., Mori, K., and Kuratsune, M.,** Polycyclic aromatic hydrocarbons in common Japanese foods. I. Broiled fish, roasted barley, shoyu, and caramel., *Gann,* 57, 133,1966.

13. **Lijinsky, W., and Shubik, P.,** Benzo (*a*)pyrene and polynuclear hydrocarbons in charcoal-broiled meat, *Science,* 145,53, 1974.

14. **Sugimura, T., Nagao, M., Kawachi, T., Honda, M., Yahagi, T., Seino, Y., Matsushima, T., Shirai, A., Sawamura, M., and Matsumoto, H.,** Mutagen-carcinogens in food, with special reference to highly mutagenic pyrolytic products in broiled foods, in *Origin of Human Cancer,* Hiatt, H. H., Watson, J. D., and Winsten, J. A., Eds., Cold Spring Harbor Laboratories, Cold Spring Harbor, N.Y., 1977, 1561.

15. **Nagao, M., Honda, M., Seino, Y., Yahagi, T., and Sugimura, T.,** Mutagenicities of smoke condensates and the charred surface of fish and meat, *Cancer Lett.,* 2, 221, 1977.

16. **Ueta, M., Kaneda, T., Mazaki, M., and Taue, S.,** Studies on mutagenicity of food. I. Mutagenicity of food pyrolysates, *J. Food Hyg. Soc. Jpn.,* 19, 216, 1978.

17. **Shimizu, H., Hashida, C., Hayashi, K., and Takemura, N.,** Mutagenicity of substance produced by combustion of some plants, *Jpn. J. Hyg.,* 32, 235, 1977.

18. **Sugimura, T. and Nagao, M.,** Mutagenic factors in cooked foods, *Crit. Rev. Toxicol.,* 6, 189, 1979.

19. **Nagao, M., Yahagi, T., Kawachi, T., Sein Seino, Y., Honda, M., Matsukura, N., Sugimura, T., Wakabayashi, K., Tsuji, K., and Kosuge, T.,** Mutagens in foods, and especially pyrolysis products of protein, in *Progress in Genetic Toxicology,* Scott, D., Bridges, B. A., and Sobels, F. H., Eds., Elsevier, Amsterdam, 1977, 259.

20. **Kosuge, T., Tsuji, K., Wakabayashi, K., Okamoto, T., Shudo, K., Iitaka, Y., Itai, A., Sugimura, T., Kawachi, T., Nagao, M., Yahagi, T., and Seino, Y.,** Isolation and structure studies of mutagenic principles in amino acid pyrolysates, *Chem. Pharm. Bull.,* 26, 611, 1978.

21. **Matsumoto, T., Yoshida, D., Mizusaki, S., and Okamoto, H.,** Mutagenic activity of amino acid pyrolysates in *Salmonella typhimurium* TA 98, *Mutation Res.,* 48, 279, 1977.

22. **Akimoto, H., Kawai, A., Nomura, H., Nagao, M., Kawachi, T., and Sugimura, T.,** Synthesis of a mutagenic principle isolated from tryptophan pyrolysate, *Chem. Lett.,* 1061, 1977.

23. **Takeda, K., Ohta, T., Shudo, K., Okamoto, T., Tsuji, K., and Kosuge, T.,** Synthesis of a mutagenic principle isolated from tryptophan pyrolysate, *Chem. Pharm. Bull,*25, 2145, 1977.

24. **Tohda, H., Oikawa, A., Kawachi, T., and Sugimura, T.,** Induction of sister-chromatid exchanges by mutagens from amino acid and protein pyrolysates, *Mutation Res.,* 77, 65, 1980.

25. **Sasaki, M., Sugimua, K., Yoshida, M. A., and Kawachi, T.,** Chromosome aberrations and sister chromotid exchanges induced by trytophan pyroysates, Trp-P-1 and Trp-P-2 in cultured human and Chinese hamster cells, *Proc. Jpn. Acad.,* 56B, 332, 1980.

26. **Takayama, S., Katoh, Y., Tanaka, M., Nagao, M., Wakabayashi, K., and Sugimura, T.,** *In vitro* transformation of hamster embryo cell with tryptophan pyrolysis products, *Proc. Jpn. Acad.,* 53B, 126, 1977.

27. **Takayama, S., Hirakawa, T., and Sugimura, T.,** Malignant transformation *in vitro* by tryptophan pyrolysis products, *Proc. Jpn. Acad.,* 54B, 418, 1978.

28. **Ishikawa, T., Takayama, S., Kitagawa, T., Kawachi, T., Kinebuchi, M., Matsukura, N., Uchida, E., and Sugimura, T.,** *In vivo* experiments on tryptophan pyrolysis products, in *Naturally Occurring Carcinogens — Mutagens and Modulators of Carcinogenesis,* Miller, E. C., Miller, J. A., Kirono, I., Sugimura, T., and Takayama, S., Eds., Japan Sci. Soc. Press, Tokyo, University Park Press, Baltimore, 1979, 159.

28a. **Nagao, M., Takahashi, Y., Yahagi, T., Sugimura, T., Takeda, K., Shudo, K., and Okamoto, T.,** Mutagenicities of α-carboline derivatives related to potent mutagens found in tryptophan pyrolysate, *Carcinogenesis,* 1, 451, 1980.

29. **Yamamoto, T., Tsuji, K., Kosuge, T., Okamoto, T., Shudo, K., Takeda, K., Iitaka, Y., Yamaguchi, K., Seino, Y., Yahagi, T., Nagao, M., and Sugimura, T.,** Isolation and structure determination of mutagenic substances in L-glutamic acid pyrolysate, *Proc. Jpn. Acad.,* 54B, 248, 1978.

30. **Wakabayashi, K., Tsuji, K., Kosuge, T., Takeda, K., Yamaguchi, K., Shudo, K., Iitaka, Y., Okamoto, T., Yahagi, T., Nagao, M., and Sugimura, T.,** Isolation and structure determination of a mutagenic substance in L-lysine pyrolysate, *Proc. Jpn. Acad.,* 54B, 569, 1978.

31. **Yoshida, D., Matsumoto, T., Yoshimura, R., and Matsuzaki, T.,** Mutagenicity of amino-α-carboline in pyrolisis products of soybean globulin, *Biochem. Biophys. Res. Commun.,* 83, 915, 1978.

32. **Setliff, J. A. and Mower, H. R.,** Mutagens in decomposition products of carbohydrates, *Fed. Proc. Fed. Am. Soc. Exp. Med.,* 36, 1304, 1977.

33. **Commoner, B., Vithayathil, A. J., Dolara, P., Nair, S., Madyastha, P., and Cuca, G.,** Formation of mutagens in beef and beef extract during cooking, *Science,* 201, 913, 1978.

34. **Miller, R. W.,** Cancer epidemics in the Peoples's Republic of China, *J. Natl. Cancer Inst.,* 60, 1195, 1978.

35. **Takahashi, Y., Nagao, M., Fujino, T., Yamaizumi, Z., and Sugimura, T.,** Mutagens in Japanese pickle identified as flavonoids, *Mutation Res.,* 68, 117, 1979.

36. **Li, M.-H., Lu, S.-H., Wang, C., Ji, Y., Wang, M., Cheng, S., and Tian, G.,** Experimental studies on the carcinogenicity of fungus-contaminated food from Linxian country, in *Genetic and Environmental Factors in Experimental and Human Cancer,* Gelboin, H. V., MacMahon, B., Matsushima, T., Sugimura, T., Takayama, S., and Takebe, H., Eds., Japan Sci. Soc. Press, Tokyo, 1979, 139.

37. **Seino, Y., Nagao, M., Yahagi, T., Sugimura, T., Yasuda, T., and Nishimura, S.,** Identification of a mutagenic substance in a spice, pumac as quercetin, *Mutation Res.,* 58, 225, 1978

38. **Nagao, M., Takahashi, Y., Yahagi, T., and Sugimura, T.,** Mutagenicities of Ordinary Foods, Proc. 7th Jpn. Environ. Mut. Soc., Mishima, 1978, 15.

38a. **Nagao, M., Takahashi, Y., Yamanaka, H., and Sugimura, T.,** Mutagens in coffee and tea, *Mutation Res.,* 68 101, 1979.

38b. **Nagao, M., Takahashi, Y., Wakabayashi, K., and Sugimura, T.,** Mutagenicity of alcoholic beverages, *Mutation Res.,* 88, 147, 1981.

39. **Uyeta, M., Taue, S., and Mazaki, M.,** Mutagenicity of hydrolysates of tea infusion, *Mutation Res.,* in press, 1981.

40. **Fukuoka, M., Kuroyanagai, M., Yoshihira, K., Natori, S., Nagao, M., Takahashi, Y., and Sugimura, T.,** Chemical and toxicological studies on bracken fern, *Pteridium aquilinum var. latiusculum.* IV. Surveys on bracken constituents by mutagen test., *J. Pharm. Dyn.,* 1, 324, 1978.

41. **Nagao, M., Takahashi, Y., Sugimura, T., and Pritikin, N.,** unpublished data.

42. **Audigier, J. C., Tuyns, A. J., and Lambert, R.,** Epidemiology of oesophageal cancer in France, *Digestion,* 13, 209, 1975.

42a. **Tamura, G., Gold, C., Ferro-Luzzi, A., and Ames, B.,** Fecalase a model for activation of dietary glycosides to mutagens by intestinal flora, *Proc. Natl. Acad. Sci. U.S.A.,* 77, 4961, 1980.

43. **Wang, C. Y., Pamukcu, A. M., and Bryan, G. T.,** Bracken fern as a naturally occurring carcinogen, *Med. Biol. Environ.,* in press.

44. **Sugimura, T., Nagao, M., Matsushima, T., Yahagi, T., Seino, Y., Shirai, A., Sawamura, M., Natori, S., Yoshihira, K., Fukuoka, M., and Kuroyanagi, M.,** Mutagenicity of flavone derivatives, *Proc. Jpn. Acad.,* 53B, 194, 1977.

45. **Bjeldanes, L. F. and Chang, G. W.,** Mutagenic activity of quercetin and related compounds, *Science,* 197, 577, 1977.

46. **Hardigree, A. A. and Epler, J. L.,** Comparative mutagenesis of plant flavonoids in microbial systems, *Mutation Res.,* 58, 231, 1978.

47. **MacGregor, J. T. and Jurd, L.,** Mutagenicity of plant flavonoids: structural requirements for mutagenic activity in *Salmonella typhimurium, Mutation Res.,* 54, 297, 1978.

48. **Yahagi, T., Mori, Y., Nagao, M., and Sugimura, T.,** Mutagenicity of quercetin and its metabolic activation (transl.), *Seikagaku,* 50, 947, 1978.

49. **Brown, J. P. and Dietrich, P. S.,** Mutagenicity of plant flavonols in the *Salmonella*/mammalian microsome test. Activation of flavonol glycoside by mixed glycosidases from rat fecal bacteria and other sources, *Mutation Res.,* 66, 223, 1979.

50. **Umezawa, K., Matsushima, T., Sugimura, T., Hirakawa, T., Tanaka, M., Katoh, Y., and Takayama, S.,** *In vitro* transformation of hamster embryo cells by quercetin, *Toxicol. Lett.,* 1, 175, 1977.

51. **Yoshida, M. A., Sasaki, M., Sugimura, K., and Kawachi, T.,** Cytogenetic effects of quercetin on cultured mammalian cells, *Proc. Jpn. Acad.,* 56B, 443, 1980.

52. **Ishidate, M.,** personal communication.

53. **Nagao, M., Morita, N., Yahagi, T., Shimizu, M., Kuroyanagi, M., Fukuoka, M., Yoshihira, K., Natori, S., Fujino, T., and Sugimura, T.,** Mutagenicities of 61 flavonoids and 11 related compounds, *Environ. Mutagen.,* in press. Mutagenicities of Flavonoids on *Salmonella,* Proc. 98th Jpn. Pharm. Soc., Okayama, 1978, 427.

54. **Herrmann, K.,** Flavonols and flavones in food plants: a review, *J. Food Technol.,* 11, 433, 1976.

55. **Ambrose, A. M., Robbins, D. J., and DeEds, F.,** Comparative toxicities of quercetin and quercitrin, *J. Am. Pharm. Assoc. Sci. Ed.,* 16, 119, 1952.

55a. **Pamukcu, A. M., Yalwner, S., Hatcher, J. F., and Bryan, G. T.,** Quercetin, a rat intestinal and bladder carcinogen present in bracken fern (Pteridium aquilinum), *Cancer Res.,* 40, 3468, 1980.

55b. **Saito, Shirai, A., Matsusima, T., Sugimura, T., and Hirono, I.,** Test of carcinogenicity of quercetin, a widely distributed mutagen in food, *Teratogen. Carcinogen. Mutagen.,* 1, 213, 1980.

56. **Int. Agency Res. Cancer,** Pyrrolizidine alkaloids, in *IARC Monographs on the Evaluation of Carcinogenic Risk of Chemicals to Man,* Vol. 10, Int. Agency Cancer Res., Lyon, 1976, 265.

57. **Schoental, R.,** Carcinogens in plants and microorganisms, in *Chemical Carcinogens,* ACS Monograph 173, Searle, C. E., Ed., American Chemical Society, Washington D.C., 1976, 626.

58. **Clark, A. M.,** The mutagenic activity of some pyrrolizidine alkaloid in *Drosophila, A. Vererbungsl.,* 91, 74, 1960.

59. **Alderson, T. and Clark, A. M.,** Interlocus specificity for chemical mutagens in *Aspergillus nidulans, Nature (London),* 210, 593, 1966.
60. **Yamanaka, H., Nagao, M., Sugimura, T., Furuya, T., Shirai, A., and Matsushima, T.,** Mutagenicity of pyrrolizidine alkaloids in the *Salmonella*/mammalian-microsome test, *Mutation Res.,* 68, 211, 1979.
61. **Furuya, T. and Hikichi, M.,** Fukinotoxin, a new pyrrolizidine alkaloid from *Petasites japonicus, Chem. Pharm. Bull.,* 24, 1120, 1977.
62. **Yamada, K., Tatematsu, H., Suzuki, M. Hirata, Y., Haga, M., and Hirono, I.,** Isolation and the structures of two new alkaloids, petasitenine and neopetasitenine from *Petasites Japonicus* Maxim, *Chem. Lett.,* 461, 1976.
63. **Hirono, I., Mori, H., and Culvenor, C. C. J.,** Carcinogenic activity of coltsfoot, *Tussilago farfara* L., *Gann,* 67, 125, 1976.
64. **Hirono, I., Mori, H., Yamada, K., Hirata, Y., Haga, M., Tatematsu, H., and Kanie, S.,** Carcinogenic activity of petasitenine, a new pyrrolizidine alkaloid isolated from *Petasites Japonicus* Maxim, *J. Natl. Cancer Inst.,* 58, 1155, 1977.
65. **Schoental, R., Fowler, M. E., and Coady, A.,** Islet cell tumores of the pancreas found in rats given pyrrolizidine alkaloids from *Amsinckia intermedia* fish and mey and from *Heliotropium supinum* L., *Cancer Res.,* 30, 2127, 1970.
66. **Vogel, E. and Sobels, F. H.,** The function of *Drosophila* in genetic toxicology testing, in *Chemical Mutagens, Principles and Methods for Their Detection,* Vol. 4, Hollaender, A., Ed., Plenum Press, New York, 1976, 93.
67. **Liu, Y. Y., Schmeltz, I., and Hoffmann, D.,** Chemical studies on tobacco smoke. Quantitative analysis of hydrazine in tobacco and cigarette smoke, *Anal. Chem.,* 46, 885, 1974.
68. **Matsushima, T.,** unpublished data, 1978.
69. **Daniels, E. G., Kelly, R. B., and Hinman, J. W.,** Agaritine; an improved isolation procedure and confirmation of structure by synthesis, *J. Am. Chem. Soc.,* 83, 3333, 1961.
70. **List, P. H. and Luft, P.,** Nachweis and Gehaltsbestimmung von Gyromitrin in Frischen Lorcheln, *Arch. Pharmacol.,* 302, 143, 1969.
71. **Wright, A. V., Niskanen,A., and Pyysalo, H.,** The toxicities and mutagenic properties of ethylidene gyromitrin and *N*-methylhydrazine with *Escherichia coli* as test organism, *Mutation Res.,* 56, 105, 1977.
72. **Hofman, J. and Hofmanova, O.,** 1,4-Benzoxazine derivatives in plants, *Eur. J. Biochem.,* 8, 109, 1969.
73. **Tipton, C. L., Klum, J. A., Husted, R. R., and Pierson, M. D.,** Cyclic hydroxamic acid and related compounds from maize. Isolation and characterization, *Biochemistry,* 6, 2866, 1967.
74. **Klun, J. A., Tipson, C. L., and Brindley, T. A.,** 2,4-Dihydroxy-7-methoxy-1,4-benzoxazin-3-one (DIM-BOA), an active agent in the resistance of maize to the European corn borer, *J. Econ. Entomol.,* 60, 1529, 1967.
75. **Hashimoto, Y., Shudo, K., Okamoto, T., Nagao, M., Takahashi, Y., and Sugimura, T.,** Mutagenicities of 4-hydroxy-1,4-benzoxazinones naturally occurring in maize plants and of related compounds, *Mutation Res.,* 66, 191, 1979.
76. **Laqueur, G. L. and Spatz, M.,** Toxicology of cycasin, *Cancer Res.,* 28, 2262, 1968.
77. **Smith, D. W. E.,** Mutagenicity of cycasin aglycone (methylazoxymethanol) a naturally occurring carcinogen, *Science,*152, 1273, 1966.
78. **Yahagi, T., Nagao, M., Matsushima, T., Kawachi, T., Nakadate, M., and Sugimura, T.,** Data on Mutation Test in the Japanese Program for Carcinogen Screening (1973-1976), Annual Report of the Cancer Research, Ministry of Health and Welfare of Japan, 1973-1976.
79. **Matsushima, T., Matsumoto, H., Shirai, A., Sawamura, M., and Sugimura, T.,** Mutagenicity of the naturally occurring carcinogen cycasin and synthetic methylazoxymethanol conjugates in *Salmonella typhimorium, Cancer Res.,* 39, 3780, 1979.
80. **Sugimura, T., Nagao, M., Matsushima, T., Yahagi, T., and Hayashi, K.,** Recent findings on the relation between mutagenicity and carcinogenicity, *Nucleic Acids Res. Spec. Publ.,* 3, 41, 1977.
81. **Hayashi, K., Nagao, M., and Sugimura, T.,** Interaction of norharman and harman with DNA, *Nucleic Acids Res.,* 4, 3679, 1977.
82. **Nagao, M., Yahagi, T., and Sugimura, T.,** Differences in effects of norharman with various classes of chemical mutagens and amounts of S-9 *Biochem. Biophys. Res.Commun.,* 83, 373, 1978.
83. **Conney, A. H., Pantuck, E. J., Hsiao, K. C., Kuntzman, R., Alvares, A. P., and Kappas, A.,** Regulation of drug metabolism in man by environmental chemicals and diet, *Fed. Proc. Fed. Am. Soc. Exp. Med.,* 36, 1647, 1977.
84. **Kada, T., Morita, K., and Inoue, T.,** Antimutagenic action of vegetable factor(s) on the mutagenic principle of tryptophan pyrolysate, *Mutation Res.,* 53, 351, 1978.
85. **Inoue, T., Morita, K., and Kada, T.,** Purification and properties of a plant desmutagenic factor for the mutagenic principle of tryptophan pyrolysate, *Agric. Biol. Chem.,* 45, 345, 1981.
86. **Lai, C. N.,** Metabolic activation of carcinogens inhibited by wheat extracts, *Univ. Tex. Syst. Cancer Cent.,* 23, 5, 1978.

87. **Yoshida, D. and Matsumoto, T.,** Changes in mutagenicity of protein pyrolysates by reaction with nitrite, *Mutation Res.,* 58, 35, 1978.

87a. **Tsuda, M., Takahashi, Y., Nagao, M., Hirayama, T., and Sugimura, T.,** Inactivation of mutagens from pyroysates of tryptophan and glutamic acid by nitrite in acidic solution, *Mutation Res.,* 78, 331, 1980.

88. **Wattenberg, L. W.,** Naturally occurring inhibitors of chemical carcinogenesis, in *Naturally Occurring Carcinogens — Mutagens and Modulators of Carcinogenesis,* Miller, E. C., Miller J. A., Hirono, I., Sugimura, T., and Takayama, S., Eds., Japan Sci. Soc. Press, Tokyo; University Park Press, Baltimore, 1979, 315.

89. **Nagao, M., Honda, M., Hamasaki, T., Natori, S., Ueno, Y., Yamasaki, M., Seino, Y., Yahagi, T., and Sugimura, T.,** Mutagenicities of mycotoxins on *Salmonella, Proc. Jpn. Assoc. Mycotoxicol.* No. 3/4, 41, 1976.

90. **Meyn, M. S., Rossmann, T., and Troll, W.,** A protease inhibitor blocks SOS functions in *Escherichia coli:* antipain prevent repressor inactivation, ultraviolet mutagensis, and filamentous growth, *Proc. Natl. Acad. Sci. U.S.A.,* 74, 1152, 1977.

91. **Umezawa, K., Matsushima, T., and Sugimura, T.,** Antimutagenic effect of elastatinal, a protease inhibitor from *Actinomycetes, Proc. Jpn. Acad.,* 53B, 30, 1977.

92. **Umezawa, K., Sawamura, M. Matsushima, T., and Sugimura, T.,** Inhibition of chemically induced sister chromatid exchanges by elastatinal, *Chem. Biol. Interact.,* 24, 107, 1979.

Chapter 11

MEDICINES SUSPECTED OF CAUSING CANCER IN HUMANS

T. A. Connors

TABLE OF CONTENTS

I. MEDICINES SUSPECTED OF CAUSING CANCER IN HUMANS

Table 1 shows those medicines for which there is some evidence from epidemiology, or from case histories, for their carcinogenicity in man.[1-3] In recent years there has been a more thorough testing of new medicines and a retesting of established ones with the result that a steadily increasing number of medicines are coming under suspicion as *potential* human carcinogens. Direct evidence for carcinogenicity in man comes from epidemiological studies, but the first indication that a chemical may be hazardous to humans may come from experiments in laboratory animals or more recently from other simpler laboratory tests which can detect substances with properties associated with carcinogens. However, in both epidemiological and laboratory studies there are many problems in interpreting the data, and neither method is sensitive enough to pick up small but very important (in terms of numbers of people affected) increases in incidence of common cancers. Cancer induction is not necessarily a simple process of interaction of the carcinogen with its target molecule, but may be dependent on a variety of other factors involving the action of promoters, proliferating agents and co-carcinogens. The selection of a group as a control to a group of people treated with a particular drug is therefore not an easy task, especially as the treated group may consist of people of different ages with different occupations and who come from different social classes and live in different areas. There have in fact been only a few systematic attempts to assess the risks involved in the use of modern medicines which may be given for long periods of time to large numbers of people.[4,5] There is not even an adequate documentation of the case histories of patients who have been reported to develop cancer after exposure to a particular drug.

There are also just as many problems in the interpretation of the results of carcino-genicity tests from whole animals or in vitro systems and in their extrapolation to humans. Any decision of the carcinogenicity of a medicine must, in the light of incomplete scientific knowledge, involve a number of assumptions, and decisions to ban it or restrict its use must also depend on its value as a medicine, the type of disease it is used to treat, and whether or not there are suitable and less harmful alternatives.

A particular problem associated with the use of some medicines is that the pathological conditions for which they are being used may actually dispose towards cancer. There is, for example, an increased risk of cancer in patients suffering from xeroderma pigmentosum and Fanconi's anemia so that, if specific drugs were developed to treat those conditions and the increased risk of cancer were not appreciated, the use of the drug might wrongly be suspected of increasing the cancer incidence. Other examples are the association between malaria and Burkitt's lymphoma, schistosomiasis and bladder cancer, and myasthenia gravis and Hodgkin's disease. Medicines may also be safe in some situations but not in others. Thus hycanthone, which has been used in programs to control schistosomiasis in the Middle East, Africa, and South America, does not cause cancer in normal mice. However, when used to treat mice infected with a schistosome, it caused a significant increase in hepatocellular carcinoma compared to mice infected with the schistosome only.[6]

II. CYTOTOXIC AGENTS USED IN THE TREATMENT OF CANCER

The strongest evidence that medicines may cause cancer comes from the use of cytotoxic agents in the treatment of malignant disease and a variety of autoimmune diseases, psoriasis, and diseases of collagen.[3,7-10] There is also evidence that they may have caused cancer in humans when used to prevent graft rejection, although not necessarily by a direct action.[11] In fact, of the chemicals listed in Table 1, five of them — cyclo-

Table 1
DRUGS ASSOCIATED WITH CANCER
INDUCTION IN HUMANS

Arsenicals	Chlornaphazine
Chloramphenicol	Oxymetholone
Cyclophosphamide	Phenacetin
DES	Phenytoin
Melphalan	Phenylbutazone
Chlorambucil	Busulphan

phosphamide, melphalan, chlorambucil, myleran, and chlornaphazine — were developed primarily for the treatment of malignant diseases. Some of the cytotoxic agents used to treat cancer seem to be more dangerous carcinogens than others, but this may be because they have been used more widely in man than others, or their effects are more fully documented. They may have also been used in instances where the patient may receive prolonged treatment, for example in myeloma or chronic leukemia or in nonlethal diseases such as psoriasis. The decision to continue to use these agents can be justified in many cases, for instance in the case of acute lymphoblastic leukemia where the prognosis is less than 1 year without treatment. In this case the possibility (not certainty, because only the risk is increased) of inducing a cancer some years later is to be preferred to immediate death. Obviously if the risks associated with each agent could be quantified, the least dangerous drugs should be used, but in practice this is not possible at present since for each type of cancer which responds to chemotherapy there is usually a best combination of drugs which has been worked out on a trial and error basis over many years. In cases where drug therapy is only of limited effectiveness, that is, there is not a large increase in survival time gained by treatment, then one must balance the effects of treatment against the acute toxic effects of the drugs rather than any of their long term effects. The decision to use chemotherapy is more difficult in situations such as the treatment of breast cancer where it is given immediately following surgery. In this case, for premenopausal women, there is a good chance of 5-year survival following surgery alone, so that the benefits of increasing the 5-year survival rate by adjuvant chemotherapy must in some way be balanced against the risk of increasing the possibility of contracting a second cancer in later years. Although there is now an extensive follow-up of many patients with cancer who have been successfully treated with chemotherapy, it is still not possible, because of the large number of variables involved and the use of drugs in combination to actually quantify the risks involved in the use of any individual agent.

The use of cytotoxic agents in the treatment of nonmalignant disease creates similar difficulties. Obviously they should not be used where there are effective alternatives which probably have less long term toxicity. However, there maybe examples where the quality of life is so poor that it is reasonable to use drugs which will successfully treat the condition but increase the risk from cancer at some later date.

The cytotoxic agents act as electrophilic reactants binding covalently mainly to sulfur, nitrogen, and oxygen atoms in a variety of molecules including macromolecules such as proteins and nucleic acids. It is generally accepted that both cytotoxicity and the initiation of cancer are dependent, in the first instance, on a reaction with DNA, which explains why this class of chemical may be effective both in the treatment of cancer and in the induction of cancer. Cytotoxicity resulting in the destruction of tumor cells (and other normal cells in the body such as bone marrow) is probably the result of an extensive binding of the carcinogen to many different sites in DNA. This reaction causes in proliferating cells an imbalance of protein and nucleic acid synthesis prior to mitosis. As a result giant cells (which have been observed in many in vitro and in vivo systems including humans) are formed followed by cell death. There is also ample evidence that DNA is the most important, if not the only target molecule in the cell, for carcinogenesis. Cancer is believed to be the result of a somatic mutation following a specific reaction of the carcinogen with DNA, and in recent years the reactions of carcinogens with DNA to give promutagenic bases have been analyzed in detail in laboratory animals.[12] Mutation is dependent on the type of reaction of the carcinogen with DNA, O^6-alkylation of guanine, for example, being more mutagenic than 7-alkylation of guanine, the persistence of the altered base (that is whether or not it is repaired before replication) being vitally important.[13] Whether or not there is cell proliferation in response to the cytotoxic properties of the agent or whether other agents are present which may cause proliferation and fix the lesion is also important. Other factors which determine whether a cancer results may be the state of differentiation of the target cell, for example whether or not it is a stem cell, and its interaction with viruses. Besides these factors the immune status of the host and probably a number of variables not yet elucidated may all be important in determining whether a mutated somatic cell eventually progresses to form a malignant tumor.

Although the many cytotoxic agents that have been used are represented by different chemical structures, the majority of them act by generation of chemically reactive species as shown by the example in Figure 1. The positively charged species will be reactive to negatively charged areas of various molecules, which explains why they readily react with sulfur, nitrogen, and oxygen atoms which may be negatively charged under physiological conditions or have areas of high electron density. There is evidence either from experiments in animals and in vitro systems or from observations in humans that members of all of the classes of cytotoxic agents, shown in Figure 2, may be carcinogenic under certain conditions.[10] Fortunately, apart from anticancer agents, very few other electrophilic reactants have been used as pharmaceuticals. The active constituent of cantharides (Spanish fly) is cantharidin, which has been employed as an irritant for the topical treatment of digital and periungal warts. Cantharidin contains a reactive acid anhydride group and has many of the properties of a very reactive cytotoxic agent, such as sulfur mustard, exerting a rubefacient and vesicant action on the skin and mucous membranes, and causing damage to the intestinal tract and bladder when taken orally. Phenoxybenzamine (Figure 3) and dibenamine are α-adrenergic blocking agents which contain a reactive chloroethylamino (nitrogen mustard) group. Their relatively slow onset of action is probably due to the time taken for them to cyclise in a similar way to aliphatic nitrogen mustards and to covalently bind to groups on or near α-adrenergic receptors. Phenoxybenzamine has been used in situations such as in the treatment of acute cardiogenic shock or over long periods in the treatment of peripheral vascular disorders. In some instances doses of up to 240 mg daily have been administered. There is no evidence from humans that phenoxybenzamine is carcinogenic, but it has been reported to cause an increase in lung tumors in mice.[14]

Scopolamine (1-hyoscine) and methoscopolamine bromide also contain an epoxy group which might alkylate under physiological conditions. These agents, like atropine, are competitive inhibitors of acetylcholine; there is no evidence that the alkylating function of scopolamine is active in vivo.

Other chemicals which act in a similar fashion to the alkylating agents described above and which are also used mainly in the treatment of cancer are the nitrosoureas, dialkyl triazenes, procarbazine and a platinum complex (cisdichlorodiammine platinum II). These drugs break down in vivo spontaneously or are metabolically converted to chemical species which react with DNA.

The other main classes of cytotoxic agent are the antitumor antibiotics and the antimetabolites. The antitumor antibiotics are a diverse group of products isolated from soil

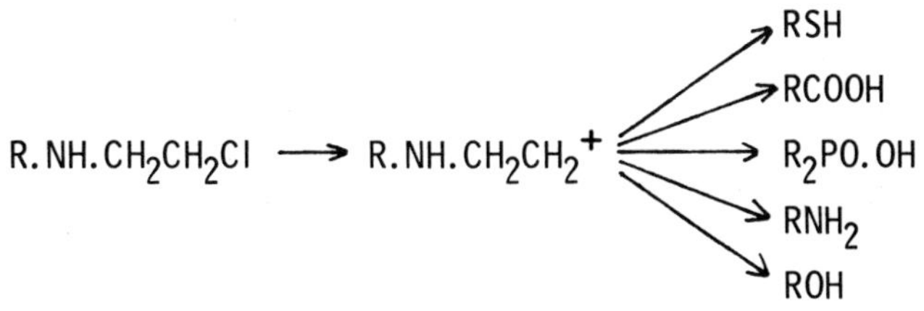

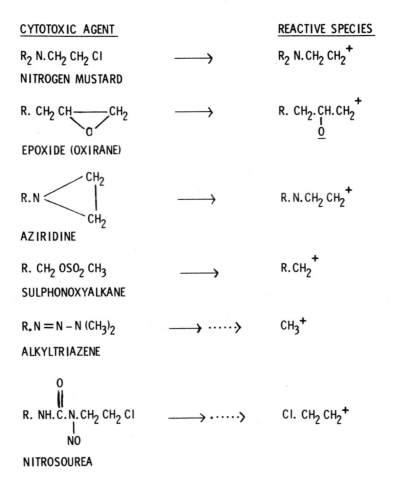

FIGURE 1. Structural formula of a nitrogen mustard and the reaction of its active species with cell constituents containing electrophilic groups.

FIGURE 2. Structural formulas of classes of cytotoxic agents used in the treatment of cancer and their reactive species. (These reactive species may not always be generated, the agent forming a transition complex with the molecule it alkylates).

microorganisms, and usually inhibit cell proliferation by some form of interaction with DNA. This may cause strand breaks in some cases, but cell death is often the result, not of covalent binding as described above, but of a very strong noncovalent binding to specific areas of DNA. The most commonly used antibiotics in the treatment of cancer are adriamycin, bleomycin, streptozotocin (which probably acts as an alkylating agent), mitomycin C, daunomycin, and actinomycin D. Although actinomycin D and bleomycin

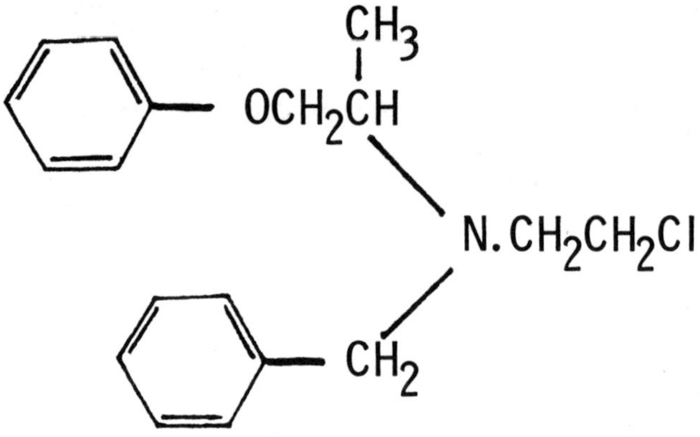

FIGURE 3.   Structural formula of phenoxybenzamine.

are negative in bacterial mutagenesis assays, which often correlate well with animal carcinogenesis assays, there is ample evidence of their carcinogenicity in rodents.[7,15] Adriamycin and its less used analogue daunomycin cause breast tumors in rats and chromosomal damage in humans. Mitomycin C and streptozotocin have also been shown to be carcinogenic in animals.[7]

The antimetabolites include analogues of purines, pyrimidines, and folic acid and are cytotoxic as a result of their interference with the *de novo* synthesis of purines and pyrimidines or with the formation of nucleic acids. Because there is less evidence that antimetabolites are carcinogenic, it has been advocated that they should be used in the place of the other agents described above in the treatment of cancer. However this would not be feasible in many cases, since some cancers, while responding to agents of the nitrogen mustard type for example, do not respond to antimetabolites. Although there is indeed less evidence that the antimetabolites are carcinogenic, methotrexate has been quite extensively used in the treatment of psoriasis, and while noncarcinogenic in rodents,[16] a number of cases of cancer have been reported in patients with psoriasis receiving methotrexate therapy.[10] Also azathioprine and 6-mercaptopurine are antimetabolites which have been widely used in the treatment, not only of cancer, but also to prevent the rejection of tissue homografts and to treat a variety of "autoimmune" diseases, and in all cases there have been reports in the literature of unusual types of cancer arising after treatment with these chemicals.[10]

III. MEDICINES WHICH ARE CONVERTED TO CARCINOGENS IN VIVO

New medicines have been introduced for the treatment of human disease in ever increasing numbers since the late 1930s and particularly since World War II, when there was a great expansion of the pharmaceutical industry. Widely used medicaments first marketed more than 15 years ago were judged to be safe if they could be given in relatively large amounts (compared to their effective dose) to rodents with no symptoms of acute or subacute toxicity. A chemical fed to animals usually at high dose levels for a period of a month or so and causing no detectable symptoms or histological damage in tissues was considered to be nonhazardous to humans. It is only relatively recently that it has been realized that chemicals which are not acutely toxic may nevertheless cause chronic effects, either as the result of prolonged administration of dose levels causing no acute symptoms or even as a result of the administration of one or very few doses followed by a latent period before the development of toxic and often irreversible symptoms. The reason for this at the molecular level is now well understood. A chemically stable drug may be metabolized in vivo to a reactive species, which like the cytotoxic agents, can bind to DNA and initiate the events leading to cancer. Since this metabolic activation may only occur by a minor pathway, there may never be sufficient produced to cause acute cytotoxic effects, but nevertheless there may be an appropriate reaction with the DNA of target cells to increase the risk of cancer. Table 2 shows that a whole variety of chemical groupings may be metabolized in vivo by pathways in which reactive chemical species may be generated. The demonstration that structures which occur commonly in drugs such as aromatic rings and methylamino groups have the potential to be converted in vivo to carcinogens, has meant that many medicines are now being reevaluated for their anticancer activity. Numbers of extensively used chemicals have now been retested in the light of current knowledge about mechanisms of carcinogenesis, and some are now suspect as carcinogens as exemplified by the nitrofurans.

A. Nitrofurans

The antibacterial properties of the nitrofurans such as nitrofurazone (Figure 4) have been known since 1940,[17] and since that time several thousand 5-nitrofuryl derivatives and analogues have been investigated for their biological activity. They represent an economically important class of compound, having been marketed for many years not only as topical and systemic human medicines, but also as veterinary products, food additives, and wine stabilizers. Table 3 lists some nitrofurans which are still in use or have been used until fairly recently as human medicines. It can be seen that the majority of the drugs are now known to be either carcinogenic in laboratory animals or have properties such as the ability to form covalent reaction products with DNA, induce DNA repair, or increase mutation rates in bacteria which are properties associated with carcinogens. In fact, the genotoxic properties of the nitrofurans were indicated as long ago as 1954 when it was found that nitrofurazone bound to DNA. There was also some early evidence that several nitrofurans were capable of inducing mutations in bacteria and phage in lysogenic *Escherichia coli*.[17] However these studies did not attract too much attention because the possibility that medicines could be converted in vivo to carcinogens had not been seriously considered. In any case it was not thought at that time that more than a few cancers in humans were caused by chemicals. The nitrofurans and many other medicaments became suspect as potential carcinogens when it was demonstrated, in studies of the mechanisms of action of some animal carcinogens, that quite often the substance administered was in effect a precarcinogen that required metabolism in vivo to the true or ultimate carcinogen, frequently via the intermediate formation of metabolites termed proximate carcinogens. The metabolic pathways for many economically important nitrofurans have now been studied,[17] and there is evidence in most cases for reduction of the nitro groups to the corresponding amine as shown by the example of nitrofurazone (Figure 4). Once formed the amine may be further metabolized, e.g., to the acetylamino derivative, or undergo ring cleavage to form the open chain nitrile. In the course of the reduction of the nitro group to the amine, it is assumed that the hydroxylamino and nitrosofuran derivatives are formed as transient reactive intermediates and that they are the ultimate carcinogens. It has been shown, for instance, that when a furyl thiazole (ANFT) is incubated under anaerobic conditions with a mammalian metabolizing system, metabolites are formed which bind strongly to RNA present in the incubation system.[18] All nitrofurans must therefore be considered as potential carcinogens since they have the ability to be metabolized in vivo to intermediates which bind to macromolecules. Many members of the class have, in addition, been shown to induce DNA repair, cause chromosome abnormalities, and be mutagenic in mammalian

Table 2

Chemical group	Metabolic pathway leading to reactive species
Aromatic ring	Epoxidation
Ethylenic group	Epoxidation
Acetylenic group	Not known
Aromatic amine	N-Oxidation (nitrosation)
Aromatic or heterocyclic nitro group	N-Reduction
Methylamino group	N-Hydroxymethylation

Table 3

Name	Usage	Duration	Toxicity G	Toxicity C
Furium	HSM	1962—1973	+	+ +
Triafur	HTM	1962—1974	NT	+ + +
Panfuran	HSM	1961—P	+	+ + +
Nitrovin	HSM	1951—P	+	—
Nifuroxime	HTM	1965—P	+	NT
Nitrofurazone	HTM	1944—P	+	+
Nifuradene	HSM	1963—P	NT	+ + +
Nitrofuratoin	HSM	1952—P	+	—
Furazolidone	HSM	1957—P	+	+

Note: G = Genotoxicity; C = Carcinogenesis.

and nonmammalian systems. In addition many have now been shown to be carcinogenic in a number of strains and species of laboratory animals. The toxic side effects seen in rodents such as immunosuppression, teratogenesis, and inhibition of spermatogenesis, as well as side effects occasionally reported in man such as chronic lung fibrosis and toxicity to the gastrointestinal tract, are all familiar side effects occurring with high dose levels of cytotoxic agents used widely in the treatment of cancer and suspected of being carcinogenic in humans. The presence of the nitrogroup of the nitrofurans is probably responsible for the carcinogenicity of these derivatives, but unfortunately the same group appears to be essential for their antibacterial activity. Mutants of *E. coli* for example, with resistance to the toxicity of nitrofurans, have lost a nitroreductase enzyme capable of reducing them to the corresponding amine.[17] It thus does not seem likely that further synthesis of nitrofurans will yield derivatives which have antibacterial properties but not mammalian toxicity, since derivatives which can be activated by bacteria will be just as likely to be activated by mammalian reductases such as xanthine oxidase, NADPH-cytochrome C reductase, and aldehyde oxidases which are abundant. There is also no reliable way of estimating whether "safe" levels of nitrofurans exist, that is, drug concentrations which may be activated by anaerobic bacteria but not by less hypoxic mammalian tissues.

The chemotherapeutic nitrothiazoles and nitroimidazoles, such as niridazole and metronidazole, presumably act by the same mechanism. Both have been shown to be carcinogenic in rodents,[5,19] although there is no evidence that their extensive use has increased the risk of cancer in humans.

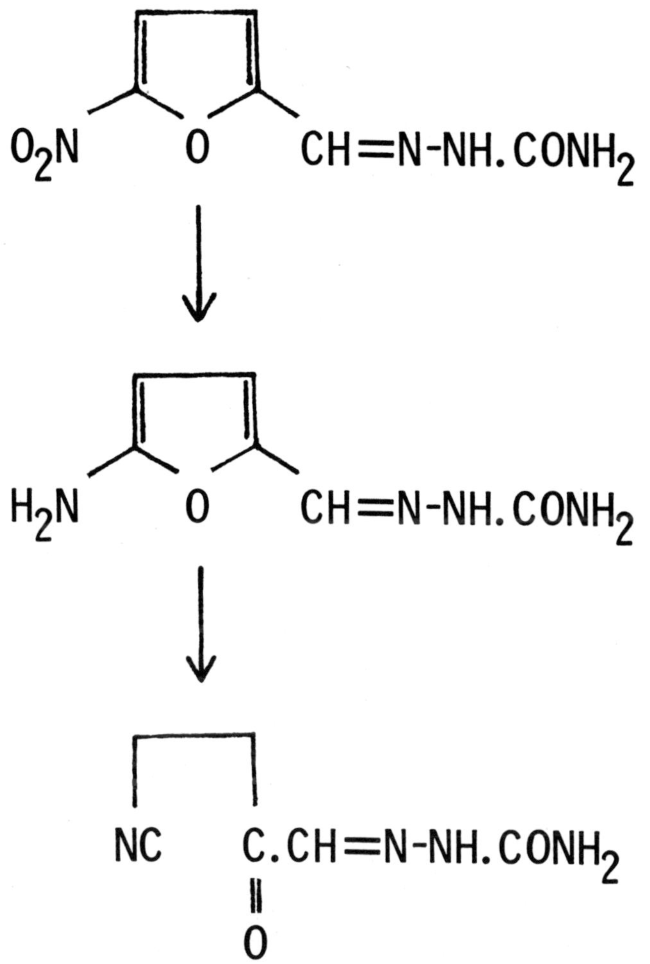

FIGURE 4.   Postulated metabolic pathway for nitrofurazone involving reduction of the nitro group and ring cleavage of the resulting amine.

B. Phenacetin and Paracetamol

Phenacetin is predominantly metabolized in humans to paracetamol, which may then be further metabolized by the scheme shown in Figure 5. Following N-hydroxylation an iminoquinone is formed which is a very reactive species. At low dose levels the metabolite is deactivated by reaction with glutathione, but at higher concentrations reserves of glutathione may be depleted and reaction may occur with macromolecules such as DNA.[20] High doses of phenacetin are hepatotoxic and N-hydroxyphenacetin, a possible metabolite, causes hepatocellular carcinoma in rats after oral administration.[21] It has also been reported recently to induce tumors of the nasal cavities in rats,[1] although other experiments have given negative results. There is also data to suggest that the heavy use of analgesics containing phenacetin is associated with necrosis of the kidneys, and Schmähl et al. have listed 38 cases of tumors of the renal pelvis associated with heavy use of phenacetin.[2] Thus there is evidence in humans that extremely high doses of phenacetin may be associated with cancer, although experimental data can be used to argue that normal doses of the drug may be safe since any of the carcinogenic metabolites produced might be detoxified by reaction with intracellular glutathione. Only when the drug is taken in doses well above the recommended dose would sufficient of the reactive

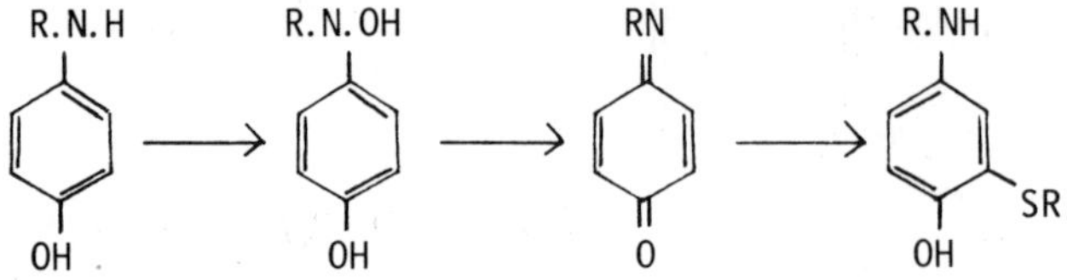

FIGURE 5.   Metabolism of paracetamol by *N*-hydroxylation followed by formation of an iminoquinone which reacts with glutathione (RS = glutathione moiety).

metabolite be formed which would saturate the intracellular glutathione. However, it has recently been shown that the protection of paracetamol toxicity by glutathione may not be a simple mopping up of the carcinogen by the thiol, but a more complicated process.[22] Although phenacetin is predominantly converted to paracetamol, there is also evidence that another metabolic pathway exists involving the formation of an intermediate epoxide and probably resulting in the generation of the same reactive species formed from paracetamol (Figure 6).[23]

Epoxides are formed, in fact, from many important drugs such as allobarbital, secobarbital, alphenal, protriptyline, carbamazepine, cyprohepatadine, and cyclobenzaprine,[24] while a number of products of drug metabolism have also been identified which suggest that an epoxide has been formed as an intermediate (e.g., diethylstilbestrol, phenytoin, phensuximide, phenobarbital, mephobarbital, methaqualone, lorazepam, imipramine, and acetanilide). However some of these intermediate epoxides have been investigated and have not been shown to have carcinogenic properties.[25]

Thus the evidence that phenacetin and paracetamol are carcinogenic in man is tenuous. Phenacetin, when abused, has been claimed to be associated with cancer, but this is based on case histories rather than the result of a properly conducted epidemiological survey. Similarly the evidence in experimental systems is again equivocal. Phenacetin has caused cancer in rodents under some conditions but not others, and although it may be metabolized in vivo to a potential carcinogen, there is evidence that this may be relevant only at excessively high dose levels of the drug.

C. Phenytoin

Phenytoin has been used for the past 40 years as an antiepileptic, and maintenance doses may be as high as 600 mg daily. However, despite the fact that this drug has been widely used to treat patients with high daily doses for the whole of their life span, it is only relatively recently that good experimental data have become available. These studies show that mice given high doses of phenytoin orally or intraperitoneally have a higher incidence of thymomas and lymphomas than controls. In vivo, phenytoin is extensively metabolized by different species by hydroxylation (in a variety of positions) of one of the 5-phenyl moieties.[26] The assumption has been made that this metabolic pathway involves the generation of a reactive and potentially carcinogenic epoxide. The teratogenicity of phenytoin and its induction of abnormal chromosomes are further evidence of its conversion in vivo to a reactive species. Evidence from case reports and epidemiological studies has also led to the conclusion that there is a positive association in epileptic patients between the occurrence of lymphomas and long term anticonvulsant therapy, in which phenytoin was administered either alone or in combination with other anticonvulsants such as phenobarbital.[26]

D. Chloramphenicol

Chloramphenicol (Figure 7) has been used to treat many bacterial infections, and for typhoid fever high doses of up to 100 g over 4 weeks may be given. Although chlor-

229

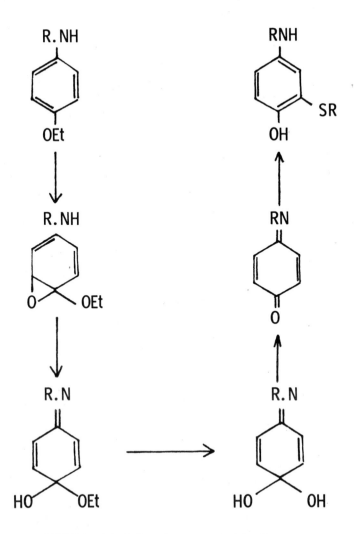

FIGURE 6.　Metabolism of phenacetin by initial formation of an epoxide, and conversion to an iminoquinone which reacts with glutathione (RS = glutathione moiety).

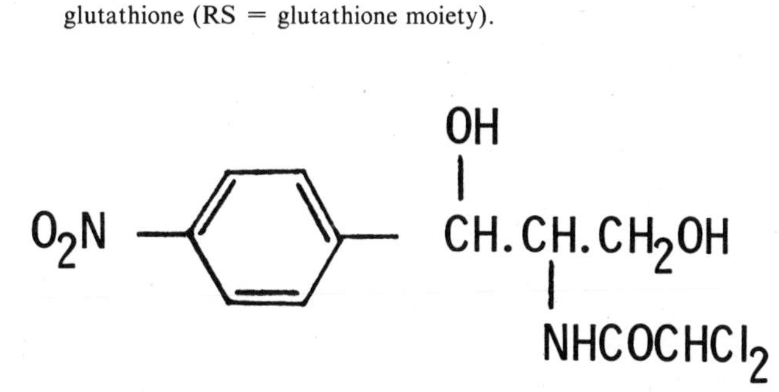

O_2N ——⟨ ⟩—— $\overset{\overset{\displaystyle OH}{|}}{CH}.CH.CH_2OH$

$\underset{NHCOCHCl_2}{|}$

FIGURE 7.　Structural formula of chloramphenicol.

amphenicol is thought to be one of the drugs for which there is reasonable evidence for its carcinogenicity in man (Table 1), there is less data to support this conclusion than is the case, for example, for phenytoin discussed above. There is no good animal data to show the drug is carcinogenic, and it caused no chromosomal abberations in the rat or in cultures of human peripheral lymphocytes. Also, although chloramphenicol is extensively metabolized, the main products are conjugates of the terminal OH group, and there is no suggestion of reduction of the nitro group to the corresponding amine (except in guinea pigs) which might proceed by formation of carcinogenic intermediates. A metabolite found in new born infants [D(-)-threo-2-hydroxyacetamido-1-*p*-nitro-phenyl-1,3-propanediol] does however suggest that the chloro groups are reactive and might be responsible for the binding of the drug to macromolecules. Chloramphenicol is undoubtedly toxic to bone marrow in some situations, and a large number of cases of bone marrow depression and aplastic anemia have been reported in subjects given the drug. There is also a suggestion from case reports that leukemia may also be associated with chloramphenicol induced aplastic anemia. A number of cases of leukemia (usually acute myeloblastic) have been described in patients receiving chloramphenicol over periods ranging from a few days to several years and subsequent to bone marrow depression or aplastic anemia. A surprising finding was that at least in seven cases, the leukemia was diagnosed within a few months of the chloramphenicol induced bone marrow depression, which itself often occurred soon after drug treatment. The latent period for cancer induction by chemicals in humans is often considered to be a minimum of several years. Where a cancer occurs within a relatively short period of exposure to a chemical, such as in the recent case reports of gastric cancer in patients who have taken cimetidine, a causal association between the drug and the cancer is highly questionable.[27] However it is an impression that leukemias and lymphomas are unusual in that they may arise after relatively short latent periods.

E. Steroidal Estrogens, Progestins, Androgens and Diethylstilbestrol

Oxymetholone is widely quoted as an example of a drug which is associated with a cancer risk in humans (Table 1) but which, like chloramphenicol, has not been adequately evaluated in animal or other experimental systems. The basis for labeling it as a carcinogen depends on a small number of reports of liver cell tumors arising in patients treated with oxymetholone alone or more frequently in combination with other adrogenic anabolic steroids and usually for several years. Many patients were suffering from Fanconi's anemia or aplastic anemia, and it could be argued that both conditions, as discussed earlier, may have neoplasia as a complication of the disease which may only become apparent when survival is extended by drugs. A large number of estrogens, progestins, and androgens have been evaluated for their carcinogenicity in animals.[1,28] Recent epidemiological studies have shown that women taking estrogens for menopausal symptoms have roughly five to ten times as great a chance of developing uterine cancer as women who take no estrogen. It has also recently been suggested that the use of menopausal estrogen may increase the risk of breast cancer 10 to 15 years after it is first taken. Particularly high breast cancer risk has been noted in estrogen users who had benign breast disease.[29] There have also been a number of case reports of hepatomas which may be associated with the use of contraceptive steroids, while there has been a suggestion that these pills may have increased the risk of breast cancer in women with benign breast disease and the rate of early cervical cancer.

The potential carcinogenicity of diethylstilbestrol was first recognized because of the occurrence of vaginal adenocarcinoma in young women aged 15 to 22 years instead of the expected age of 50 years or more.[30] Sixty-four cases of diethylstilbestrol-related carcinoma of the vagina had been recorded by 1972, and by 1976 this number had increased to 154.[31] Since diethylstilbestrol was probably taken by large numbers of pregnant women in the U.S. between 1950 and 1970, it has been predicted that there will still occur many more cases of vaginal cancer in the offspring of women treated with this drug. However, a recent report has indicated that the risk of cancer among these women may not be as high as earlier studies have indicated. In a study of 3339 women whose mothers took diethylstilbestrol to prevent miscarriage, only four cases of cancer of the vagina were found. Furthermore, the incidence of vaginal adenosis, which may represent a precancerous lesion, was also much lower than previously reported, indicating that the hazard is less than was once expected.

Little is known of the possible mechanism by which the synthetic steroids and diethylstilbestrol may cause cancer. It is well known that some steroids are metabolized to excretory products via chemically reactive epoxides and semiquinones, and some of these intermediates have been shown to bind to macromolecules.[32,33] A reactive epoxide of diethylstilbestrol has also similarly been claimed to be the carcinogenic intermediate of this chemical.[34] A number of synthetic estrogens and progestins contain an acetylenic group in the 17 position to prevent further metabolism. It has recently been demonstrated that the abnormal porphyrin pigments that accumulate in rats following the injection of high doses of norethyndrone are associated with the presence of the acetylenic group[35] which is metabolized by liver microsomes to an as yet unidentified metabolite. There are thus a number of pathways by which these steroids can form active products which could covalently bind to DNA and initiate cancer. However, there is also the possibility that this class of drug, with its complicated effects on cell growth and differentiation, could act as carcinogens by mechanisms other than by formation of metabolites capable of reacting with DNA. Thus it has been argued that diethylstilbestrol, which has recently been shown to be teratogenic and carcinogenic in rat offspring after transplacental and transmammary exposure,[34] might interfere with the normal development of the uterovaginal tract in the embryo. The increased estrogen stimulation during puberty may then cause hyperplasia, which itself may lead to malignant transformation or which may make the tissue sensitive to exogenous carcinogens or perhaps activate dormant viruses. It has been shown, for example, that diethylstilbestrol causes hyperplasia in rodents at the age of puberty, but that these changes can be prevented if they are castrated before puberty.

IV. ARSENIC

The carcinogenic action of "arsenic" in workers exposed to high levels of the metal were recognized more than 150 years ago. There is also an association between skin cancer and exposure to arsenic (as its oxides or sodium potassium and calcium salts) in drinking water and insecticides. Arsenic salts and oxide have also been used until fairly recently in the treatment of a number of skin conditions, particularly psoriasis vulgaris. Schmähl et al. recorded the case histories of 226 patients who developed cancer after being treated with arsenic for a variety of skin diseases.[2] The mechanism of action of arsenic is quite obscure, and it is widely quoted as one of the few examples of a human carcinogen which has not been shown subsequently to be carcinogenic in animals. Arsenic causes primarily skin cancer in humans and it often occurs in people exposed to sunlight (e.g. in vineyard workers using arsenic as a pesticide). Since arsenic has also been claimed to inhibit DNA polymerases, some of which might be involved in repairing damaged DNA, its mechanism of action may not be a direct one. It might, for example, prevent the repair of UV induced DNA damage and increase the incidence of skin cancer, especially of people exposed to sunlight in the same way as subjects with xeroderma pigmentosum, and, having impaired ability to repair DNA damage by UV, may have an increased risk of skin cancer.

V. PHENYLBUTAZONE

Although phenylbutazone is an effective anti-inflammatory agent, its toxicity has prevented its use in long term therapy. Apart from some case histories of patients treated with phenylbutazone, usually for inflammatory joint pain, and who subsequently developed leukemia, there is very little evidence for its carcinogenicity. Like chloramphenicol it may cause bone marrow depression and aplastic anemia. No experiments have been carried out to assess its carcinogenicity in animals, but it has been inactive in a variety of bacterial mutation assays and did not cause chromosome abnormalities in bone marrow cells of hamsters.

VI. OTHER PHARMACEUTICALS

Besides the classes of agents described above, a number of other pharmaceuticals have given some evidence of carcinogenicity in animals (Table 4). In fact, of some 84 medicines evaluated in a recent review,[1] well over half showed some evidence of carcinogenicity. Also, for some chemicals for which the data were not considered sufficient for evaluation, such as reserpine, more recent evidence has now indicated that it may increase the incidence of breast cancer in female mice and of the adrenal in rats. Furthermore, other drugs, such as the H_1 blocking antihistamine methapyrilene not previously evaluated, has now been shown to cause liver cancers in mice. A possible activation pathway could involve conversion of the methylamine moiety to an N-methylol, which if demonstrated, would lead to evaluation of a whole range of H_1 receptor antagonists structurally related to histamine and containing N-dimethylamino groups such as diphenylhydramine, chlorpheniramine, chlorocyclizine, and promethazine. Diazepam similarly contains an N-methyl group which is known to be metabolized and has caused liver cell adenomas in mice (Figure 8).

Isoniazid has been shown in a number of experiments to be carcinogenic in mice. More recently it has been shown to be metabolized in vivo to unstable intermediates which may break down to reactive chemical species (Figure 9). On the other hand, isoniazid and its analogues have been used in large amounts as antitubercular and antileprotic agents, and yet there is no evidence despite their widespread use that they are carcinogenic in humans.[5]

Other areas of research relatively unexplored have indicated that drugs may also be indirectly involved in carcinogenesis. Many nitrosamines have been shown to be potent carcinogens, and it has been demonstrated that exogenous amines, including drugs such as tetracyclines, may under certain conditions undergo nitrosation in the gastrointestinal tract by interaction with dietary sodium nitrite.[2] Futhermore, with increasing knowledge of the complicated nature of carcinogenesis including promotion and alterations of metabolism of xenobiotics, it seems likely that drugs may cause cancers by pathways not involving reaction with DNA directly.

VII. EVALUATION OF RISK

Increased knowledge of mechanisms of carcinogenicity and the evaluation of the safety of medicines by experimental and epidemiological methods has been valuable in that it has identified potentially dangerous products which, if they are of no great importance, may be withdrawn from use. However, these studies have also created problems, inasmuch as they have identified as possible human carcinogens valuable products used to treat potentially lethal conditions or to greatly improve quality of life. Using present day methodology one can indicate suspicion of carcinogenicity, but in most cases cannot quantitate the level of risk and whether situations exist where useful medicines may be used safely and effectively. Since cancer is most probably the result of a single cell mutation which in theory may be the result of a single molecular interaction of the carcinogen with DNA, then conceptually no absolutely safe level of carcinogen can exist. However, it can be argued in pragmatic terms that for some carcinogens the level of risk

233

Table 4
PHARMACEUTICALS SHOWING SOME EVIDENCE OF
CARCINOGENICITY IN ANIMALS

Aurothioqlucose	Oxazepam
Azaserine	Phenoxybenzamine
Alkylating agents	Pyrimethamine
Antitumor	Phenobarbital
antibiotics	
Contraceptive	Pronetalol
steroids	Propyl thiourea
Cantharidin	
Dithranol	Methyl thiouracil
Ethionamide	Thiouracil
Griseofulvin	Tannic acid
Hycanthone	Urethane
Iron dextran	
Isoniazid	
Metronidazole	
Niridazole	
Nitrofuran	

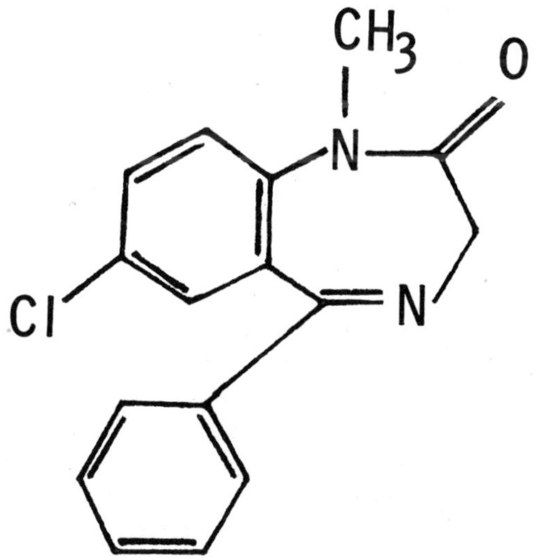

FIGURE 8. Structural formula of diazepam.

when the drug is used at recommended doses is so low as to be acceptable. For some drugs the useful effect is mediated by the same pathway by which cancer is induced, e.g., cytotoxic agents which rely on their anticancer and immunosuppressive properties by covalent binding to DNA, and for this class of agent there must always be a risk of carcinogenicity with its use. For other drugs such as the nitrofurans, the generation of a potentially carcinogenic metabolite appears to be necessary for biological activity, and presumably there will always be some risk at effective dose levels, unless it can be demonstrated that the target bacterial or protozoal cell can activate the drug at levels which are not metabolized by the host. However, for the great majority of medicines, the formation of a potentially carcinogenic metabolite is not necessary for the pharmacological properties of the agent. Quite often the carcinogenic metabolite is only formed in minute amounts by a minor metabolic pathway, and in these cases it can be

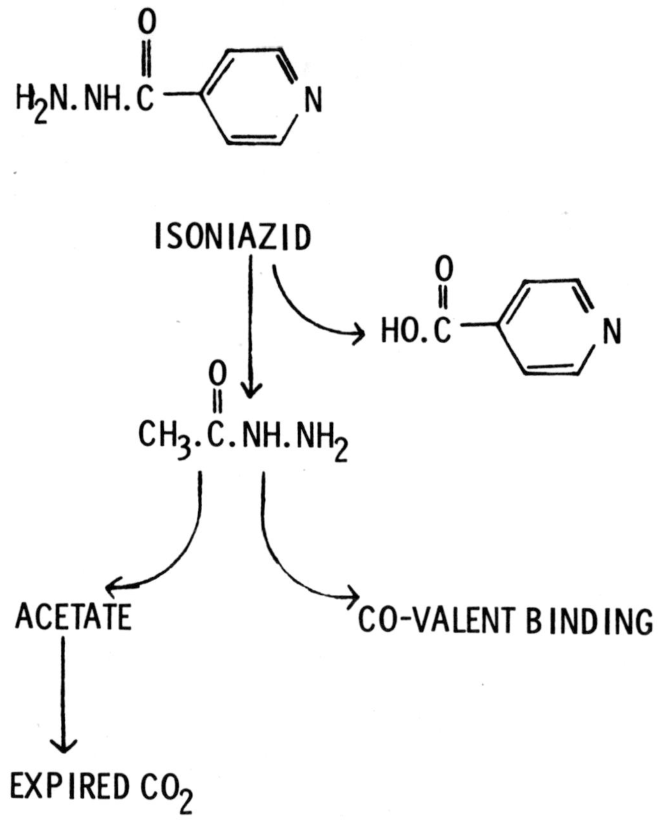

FIGURE 9.   Breakdown of isoniazide to form reactive intermediates.

argued that at some dose levels the chances of an active metabolite reacting with DNA are so low as to be acceptable. The drug may be excreted unchanged or as an inactive metabolite (Figure 10). Even if a carcinogenic metabolite is formed it may be handled by a number of pathways in preference to reacting with DNA. It can, for example, be further metabolized to inactive metabolites, or it may interact with cellular macromolecules such as proteins, which are present in high concentration and which may not be involved in carcinogenesis. There are also small molecular weight materials in the cell, such as glutathione, which react readily with carcinogenic metabolites with electrophilic properties and can prevent reaction with DNA. Even if binding to DNA takes place, there are, as previously discussed, many factors such as repair mechanisms which may prevent the induction of cancer.

Unfortunately present day techniques are not yet sensitive enough to detect small levels of carcinogenic metabolites and to determine whether or not they are formed when a drug is being used under recommended conditions. If it were possible to show that at these levels no carcinogenic metabolites were formed, then presumably a drug would be assumed to be safe even if it were known to be carcinogenic when it was abused or tested in high dose levels in animals. Epidemiological methods are not sensitive enough to determine small but important increases in cancer incidence; while to determine low levels of risk experimentally in rodents, very large numbers of animals need to be used at each dose level. A few experiments on large numbers of animals have been carried out in recent years, but sufficient data are not available to indicate whether or not a threshold exists for carcinogens in rodents under experimental conditions.

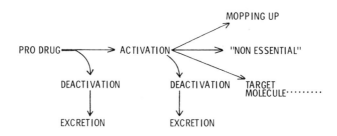

FIGURE 10. Variables influencing the reaction of an active metabolite with its target molecule.

Attempts to evaluate risks are vital but must necessarily be based on incomplete evidence and may lead to equivocal results. β-Naphthylamine is a potent carcinogen in humans and its effects have been studied in detail, once it was realized that workers involved industrially in the distillation of this chemical had a greatly increased risk of bladder cancer.[36,37] Figure 11 shows that workers exposed to high doses of the chemical for 5 years or more have a great increase in bladder cancer incidence, although only after a latent period of about 10 years. Workers exposed for periods of 4 years also have a high bladder cancer incidence, but this occurs only after a latent period of some 15 years. The shape of the curve is quite different in workers exposed to shorter periods of no more than 2 years. Although there are (after a latent period of 15 years) an increased number of workers with cancer, this does not rise until a further 10 years. The extension of this argument is that a dose level exists which may not increase the incidence of cancer until a very long latent period, such that old age and death would occur before the induction of the cancer. The results obtained with this human carcinogen are very similar to the results obtained with the use of cytotoxic agents in the treatment of Hodgkin's disease.[38] Figure 12 shows that patients with Hodgkin's disease and treated in recent years (between 1968 and 1972) have an increased probability of developing cancer compared with controls. This was the period when cytotoxic agents began to be used intensively at high dose levels and in combination in the treatment of this disease. Earlier treatments (e.g. from 1960 to 1964) were less intensive, and there is an indication that there was an increased latent period before second primary malignancies occurred. In the early days of chemotherapy (1950 to 1954), drugs were used much more cautiously, and there was clearly a longer latent period and a decreased probability of contracting a second cancer. Thus in both the cases of β-naphthylamine and cytotoxic agents the lowest exposure dose had a long latent period and probably decreased incidence of cancer. The lowest exposure levels in these cases still represent very high exposure levels when compared with most drugs used under recommended conditions, and it could be argued that if these results are extrapolated, then for most medicines (even if there is a risk of cancer) the risk is low and the latent period so long that most exposed persons will be dead from other causes before the cancer would be expected to appear. However, in arguments such as these there is always conflicting evidence again based on incomplete data and involving a number of assumptions. Figure 13 shows the mutagenicity to *Salmonella Typhimurium* and *E. coli* of the urine of patients treated with cytotoxic agents compared with the urine of nurses giving the treatment and with controls (hospital workers not exposed to the drugs). Bacterial mutagenicity is associated with carcinogenicity and, as expected, the urine of patients was much more mutagenic to bacteria compared to controls. However, the nurses handling the drugs and presumably only exposed to very small amounts nevertheless had a significantly higher level of mutagens in their urine than controls. This was also probably associated with their

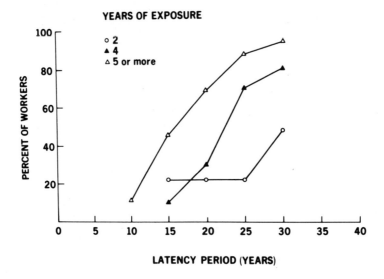

FIGURE 11.   Bladder cancer in distillers of aromatic amines exposed for different periods.[29]

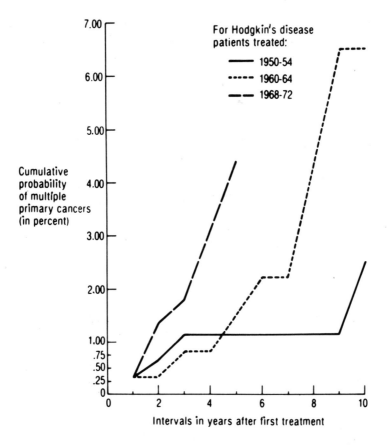

FIGURE 12.   Second primary cancer incidence in patients treated for Hodgkin's disease for different periods. (From Brody, R. S., Scottenfeld, D., and Reid, A., *Cancer,* 40, 1917, 1977. With permission.)

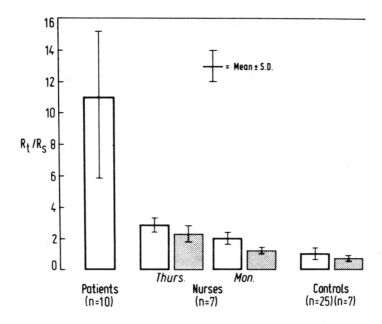

FIGURE 13.   Mutagenicity of urine samples of patients and nurses exposed to cytotoxic agents. (From Falck, K., Grohn, P., Sorsa, M., Vainio, H., Heinonen, E., and Holsti, L. R., *Lancet,* i, 1250, 1979.

exposure to cytotoxic agents, since their urine was more mutagenic on the days that they handled the drug than on the days they did not.[39]

As medicines are more thoroughly investigated, it seems from past experience, that the majority will come under suspicion as potential carcinogens if one considers the evidence from all sources. Hence there must be some attempt to evaluate risk, and this will be possible scientifically only when a lot more is known about the mechanism of action of these drugs in humans and their metabolic pathways, and when some means is devised of measuring the interaction of small amounts of drugs or their metabolites with DNA in vivo.

In the meantime, the decision to use a particular medicine cannot depend on scientific arguments alone but on some wider form of judgment taking into consideration the social value of the chemical.

REFERENCES

1. **Tomatis, L., Agthe, C., Bartsch, H., Hutt, J., Montesano, R., Saracci, R., Walker, E., and Wilbourn, J.,** Evaluation of the carcinogenicity of chemicals: a review of the International Agency for Research on Cancer, *Cancer Res.,* 38, 877, 1978.
2. **Schmähl, D., Thomas, C., and Auer, R.,** *Iatrogenic Carcinogenesis,* Springer-Verlag, New York, 1977.
3. **Connors, T. A.,** Alkylating agents, nitrosoureas and dialkyltriazenes, in *Cancer Chemotherapy Annuals,* Pinedo, H. M., Ed., Excerpta Medica, Amsterdam, 1979.
4. **Jick, H. and Smith, P. G.,** Regularly used drugs and cancer, in *Origins of Human Cancer,* Hiatt, H. H., Watson, J. D., and Winsten, J. A., Eds., Cold Spring Harbor Laboratory, Cold Spring Harbor, New York, 1977, 389.
5. **Goldman, P., Ingelfinger, J. A., and Friedman, P. A.,** Metronidazole, isoniazid and the threat of human cancer in *Origins of Human Cancer,* Watson, J. D., and Winsten, J. A., Eds., Cold Spring Harbor Laboratory, Cold Spring Harbor, New York, 1977, 465.

6. **Hease, W. H., Smith, D. L., and Bueding, E.,** Hycanthone-induced hepatic changes in mice infected with schistosoma mansoni, J. Pharmacol. Exp. Ther., 186, 430, 1973.

7. **Connors, T. A.,** Induction of cancer by drug therapy, in *Drug Toxicity,* Gorrod, J. W., Ed., Taylor and Francis, London, 1979, 161.

8. **Einhorn, N.,** Acute leukaemia after chemotherapy (melphalan), *Cancer,* 41, 444, 1978.

9. **Li, P. F.,** Second malignant tumors after cancer in childhood, *Cancer,* 40, 1899, 1977.

10. **Sieber, S. M. and Adamson, R. H.,** Toxicity of antineoplastic agents in man: chromosomal aberrations, antifertility effects, congenital malformations and carcinogenic potential, *Adv. Cancer Res.,* 22, 57, 1975.

11. **Hoover, R.,** Effect of drugs — immunosupporession, in *Origins of Human Cancer,* Hiatt, H. H., Watson, J. D., and Winsten, J. A., Eds., Cold Spring Harbor Laboratory, Cold Spring Harbor, New York, 1977, 369.

12. **Frei, J. V., Swenson, D. H., Warren, W., and Lawley, P. D.,** Alkylation of deoxyribonucleic acid in vivo in various organs of C57BL mice by the carcinogens N-methyl-N-nitrosourea, N-ethyl-N-nitrosourea and ethyl methanesulphonate in relation to the induction of thymic lymphoma, *Biochem. J.,* 174, 1031, 1978.

13. **Swenberg, J. A., Cooper, H. K., Bucheler, J., and Kleihues, P.,** 1,2-dimethylhydrazine-induced methylation of DNA bases in various rat organs and the effect of pretreatment with disulfiram, *Cancer Res.,* 39, 465, 1979.

14. **Stoner, G. D., Shimkin, M. B., Kniazeff, A. J., Weisburger, J. H., Weisburger, E. K., and Gori, G. B.,** Test for carcinogenicity of food additives and chemotherapeutic agents by the pulmonary tumor response in strain A mice, *Cancer Res.,* 33, 3069, 1973.

15. **Adamson, R. H., and Sieber, S. M.,** Antineoplastic agents as potential carcinogens, in *Origins of Human Cancer,* Hiatt, H. H., Watson, J. D., and Winsten, J. A., Eds., Cold Spring Harbor Laboratory, Cold Spring Harbor, New York, 1977, 429.

16. **Rustin, M. and Shubik, P.,** Life span carcinogenicity tests with 4-amino-N^{10}-methylpteroylglutamic acid (methotrexate) in Swiss mice and Syrian golden hamsters, *Toxicol. Appl. Pharmacol.,* 26, 329, 1973.

17. **Bryan, G. T.,** *Nitrofurans: Carcinogenesis, a Comprehensive Survey,* Vol. 4, Raven Press, New York, 1978.

18. **Swaminathan, S., Wong, R. C., Lower, G. M., and Bryan, G. T.,** Binding of 2-amino-4-(5-nitro-2-furyl)-2-^{14}C-thiazole (ANFT) to yeast transfer RNA, using rat liver microsomes, *Proc. Am. Assoc. Cancer Res.,* 18, 187, 1977.

19. **Urman, H. K., Bulay, O., Clayson, D. B., and Shubik, P.,** Carcinogenic effects of niridazole, *Cancer Lett.,* 1, 69, 1975.

20. **Hinson, J. A., Mitchell, J. R., and Jollow, D. J.,** Evidence for N-oxidation of acetanilide derivatives, *Fed. Proc. Fed. Am. Soc. Exp. Biol.,* 33, 573, 1974.

21. **Nery, R.,** The possible role of N-hydroxylation in the biological effects of phenacetin, *Xenobiotica,* 1, 339, 1971.

22. **Wendel, A., Feverstein, S., and Konz, K. H.,** Acute paracetamol intoxication of starved mice leads to lipid peroxidation in vivo, *Biochem. Pharmacol.,* 28, 2051, 1979.

23. **Gorrod, J. W.,** Toxic products produced during metabolism of drugs and foreign compounds, in *Drug Toxicity,* Gorrod, J. W., Ed., Taylor and Francis, London, 1979.

24. **Oesch, F.,** Metabolic transformation of clinically used drugs to epoxides: new perspectives in drug-drug interactions, *Biochem. Pharmacol.,* 25, 1935, 1976.

25. **Glatt, H. R., Oesch, F., Frigerio, A., and Garattini, S.,** Epoxides metabolically produced from some known carcinogens and from some clinically used drugs. I. Differences in mutagenicity, *Int. J. Cancer,* 16, 787, 1975.

26. International Agency for Research on Cancer, Monographs on the evaluation of carcinogenic risk of chemicals to man: some miscellaneous pharmaceutical substances, IARC, Lyon, 13, 201, 1977.

27. **Ruddell, W. S. J.,** Gastric cancer in patients who have taken cimetidine, *Lancet,* i, 1234, 1979.

28. **Lingeman, C. H.,** Carcinogenic hormones, in *Recent Results in Cancer Research,* Vol. 66, Springer-Verlag, New York, 1979.

29. **Upton, A. C.,** Cancer and Estrogen Use, Natl. Cancer Institute, special communication, May 22, 1978.

30. **Herbst, A. L. and Scully, R. E.,** Adenocarcinoma of the vagina in adolescence, *Cancer,* 25, 745, 1970.

31. **Herbst, A. L., Scully, R. E., Robboy, S. J., Welch, W. R., and Cole, P.,** Abnormal development of the human genital tract following prenatal exposure to diethylstilbestrol, in *Origins of Human Cancer,* Hiatt, H. H., Watson, J. D., and Winsten, J. A., Eds., Cold Spring Harbor Laboratory, Cold Spring Harbor, N.Y., 1977, 399.

32. **Horning, E. C., Thenot, J. P., and Helton, E. D.,** Toxic agents resulting from the oxidative metabolism of steroid hormones and drugs, *J. Toxicol. Environ. Health,* 4, 341, 1978.

33. **Kappus, H. and Bolt, H. M.,** Irreversible protein binding of norethisterone (norethindrone) epoxide, *Steroids,* 27, 29, 1976.

34. **Vorherr, H., Messer, R. H., Vorherr, U. F., Jordan, S. W., and Kornfeld, M.,** Teratogenesis and carcinogenesis in rat offspring after transplacental and transmammary exposure to diethylstilbestrol, *Biochem. Pharmacol.,* 28, 1865, 1979.
35. **White, I. N. H.,** Metabolic activation of acetylenic substituents to derivatives in the rat causing the loss of hepatic cytochrome P450 and Haem, *Biochem. J.,* 174, 853, 1978.
36. **Harris, C. C.,** The carcinogenicity of anticancer drugs: a hazard in man, *Cancer,* 37, 1014, 1976.
37. **Williams, M.,** Occupational tumours of the bladder, in *Cancer,* Raven, R., Ed., Butterworths, London, 1958, 337.
38. **Brody, R. S., Scottenfeld, D., and Reid, A.,** Multiple primary cancer risk after therapy for Hodgkin's disease, *Cancer,* 40, 1917, 1977.
39. **Falck, K., Grohn, P., Sorsa, M., Vainio, H., Heinonen, E., and Holsti, L. R.,** Mutagenicity in urine of nurses handling cytostatic drugs, *Lancet,* i, 1250, 1979.

Appendix 2

PREVENTION OR CURE?
USE OF TOXIC HERBS AND GEOGRAPHIC PATHOLOGY*

R. Schoental

It is suggested that certain of the childhood disorders, sometimes masquerading as "malnutrition," as well as some of the tumors encountered in developing countries, maybe due to toxic and/or carcinogenic constituents present in the diet or in herbal remedies used by women during pregnancy and lactation or given to the babies.

The occurrence of specific types of tumors in distinct geographical areas points to their relation to the local floras that vary depending on the geographical and climatic conditions. The chances of the identification of the causative agents of certain diseases and tumors that occur in young children are better than in the case of adults. The importance of protecting pregnant women and young children from the ill effects of insidiously acting "medicines" is discussed.

INTRODUCTION

In spite of great efforts devoted to the finding of a *cure* for cancers, this aim is still as elusive as ever, though some beneficial results are being obtained in certain specific forms of cancer. Some new discovery made tomorrow, next month, next year, or next hour — may change completely the situation, but at the moment there is no definite lead to suggest a particular approach that would give promise of success.

The position as regards cancer *prevention* is quite different and more hopeful. Enough is already known about agents that can induce tumors and certain other incurable diseases in experimental animals to suggest the possibility that prevention of such diseases could be achieved now. A fraction of the efforts and expenditure that go into the task of finding "cures" could reduce considerably the incidence of a number of incurable diseases, if applied to prevention. A few random examples may be sufficient and indicate the benefits that would result if these problems could be dealt with appropriately.

1. High quality grains could be grown in place of tobacco.
2. Introduction of better methods of combustion would prevent air pollution and give better caloric returns.
3. Freely available "on demand" surgical abortion would prevent the use of risky, inefficient abortifacients and the birth of unwanted, hence unhappy individuals, sometimes crippled in body or mind.

No country can afford large numbers of chronically ill and incurable people. Disease is a costly luxury, in terms of hospital facilities, medical personnel and umemployability, and unproductivity of the ill. Prevention of illness is urgent not only from pure humane considerations, but also on economic grounds. However, among the problems mentioned some require legislation or some other action by official authorities which are usually slow; the action which can be taken by an individual and which depends on his or her own decision, can be immediate, but the person must know what action to take.

The individual who smokes has to decide whether the pleasure of smoking is worth paying for with illness such as bronchitis and/or lung cancer, which can follow the smoking of tobacco in the years to come. Such decision making is the right of any individual. Quite a different moral problem is presented however by the use of dangerous

---

*   From Schoental, R., *Trop. Geogr. Med.,* 24, 194, 1972. With permission.

medicines or inefficient abortifacients by pregnant or lactating women. The thalidomide tragedy is a striking example. Such materials may not be dangerous to the adult woman, but if abortion is not accomplished and the child is born, it will be subject to the ill effects of the abortifacient used; similarly, the suckling baby can be poisoned by his mother's milk, if carcinogenic or hepatotoxic ingredients to which the adult female may be relatively resistant, are present in her diet or in other products she uses. It is not right to expose the innocent young to hazards that can be avoided.

TOXIC SUBSTANCES IN GEOGRAPHICAL PATHOLOGY

In Africa as in many other developing countries, certain diseases predominate which are rare in the Western Countries. To these belong marasmus, kwashiorkor, certain tumors of childhood and of young age, and various liver disorders including primary liver cancer. It is known from epidemiological studies in man and from experimental work in animals, that cancer has a long latent period before it becomes apparent. Cancers that occur at an early age might have been initiated *in utero* or soon after birth.

In trying to trace the causes of such incurable diseases as cancers, it would be necessary to obtain the life histories not only of the patients, but also as regards the health conditions and treatments of their mothers at the time of conception, during pregnancy and during the suckling of the patient. It is known that certain toxic substances when ingested by the pregnant female will affect the fetus *in utero;* when taken during lactation these (or their metabolic products) will be excreted and poison the milk. Moreover, the fetus and the very young are more sensitive to certain poisonous materials than adults and it is exactly during pregnancy, parturition and lactation that women often require some medication. Only in the present century have synthetic chemicals supplemented or replaced "natural" herbal medicines in the West. In developing countries, herbal remedies are still the rule, especially in remote rural districts, where plants which grow locally are the only available "medicines."

Plants that are acutely poisonous are usually known as such by the local people; however, nobody could be aware of the hazard of plants which do not show immediately toxic effects, but which act insidiously and cause chronic disease and eventually death only after a long latent period. Such insidious action has only recently come to be recognized, and can only be detected by screening the plant materials in long term animal experiments.

It is about 31 years since the first hepatomas were found among rats given intermittently extracts from *Senecio Jacobaea* L (ragwort) in drinking water, and almost 25 years since a single dose of a pure Senecio (pyrrolizidine) alkaloid proved sufficient for the induction of chronic liver disease and liver tumors in rats. Since then many natural products of plant and microbial origin, of diverse chemical structures, proved to be carcinogenic; cycasin, macrozamin, aflatoxins, streptozotocin, elaiomycin etc., and many more will no doubt be discovered in the near future. These natural carcinogens (as well as some synthetic ones, notably the nitroso-compounds) have been shown to induce tumors even with a single dose. The implications of this finding are very important, but have not yet penetrated into the clinical considerations of the etiology of human and livestock diseases. The seriousness of such situations and their applicability to man has still to be demonstrated.

"NATURAL PRODUCTS" AND DISEASE

The realization that chronic disease and cancer can be caused by "natural" products (whether of plant, microbial, or viral origin) is relatively new and the Health Services have still to make appropriate deductions and practical recommendations.

However, elimination of viral and microbial toxins would present great difficulties, particularly in developing countries, where food and other resources are scarce. On the other hand, it should not be impossible by appropriate propaganda to stop people from using as medicines, particularly dangerous plants, which could be replaced by others, less harmful and possibly more effective. As example, can serve the decrease in Jamaica of the incidence in children of "veno-occlusive" liver disease following a successful educational campaign against the use in "bush teas" of the toxic *Crotalaria fulva* L which contains fulvine, a pyrrolizidine alkaloid (G. Bras, personal communication).

In Africa, certain specific tumors (esophageal, nasopharyngeal, liver, Burkitt lymphomas etc.,) rare in the Western countries show a strikingly high incidence, confined to distinct localized pockets.[5] The reasons for the local differences in type and incidence of tumors are not known, as the etiology of these tumors is still obscure. Can there be some relation between the type of tumor and some particular plants that grow in these localities and are ingested by the local people as food or as medicine? This possibility has yet to be explored. The vegetation of Africa is known to be very rich and varied and some systematic studies on the distribution of various species have already been published and others are in preparation (Flora of tropical E. Africa).[2]

The vegetation varies depending on altitude, on climatic and soil conditions, and these factors can affect the content and the particular structures of toxic plant constituents, even in closely related species.

In East Africa can be found more than 200 species of Crotalarias and large numbers of species of the genera Senecio, Heliotropium, Cynoglossum, Trichodesma etc. (J. Gillett, personal communication). In plants of these genera, more than 100 pyrrolizidine alkaloids have already been identified.[13] Not all are toxic, but their biological effects cannot be recognized until the plants are appropriately studied.

Pyrrolizidine alkaloids have been investigated pharmacologically already, about 35 years ago by Harris, Chen and their colleagues at the Eli Lilly Co.[8] and found not to possess significant medicinal value. Many of the alkaloids have, however, hepatotoxic and carcinogenic action[4,9-12] and are able to induce tumors in rats even with a single dose.[11] Such an oral dose of the order of LD_{30-60} will cause in some of the rats, liver lesions resembling hepatitis with jaundice etc.; others of the treated rats that survive longer will develop more chronic effects, like liver cirrhosis or primary liver tumors, which take time to "ripen," and become apparent after long latent periods. The end effects depend on the structure of the alkaloids, on the size of the dose (when a single one is given), on the dosage schedule (when small repeated doses are given) and in particular on the susceptibility of the individual, which is related to sex, diet, etc. but most strikingly to age. New-born rats are about 15 times more sensitive than adult females to the toxic action of pyrrolizidine alkaloids.[10] Certain of the pyrrolizidine alkaloids can affect besides the liver, also other organs, the lung, the heart, the vascular system, the pancreas, brain, kidneys etc.[4,6,7,9,11,12]

In the industrially developing countries which still rely mostly on natural products for their traditional medicines,[14] liver disease and primary liver tumors occur with great frequency. Moreover, liver lesions are encountered among young children, either in the form of liver cirrhosis, kwashiorkor, or marasmus which are considered as due to malnutrition. Most of the cases due to genuine malnutrition recover or improve on appropriate refeeding, but a core of about 20% of hospital admissions of "malnutrition" children (often still on the breast) die in the hospitals. The proportion of the incurable "malnutrition" remained almost the same in spite of the various nutritional regimens that have been tried in the course of the last 40 years.

TOXINS AND INCURABILITY

The incurable cases of marasmus and liver cirrhosis are probably of toxic origin, the children having been exposed to hepatotoxins, whether taken by their mothers during pregnancy or lactation, or given to the babies as remedies for childhood disorders. It is significant that measles — a comparatively mild disease in the Western countries — leads often to "malnutrition" of the severe type in African children. Could this be the consequence of treating measles by the application of fresh juice from Crotalaria plants to the affected skin?[14]

In the case of yound children suffering from liver disease or cancer, some chance exists of tracing the etiological factors of these disorders. The mothers may still remember whether and which remedies they used themselves during pregnancy, parturition or lactation and which they gave to the child. Even a few well-documented cases could give a lead, which would be of great importance for the understanding of the etiology of such disorders, not only in children, but probably in adults as well and open possibilities for their prevention.

THE INFORMATION GAP

The difficulty in obtaining reliable information from mothers of ill children cannot be underestimated. The majority of women will not admit having used any of the traditional remedies either for themselves or for the children. Only when several plants, some toxic and some innocuous ones are shown to a group of women, comprising mothers of both healthy and ill children, it is usually possible to start them discussing the plants, and the conditions for which these would be used, etc. With the help of interpreters, much patience, and observing the reactions of the mothers of the ill children, the true situation can be gathered and the particular plant(s) that has been used might be identified. Such enquiries have to be done with much tact and caution, as the realization that the child's illness might have been caused inadvertently by their own actions would cause great anguish to the mother.

The possibility that toxic plants might sometimes be included in childhood "medicines" receives support from the report of two fatal cases of children that were treated with some unidentified herbs.[1]

In a recent paper Frood *et al.*[3] drew attention to the observation that illness in children that subsist on low protein diet appear to have serious consequences. The effects of toxic "medicines" are also likely to be more serious under such conditions.

ACKNOWLEDGMENTS

I am greatly indebted to the scientists, doctors, nurses, patients etc, too many to be mentioned by name, who helped during my visits to Africa and Asia to obtain the information which led to the ideas expressed in this paper.

My thanks are due to the Medical Research Council for leave of absence during these visits and to the British Council for sponsoring the visits to East Africa during 1970.

REFERENCES

1. **Bwibo, N. O.,** *Br. Med. J.,* 4, 601, 1969.
2. Flora of Tropical East Africa, Government Printer, Nairobi, Kenya.
3. **Frood, J. D. L., Whitehead, R. G., and Coward, W. A.,** *Lancet,* 2, 1047, 1971.
4. Harris, P. N. and Chen, K. K., *Cancer Res.,* 30, 2881, 1970.
5. **Hutt, M. S. R. and Burkitt, D.,** *Br. Med. J.,* 2, 719, 1965.
6. **Kay J. M. and Heath, D.,** *"Crotalaria Spectabilis," the Pulmonary Hypertension Plant,* Charles C. Thomas, Springfield, Ill., 1970.

7. **McLean, E. K.,** *Pharmacol. Rev.,* 22, 429, 1970.
8. *Research Today,* Eli Lilly & Co., Indianapolis, Ind., 1949, 5.
9. **Schoental, R.,** *Cancer Res.,* 28, 2237, 1968.
10. **Schoental, R.,** *Nature (London),* 227, 401, 1970.
11. **Schoental, R. and Bensted, J. P. M.,** *Br. J. Cancer,* 17, 242, 1963.
12. **Schoental R., Fowler, M. E., and Coady, A.,** *Cancer Res.,* 30, 2127, 1970.
13. **Warren, F. L.,** *"Senecio Alkaloids" in the Alkaloids,* Vol. 12, Manske, R. H. F., Ed., Academic Press, London, 1970, 245.
14. **Watt, J. M. and Breyer-Brandwijk, M. G.,** *Medicinal and Poisonous Plants of Southern and Eastern Africa,* 2nd ed., Livingstone, Edinburgh, 1962.

INDEX